B1

Sport and Medicine

Dedicated to
Lorna
James, Fiona, John

Sport and Medicine

Peter N. Sperryn

MB BS, FRCP(Glasg), DPhysMed, FACSM
Consultant in Physical Medicine, Hillingdon Hospital;
Vice President, British Association of Sport and Medicine;
Honorary Medical Adviser, British Amateur Athletic Board;
President, London Athletic Club and University of London Athletic Club

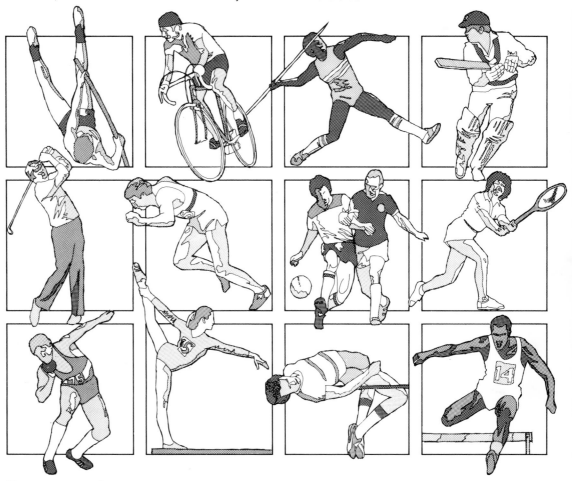

Butterworths

London Boston Durban Singapore Sydney Toronto Wellington

First published, 1983

Reprinted 1985

© Dr P. N. Sperryn, 1983

British Library Cataloguing in Publication Data

Sperryn, Peter N.
  Sport and medicine.
  1. Sports medicine
  I. Title
  617′.1027   RC1210

  ISBN 0-407-00270-7 (Cased)
  ISBN 0-407-00413-0 (Soft cover)

Library of Congress Cataloging in Publication Data

Sperryn, Peter N. (Peter Neville)
  Sport and medicine.

  Includes index.
  1. Sports medicine.   I. Title
  RC1210.S626   1983   617′.1027   83-6388

  ISBN 0-407-00270-7 (Cased)
  ISBN 0-407-00413-0 (Soft cover)

Photoset by Butterworths Litho Preparation Department
Printed and bound by Robert Hartnoll Ltd, Bodmin,
Cornwall

Foreword 1

This is a very interesting and challenging book; it is also remarkably comprehensive. The significance of the title – *'Sport **and** Medicine'*, I would suggest, singles it out from the many previous books on 'sports medicine'. It is obviously intended for the intelligent layman (physiotherapist, coach, trainer, team manager, etc.) as much as for the doctor with a particular interest in sports medicine and sports injuries.

The author is more than qualified to deal with this complex and extensive field. An accomplished athlete himself, he is also a mature doctor and an experienced administrator. Sports medicine is not really a clear cut specialty: it comprises applied multidisciplinary general practice with a modicum of surgery where required. However, dealing with what are largely minor ailments and complaints requires more than straightforward common sense combined with a sound basis of medical knowledge. There has to be an understanding of body function and an appreciation of the fact that anyone indulging in sport and recreation needs their medical 'troubles' diagnosed, treated and cured as expeditiously as possible so that they may continue those activities – be they entertaining, beneficial or competitive – with minimal interruption. It is a great pity that when the British Government set up the Sports Council which generated the excellent slogan 'Sport for All', it was not appreciated that this would also involve 'more sport injuries for all'. Sadly, in this country we lag a very long way behind our colleagues in Europe and America. I hope that this excellent book will help to further a rapid improvement in this state of affairs. It contains a mass of information presented in a clear, simple and practical style, assisted where necessary by straightforward, intelligible line drawings.

The first part of the book provides a simple but in-depth exposition of the function of the various organs of the body, and links this physiology to ailments associated with participation in sport as well as the medicaments used to deal with them. This precedes a description of sports injuries of various parts of the body and their treatment, including surgery.

Interspersed are excellent little articles on such continuing controversial subjects as age, alcohol, diet, doping, footwear, participation of women in sport – and the very important psychological factors involved in recreational and athletic competitions.

There is something for everyone who is interested in this field. I would suggest that it should not at first be read from cover to cover; the index will assist selective reading. I have no doubt it will prove of great value to all concerned with sport *and* medicine and I wish it well.

The Rt. Hon. The Lord Porritt, GCMG, GCVO, CBE, MCh, FRCS
Formerly President, Royal College of Surgeons of England; President, British Medical Association; President, Medical Commission of the IOC; President, British Association of Sport and Medicine

Foreword 2

I strongly suspect that Peter Sperryn chose with great care the title of his latest book *Sport **and** Medicine*, the strong implication being that there are two separate broad general disciplines that are interrelated, the book being about that relationship. Of course, it is acknowledged that there are several other more specific disciplines involved, ranging through sound clinical diagnostic medicine, exercise physiology, biomechanics, coaching, psychology and education. The only assumption made, which few will deny, is that nowadays medical support is essential for the realization of the athlete's natural capacity for optimum performance.

I am certain that it is my own hypersensitivity, stemming from a deprived background, which makes me rejoice that the title is not *Sports Medicine*. A subtle difference perhaps, but under its banner, I often sense a glamour and mystique behind which many things are both promoted and justified, bringing with them a new breed of scientists who feel that through sport many of their own barriers may be quickly crossed or conquered. My own involvement in sport as an athlete, teacher, coach and mere observer for more than 30 years, convinces me that in the relationship between sport and medicine, sport has always made the more generous contribution in the past.

Of course, as coaches, we adopted and adapted Newton's laws and have been eternally grateful for A. V. Hill's work on acceleration in the 1920s, which seemed to be uniquely related to the needs of sport. It is little, however, compared with the generations of athletes who have given blood, sweat, urine, muscle biopsies and personality inventories, have often been immersed in tanks, and photographed naked in three dimensions at altitude. So often we were motivated to help by the assumption, if not the fact, that in other countries such as Cuba, East Germany and the Soviet Union, this was how their athletes were selected, trained, monitored and even manipulated in the pursuit of excellence. Without real knowledge we cannot make comparisons, cast aspersions or have any real confidence in our own teachings.

If I have been hypercritical of our medical colleagues, let me redress the balance by expressing my growing concern over recent observations within sport. Although generally there can be no doubt that standards of performance relate specifically to both the quality and quantity of training, the ground rules have now changed. We cannot assume that the old adage 'no amount of exercise will damage a healthy body' still applies. Many of our most serious medical problems occur directly through stress and overuse. There may well be biomechanical factors involved but bad techniques and imbalanced training programmes are more commonly the perpetrators. Too much, too soon; the nonsense of running through pain barriers; unsupervised weight training – we have all been guilty and often responsible for converting minor problems into major injuries. Osteochondritis and Achilles tendinitis are the bane of athletics, yet their specific cause is unknown and we have never monitored our training programmes to find related factors.

The mass of inexperienced joggers now joining our

club ranks pose an additional responsibility, for they are most vulnerable. Very often they jog seeking good health, but lose it when tempted into marathon mania. Specific fitness must not be 'sold' as the panacea for all ills, or confused with being healthy, despite the known relationships.

At last it seems that the message is getting through. Education, change, innovation, feedback and dissemination are now the commonsense practices which govern the relationship between sport and medicine. The coach must fully accept his role as the synthesizer or catalyst, choosing with care from the multitude of new ideas, science, innovation or research which comes his way. His own empirical knowledge is a vital part of the feedback of information. He frequently will have to make the ethical decisions, and make it clear that he accepts the responsibility.

The scientist has at last climbed from his lofty academic pedestal. There is a genuine desire to help and educate, as well as to look sympathetically at the jungle of panaceas, short-cuts, aids, props, etc. What is more, the help is all the more generous when one appreciates that, in Britain at least, it is freely given without reward and without institutional back-up.

The complex mosaic of human performance is a marvellously stimulating and fascinating field. It deserves the greatest care that all concerned are capable of. It is therefore a pleasure to welcome this most recent work of Peter Sperryn, whose writing not only conforms to my own personal and simplistic requirements, but also is actually the result of years of practical work in the field, of countless hours helping hosts of athletes from a wide range of sports, in an honest and earnest belief in the need for the dissemination of ideas and the minimum of bureaucracy and professional jealousy. Both Sport and Medicine can only be the richer for that.

Ronald J. Pickering, MEd, DPE
Former AAA National Coach; Fellow of the Physical Education Association; Fellow of the Institute of Leisure and Amenity Management

Preface

Sport in the 1970s brought greater demands on the champions and an explosive growth of public interest in mass participation. However, 'Sport for All' inevitably leads to 'Sports Injuries for All'. So we need 'Sports Medicine for All'.

Sadly, medicine has been slow to respond to the changing needs of society as it replaces its old afflictions with the new challenges of fitness and exercise. Twenty years after publication of the first major textbook on sports medicine in Great Britain, for instance, the National Health Service still discouraged provision of sports medical services; few medical and paramedical students received instructions in the subject; few sports organizations made substantial provision for their members.

Sports medicine is not a clear-cut medical specialty but is well defined as the medicine and science of exercise and sport – a wide interest, in which many different professions meet on the common ground of sporting endeavour.

Over my years in sport and medicine the gap between narrow specialist knowledge and its widespread dissemination seems to have widened. This book is written with the aim of bringing together in one volume the many strands of sports medicine in a clear, concise, factual and readable form. It is aimed at all sports enthusiasts interested in sports medicine and at those professional readers seeking to apply their medical knowledge to sport.

Considerations of space and economy dictate an emphasis on essential principles. I have tried to recruit relevant aspects of medicine and science to the immediate and practical aid of the doctor, therapist, physical educator and coach – and the player – puzzled by the problems of, and seeking answers to, the fascinating challenges of sports medicine. The index is designed to facilitate cross-reference to relevant subjects and thus keep the main text as concise as possible. I have not tried to include first aid or detailed traumatology, for which many good books exist.

Nobody can write such a book unaided. I thank my many colleagues around the world for their constant help and encouragement over the years of our continuing efforts to establish sports medicine in its proper place. My knowledge draws on the sum of theirs; my mistakes are my own. I am particularly indebted for detailed comments on chapters to Dr Carolyn Ritchie, PhD, Dr Denise Yeldham, BSc, MRCPsych and to Dr Craig Sharp, BVMS, PhD, MRCVS.

I thank Sheila Galbraith warmly for preparing the artwork from my thumb-nail sketches and my publishers for accepting so readily my suggestion of a second colour. My intention is to rely on simple line diagrams to highlight essentials and avoid confusion.

Most of all I thank Brian Banks, who responded to the challenge of such a text and initially commissioned me to produce this book. Since then he has relentlessly goaded me out of my sloth and shouldered all the heaviest burdens of subediting, labelling and planning. His constant encouragement and discipline have made a book come out of an idea.

Peter Sperryn

Contents

1 The case for exercise

There is much evidence that inactivity is related to physiological deterioration, illness and death. On the other hand, there is little evidence that specific levels of fitness or athletic participation give specific benefits in terms of longevity. Physical activity is beneficial to health in a general way and, while not necessarily guaranteeing the individual a longer life, can improve the quality of his daily life and delay deterioration in fitness due to age and inactivity.

Men and women of all ages can improve cardiac, respiratory and muscular functions by regular activity. Moderate levels of rhythmic exercise of the large muscle groups of the trunk and limbs produce the safest consistent improvement in oxygen uptake and cardiovascular function. The muscles become more efficient through chemical enzyme changes and increases in the capillary circulation. The optimum level of exercise is about three sessions weekly of 20 minutes each and sufficiently severe exercise should be taken to raise the pulse to between 140 and 160 beats per minute (beats/min). Harmful effects are unlikely, provided that exercise levels increase gradually from modest beginnings.

Psychological benefits develop hand in hand with increasing physical fitness and increased extroversion, self-confidence, self-awareness and well-being have all been demonstrated. Memory improvement has been shown in elderly subjects on an exercise programme. Training effects tend to be specific to the functions being trained and this event specificity, e.g. swimming/jogging/cycling, should be taken into account when activities are planned.

Childhood and adolescence

Children are spontaneously active and playful but become lazy and obese as they grow into conformity with the Western adult lifestyle. The instillation of positive attitudes to exercise and games in the young is more likely to create life-long commitments to enjoyable physical activity and this may be even more important for mentally or physically disabled or deprived children whose development lacks the stimulus of normal spontaneous play.

Pregnancy

Fit mothers have easier pregnancies and deliveries. Moderate exercise throughout pregnancy should be encouraged in the absence of specific medical contraindications. Smoking is associated with the birth of smaller-than-average babies.

Obesity

Forty per cent of the British adult population is obese to a degree which is associated with increased chances of cardiovascular disease, diabetes and complications from surgery. While dieting is generally boring for most people, exercise has a considerable anti-obesity effect because it speeds up the body's chemical activity in a way which allows it to burn off more fat than would be expected from the exercise itself.

1

Moderate exercise does not increase the appetite disproportionately so that regular exercise, despite some increase in appetite, does not lead to weight gain. Diabetic patients may find control easier if they take regular exercise.

Exercise and coronary heart disease

Physically active people have fewer fatal heart attacks than the lazy. It is thought that the heart is protected by long-term regular exercise, including regular amounts of fairly intensive work such as sport participation or garden digging. Exercise also improves other cardiac risk factors such as blood pressure, the level of circulating fats in the blood and the efficiency of the blood's clotting mechanisms.

Exercise and chronic disease

Most sick people show physical underachievement due to unfitness over and above the specific effects of their diseases. Regular exercise generates extra physical work capacity. This has been well shown in exercise programmes for heart-attack victims and is the basis for rehabilitation in locomotor and chronic respiratory disease. The aim in these circumstances is to improve the patient's quality of life by allowing daily functions to be performed with greater control and less fatigue.

Old age

Old people become unfit by letting their daily level of physical activity fall. Much of this age-related deterioration is readily corrected by simple exercise programmes. Muscle power, tendon strength and cardiorespiratory efficiency all improve considerably, even with simple walking programmes which are safe for most people. Much of the physical decline after the age of 60 can be delayed and partly prevented if substantial physical activity is maintained. Apart from the physical benefits, which also include reduction in joint stiffness and improved neuromuscular co-ordination, mental benefits such as increased concentration and memory and brightening of mood are all useful in the elderly. It is also possible that the increased heat production of the physically active body may play a part in the prevention of hypothermia, a common cause of death in the elderly.

Cardiac risk factors

The concept of risk factors is crucial to any discussion on exercise and health. Several factors have been clearly related to the incidence of cardiovascular disease. These include exercise, or lack of exercise, age, sex, family history, smoking, hypertension, hyperlipidaemia, diabetes and personality type. Each of these factors plays a part in the individual's tendency to suffer from heart disease. Different people have different degrees of liability to these diseases according to their individual constitution and habits.

All risk factors interrelate so that, for instance, the risks of smoking are added to those of high blood pressure or diabetes but are not simply corrected by an appropriate dose of hard exercise. This explains the difficulty in assessing the precise benefits of exercise of any sort in communities and even more so in individuals. It is simply impossible to relate a given amount of sport or exercise to a clear risk of heart attack or extra number of years to be lived. This may be surprising, particularly when surveys have suggested that the risks of smoking may be expressed as 5 minutes' loss of life per cigarette smoked. A 5 minute risk per cigarette is, however, an overall average figure which may be drastically modified in any individual by his other risk factors. Briefly, cardiac risk factors operate as follows.

In general, the risk of vascular illness increases with age and affects males more than females. Premature cardiac deaths are usually related to extra risk factors or structural abnormalities such as abnormal heart vessels. Family history dictates the general liability of the individual to various diseases, particularly those affecting the blood vessels; a strong family liability to hypertension, hyperlipidaemia and diabetes is often evident. In hyperlipidaemia, the circulating fats (cholesterol and lipids) in the blood exceed normal levels and this condition is related to premature formation of atheroma, or fatty plaques, in the blood vessel and heart linings which cause coronary thrombosis.

Hypertension, or raised blood pressure, increases the general risk of stroke and heart disease. Many large-scale surveys have suggested that long-term prophylactic treatment as a result of screening programmes may have some benefit. Unfortunately, this benefit is best shown in population studies and the detailed benefit to a given individual with high blood pressure is uncertain. The statistical benefit must be weighed against the great inconvenience of life-long daily medication. While exercise tends to lower blood pressure, this is neither dramatic nor therapeutically significant and it should be remembered that extreme exercise, or exercise associated with mental stress, will still cause a sharp temporary increase in blood pressure.

Risks of exercise

Death may occur during exercise. This sometimes happens simply because a very ill person happens to be exercising. On the other hand, the cause and effect relation may be more direct. It is difficult to interpret the published work on exercise related to death. This is partly because widely varying populations have been studied and widely differing results would therefore be expected.

For instance, military conscripts in one study showed 45 exercise-related deaths in a total of 660 000 man years of exposure to exercise programmes; 36 per cent of these deaths were due to cardiovascular causes. In contrast, a well-quoted study has shown the risk of exercise-related deaths for rugby referees to be as high as one per 3000 hours of exposure compared with one per 50 000 hours in the players themselves. This might be anticipated to some extent, bearing in mind that many rugby referees summate their risk factors of hypertension, obesity and smoking quite dramatically.

At the other end of the scale, experience of carefully supervised post-coronary rehabilitation programmes has been gained from North America in the 1970s. A summary of results from 25 different programmes involving over 8000 cases and over 80 centres showed 10 deaths, giving an overall risk of about one death per 30 000 hours of exposure to an exercise programme. The risk in the most experienced of all the North American coronary rehabilitation programmes was only one death per 216 000 hours of exposure. Thus it is evident that while there can be no dramatic individual promise related to an exercise programme, there is no disagreement about the general benefits to long-term health, and particularly well-being, in participants as a group and the risks associated with regular exercise are very small.

Two important factors should be remembered: first, exercise-related risks are to some extent dependent upon detection of obvious risk factors; and secondly, risks should be related to the overall hazards of life. For instance, the relative risks of death for various activities show four in 100 000 people to be at risk per year from playing football, compared with two in 100 000 from taking oral contraceptives, six in 100 000 from being run over, 20 in 100 000 from influenza and 500 in 100 000 from smoking over 20 cigarettes per day. Obviously, a sense of perspective is important!

Political aspects

The spread of 'Sport for All' shows that governments have gradually come to recognize that the state of a nation's health can be improved if a reasonably high level of physical activity can be achieved in the

3

population. Some countries have gone much further than others. For instance, in the German Democratic Republic, there is a constitutional commitment to physical activity throughout the population. In many other countries there has been a marked ambivalence at Government level about the strength of commitment to public fitness. The British Government's failure to bring about drastic reductions in smoking, because of largely financial considerations, should also be kept in perspective. For instance, figures quoted in 1979 showed that the British Government gained about £1000m in revenue from tobacco taxation, but spent only about £15m on its grant to the Sports Council whose motto is 'Sport for All' and just £1m on its anti-smoking campaign through the Health Education Council. This David faced the Goliath of a £100m promotional budget by the tobacco industry, including sports-related advertising. So strong is the influence of the smoking lobby and its selective advertising-based subsidy of certain sports activities, that the Sports Council was unable, even after two debates, to recommend a ban on tobacco advertising in sport. Ironically, the Government in the same year gave over £10m in capital grants for the development of cigarette factories in Durham and Northern Ireland.

Perhaps the 'political' factor should be added to the other cardiac risk factors outlined above.

2 Medical screening of fitness

Some of the dangers to health and life may be predictable by medical examination, others are unforeseeable. Between these two extremes the concept of risk factors, outlined in Chapter 1 with respect to heart disease, applies and the accuracy of risk prediction depends to some extent on the elaborateness (and hence expense) of assessment undertaken.

Who is eligible for an exercise programme? Virtually everybody in the population would benefit by regular exercise. This includes many disabled persons who are living second-rate lives because of underactivity, often because of preventable social factors further reducing their degree of independence.

Do we need a medical examination before a training programme? This is a difficult question to answer. Probably, the main motivation is the question of medicolegal protection for those leading the exercise programme, coupled with the benefit of picking up the more obvious risk factors in potential patients. This slightly sidesteps the issue however. An ideal state of affairs would be for the entire population to have regular health screening programmes, coupled with a regular exercise commitment.

Absolute contraindications to exercise

Patients suffering from active cardiovascular and respiratory disease should not be actively exercised before completion of adequate medical treatment.

Active infections, fever, gross anaemia and metabolic disorders such as thyroid, adrenal or kidney diseases preclude athletic exercise until cure is achieved because all these conditions may cause sudden death, usually through the final mechanism of cardiac failure.

Relative contraindications to exercise

Recent recovery from the above disease states, chronic disabilities from lesser degrees of these conditions, uncontrolled hypertension and musculoskeletal disease all call for expert medical assessment. One aspect calling for particular professional attention is the part which drugs may play in disease and exercise. Many drugs have primary or secondary effects which may alter the safety of, or capacity for, exercise and a temporary restriction of exercise may be necessary.

Medical examination for fitness programmes

A clinical history and physical examination are required. The most frequent extension of this simple protocol, similar to the short Life Assurance type of examination, is the electrocardiograph (ECG). Beyond that, more sophisticated testing involves blood tests and other tests designed solely to check up on risk factors, e.g. circulating blood lipids.

Clinical history

This may be combined with a computerized *pro-forma* seeking details of the subject's previous medical symptoms, relevant family history and medication.

It is axiomatic that the proposed nature of the training programme must be carefully considered and related to the whole medical examination.

Physical examination

The routine clinical examination includes examination of the height, weight, degree of obesity, skin features, breasts, arm-pits, neck and groin for palpable lymph nodes indicating possible infection, and the superficial appearances of the hair and scalp, eyes, ears, nose and mouth, including teeth and gums, tonsils and throat. The blood pressure is measured and the heart and lungs are listened to for abnormal sounds.

While the range of normal heart sounds, as well as those relating to diseased valves, is well established, there may still be considerable difficulties in interpretation of findings. The most common single problem lies in the assessment of cardiac murmurs which are caused by high rates of blood flow through the valves lying between the chambers of the heart. This may be due to diseases like rheumatic fever which may, in some instances, call for care or even prohibition of exercise. Simple murmurs often reflect only the increased rate of blood flow in fit subjects however, and the presence of 'murmur' is not necessarily a sign of disease.

The pulse rate and rhythm are examined. Increasing fitness leads to slowing of the pulse and the normal sinus arrhythmia with its slight acceleration of pulse rate during inspiration may be mistaken for fibrillation by the inexperienced. A grossly irregular pulse calls for full medical assessment.

In cases of doubtful murmurs, it is often helpful to re-examine the heart carefully after exercise. This is useful to confirm that slight irregularities of heart sounds and pulse are normal if they become entirely regular during the test exercise.

The abdomen is palpated for the obvious landmarks of the liver and spleen margins as well as for any unexpected findings of disease or unusually palpable or anatomically abnormal kidneys. The inguinal area in the groin is examined for the presence of hernias, particularly if vigorous exercise involving straining or lifting is envisaged. This is combined with external examination of the genitalia.

The central nervous system examination is usually limited to assessments of the response of the eyes to light and of the reflexes elicited by tapping tendons at the elbow, wrist, knee and ankle with a small rubber-capped reflex hammer.

Further examination

Further examination is indicated if the clinical history or routine physical examination suggests any form of disease calling for more specific examination, such as tests of hearing, examination of the interior of the eyes with the ophthalmoscope, or internal pelvic examination indicated in certain alimentary or genitourinary conditions.

Sport-specific examination

Clearly, a fitness certificate does not let a blind man play cricket or a child with deformed feet run very far, although both subjects are in all other normal respects 'fit'. The purpose of a sports medical examination is, in the light of medical findings, to guide the subject towards suitable forms of exercise. The physician should not encourage either false hopes or apply the, regrettably, more usual medical response of absolute prohibition, without further thought.

More specific examination is needed of those parts of the body most involved in particular sports. For instance, marksmen clearly need normal or properly corrected visual acuity as part of their fitness, runners need healthy feet, and swimmers need to have their sore throats and ears put right before they are fit for their endeavours. It is the responsibility of sporting bodies to define the levels of fitness required for their particular sports and medical officers will bear these obvious criteria in mind whenever they examine potential sportsmen and sportswomen.

Tests

A normal part of routine clinical examinations is to test a small sample of urine with a chemically impregnated dipstick which indicates the presence of blood, protein or sugar. Positive findings may indicate that there is a need for further blood or urine tests and X-rays.

It is not normal to have X-rays as part of a routine medical examination of fitness. There may, however, be reasons why the individual should have an X-ray. These include relevant past or present illnesses or injuries. Routine chest X-rays are not now encouraged on a nationwide basis in the UK for the detection of tuberculosis as that disease has been gradually brought under reasonable control. As many conditions, including tuberculosis and some forms of cancer, may be easily detectable in their early stages with a chest X-ray, it is sound practice to include a chest X-ray in subjects of any age known to be in contact with tuberculosis or from the immigrant communities which are now the main source of tuberculosis in the UK.

Blood tests Blood tests are not normally required as part of a routine medical examination. Anaemia is so common in women of childbearing age, however, that a simple finger-prick haemoglobin test is desirable.

Further blood tests would be indicated only by abnormal findings of the medical history or examination.

The application of automated blood testing systems in recent years has allowed mass screening of small blood samples for many substances. The usual screening programme involves checking the levels of about a dozen substances in the blood but, unfortunately, these are mostly indicative of disease states and there are no positive blood tests indicating fitness. Unfortunately, the relevance of automated blood screening tests to the fit athlete or even the middle-aged would-be jogger is unclear. They are expensive and sometimes throw up unexpected results which are frankly inexplicable – as well as, occasionally, the presence of unsuspected disease.

More specific blood testing on a large scale for blood lipid levels may be desirable as a preventive measure, especially where there is a strong family history of cardiac disease and a major cardiac risk factor may thus be detected and treated. The main deterrents to such screening programmes are expense and lack of availability, although the theory is sound.

Electrocardiograph (ECG) The ECG measures electrical potential differences between different parts of the heart as viewed from different angles. It is, in effect, an electrical three-dimensional picture of the heart. It is entirely painless as it simply measures the body's natural electricity through electrodes placed on the four limbs and the front of the chest.

The place of the routine ECG in clinical examination is much debated. It is probably unnecessary in the overwhelming majority of examinations. While, theoretically, it should be most useful in detecting heart abnormalities, its value is limited mainly by the ignorance and inexperience of the tester. Very fit athletes often have bizarrely abnormal ECGs and, if these are misinterpreted as signs of disease, the resulting prohibitions are unfortunate!

On the other hand, simple electrocardiography by an experienced practitioner is invaluable in the assessment of irregular heart rhythms and in the early detection of cardiac abnormalities precipitated or exacerbated by exercise. It is most valuable when performed during one of the many exercise tests protocols.

Summary

The routine medical examination for fitness therefore consists of a simple clinical history and physical examination, together with dipstick analysis of the urine. All further procedures are dictated by clinical findings or by more elaborate demands or protocols adopted by the parties involved. The role of the ECG is debatable on the mass scale but highly important in training programmes associated with cardiac disability.

Fitness testing

There are two levels of exercise testing. First, simpler protocols are used in medical practice to get an overall idea of exercise capacity and fitness as well as to assess the cardiac response to exercise, particularly if there is doubt about cardiac disease as a limiting factor. Secondly, more sophisticated protocols are used for highly trained subjects and many of these are closely linked with current research methods in fitness testing.

While the problems of assessing the precise degrees of fitness of elite sportsmen have always been matters for debate and continuing research, the practical use of simple exercise tests brings them within reach of the club sportsman as well as the general practitioner. It is true that many elaborate tests can be suitably modified to serve the needs of the simplest rehabilitation patient or 'man in the street'.

There are four levels of exercise testing which can be considered – step tests, bicycle ergometry, treadmill studies and actual sport-specific protocols.

Step tests

There are numerous step-test protocols including the Harvard, Masters and Kasch and their various modifications. The principles are similar, the details vary.

It is vital that, whatever test is followed, the protocol is standardized because only if all subjects are given the same test can the results be comparable. In the basic test, the subject steps up and down from a standard-height step or bench at a predetermined rate, most simply governed by a stopwatch or metronome. For instance, one modification of the Harvard step test recommends 5 minutes of continuous stepping up to a height of 15¾ inches (40 cm) for men and 13 inches (33 cm) for women at the rate of 22½ steps/min, which corresponds to a metronome count of 90 beats/min. The subject faces the bench and leads with one leg ('up'), then steps up with the other leg ('two'), steps down with the leading leg ('three') and finishes the cycle by bringing down the second leg ('four'). Thus, the 'up–two–three–four' rhythm is repeated on the beat. Another modification (Gallagher) involves the same rhythm set at the faster rate of 30 cycles/min instead of 22½ for the shorter period of 4 rather than 5 minutes.

The pulse rates are then counted accurately at specified intervals after the cessation of exercise. In the simplest protocol, the pulse rate half a minute after exercise is taken as the determinant of fitness. In the more complex protocol (Gallagher), the pulse is measured at intervals of 1, 2 and 3 minutes after exercise and an index of fitness calculated from these three counts. The comparative fitness of the subject is then determined by reference to standard tables.

The would-be practitioner in this field has two choices. He can copy exactly one of the many existing protocols, including any exact bench heights specified, or he can modify the technique to suit his own circumstances. It is important that the shortcomings of these tests be remembered. Theoretically, all subjects should be put through the same workload. As this means an infinitely adjustable bench height for the different heights of subjects, this is obviously more complicated. Well-trained endurance athletes do unduly well in this test which is physiologically slanted towards aerobic capacity such as is necessary for moderate-intensity middle-distance running. For practical purposes, the taller endurance sportsman will tend to be flattered by his fitness index; in contrast, the shorter, fatter power-event person will seem disproportionately unfit. Because of these disadvantages, more sophisticated physiological testing has been developed.

Bicycle ergometry

This consists of a modified bicycle with seat, pedals and variable-resistance drive wheel. The resistance of the drive wheel is adjusted to set a predetermined standard workload for the subject. He then has to sustain this workload either by faster pedalling against a smaller resistance or slower, harder pedal work against a bigger resistance. Thus, not only can overall workload be set, but the different aspects of stamina or power fitness can be considered.

In simple bicycle ergometry, the pulse rate can be plotted at the end of exercise and the fitness index compared with standard tables.

More sophisticated bicycle ergometry gives more information. The commonest extension is to combine this procedure with analysis of the gases breathed in from the atmosphere and exhaled from the lungs. In this test, the subject has his nose clamped and breathes in and out through a closed tubing system. This is easily managed with practice. The differences between the amounts of oxygen and of carbon dioxide breathed in and out are measured, the oxygen consumption is calculated and, by comparison with the workload at different rates, the maximum oxygen uptake ($\dot{V}O_{2_{max}}$) can be determined. This gives a comparison with other subjects as well as providing a measure of the individual's fitness compared with his own personal capacity, especially on repeated testing.

Treadmill tests

There are many types of treadmill available. The more expensive varieties have to be built into laboratory floors for stability; simpler ones are small and portable. They may operate only in the horizontal plane or they may be capable of being raised through various gradients, thus increasing the workload required of the subject.

The standard test protocols all follow assessment of standard measurements, e.g. pulse, at rest followed by continuous walking or running at progressively harder resistances. The subject starts by walking on the level. At least 3 minutes is usually allowed for each gradient so that physiological function can stabilize fully before the next increase in workload. At each stage, the treadmill gradient is raised one unit.

The advantage of this scheme is that the progressive increase in intensity of workload required is such that, despite its complexity, few tests last longer than about 20–25 min and the end point of the test coincides with the subject's maximum exercise capacity, thus giving the most useful information. Naturally, modified treadmill tests for medical purposes remain safely at the much lower submaximal levels which give relevant clinical information without needing to go to the length or severity of the tests required for trained athletes.

The practical difficulty is that, in order to gain maximum information from the treadmill tests, a considerable expense and degree of mechanization is required. It is difficult for inexperienced personnel to measure pulse and blood pressure accurately during locomotion, particularly when the rhythmic thumping of the running action or fast walking continues. The bicycle ergometer is much easier to use in this respect.

Sport-specific tests

For the moderately fit or unfit subject a test run of 1½ miles (2.4 km) gives a time which correlates well with aerobic capacity, or endurance fitness. This is one of the basic assessments associated with 'Aerobics', originally pioneered by Bruno Balke. The disadvantages of the actual test run are that it tends towards maximal exercise for the individual and therefore may introduce risk factors. Secondly, it requires a certain amount of training and fitness above the beginner's level and is therefore more suited to trained subjects than novices, particularly over the age of 30 when cardiac risk factors increasingly suggest submaximal rather than maximal effort. Thirdly, it may be misleading in highly trained subjects who may be too fit for this test as an aerobic indicator and who go into the anaerobic state of oxygen debt as they get nearer their maximum effort.

Perhaps the best use for this test is as a long-term, simple, pleasant and reliable indicator of progress and fitness in those committed to their jogging or running programmes.

Rowers and canoers can be tested in special tanks in which the competitive movements are reproduced in a fixed boat against which the water current is directed at variable speeds.

Swimmers may also be tested in such a 'flume' or accompanied by a mobile bathside trolley – or overhead gantry – which receives the testing tubes and leads, although a brief pause is necessary for blood testing.

Most athletes may be tested by radiotelemetric methods. These are often used for ECG data recording and transmission. Surface electrodes lead to a compact recorder or transmitter strapped on to the body or clothing. A modification of this is available in lightweight pulse-meters which give a digital reading of pulse rate to the athlete. More sophisticated models include an audible signal which may indicate pulse rates below or above a predetermined range and thus give a simple indication to the user of his physiological state.

Radiotransmitting capsules may be swallowed and give accurate readings of body-core temperature during exercise – a more comfortable method than older rectal electrodes with accompanying wires.

Practical problems of all fitness tests

Technical factors limit the amount of information to be gained by these tests. For simple purposes, the step tests are admirable and have the virtue of simplicity,

cheapness and reproducibility. It is not practical to count the pulse during the test and only with sophisticated equipment can reliable interference-free ECGs be obtained. If, therefore, the step test is the basis of a medical assessment as opposed to an athletic one, it is best to take the ECG tracings during brief pauses in the exercises. The small deviations of the ST segment can then be seen more clearly.

Bicycle ergometry allows all severities of exercise to be tested. Its smoothness allows easier measurements of pulse and blood pressure during exercise by the average technician and this makes it suitable for more detailed measures of high-level fitness in athletes than the step test and at a considerably lower cost than with treadmills. A serious limitation of bicycle ergometry, however, is that although it is a good indication of cycling capacity, it is a far less satisfactory test of any other type of activity such as swimming or running. Ideally, the most relevant test information can only be gained by measuring the exact type of exercise for which each subject is trained. All other tests are less relevant, because of the subject's unfamiliarity with, and lack of training on, the different equipment.

The treadmill is probably the best all-round laboratory testing system because running is more widely applicable to subjects than is bicycling. Much practice is needed for pulse and blood-pressure determinations during exercise and the same remarks apply to ECG tests as for step tests. As laboratories with good treadmills usually have the most sophisticated ECG and gas analysis equipment, however, these practical problems can be overcome. Thus, with both bicycle and treadmill ergometry, extremely accurate and reproducible functional fitness assessments can be made involving pulse rates, blood pressure, continuous ECG recording and respiratory gas exchange. Blood tests are easily performed during or between bouts of exercise as the subject is static and both methods allow an exact measurement of the work actually being done.

It is thus possible to obtain an extremely detailed analysis of the physical, cardiac, respiratory and biochemical responses to exercise at all grades of severity.

Warnings

While the overwhelming majority of exercise tests are carried out uneventfully, a note of warning should be sounded. A complication rate of one cardiac emergency in 216 000 patient hours has been quoted in post-coronary supervised exercise programmes compared with a chance of one heart attack per 364 000 patient hours in the same (Toronto) general population, which indicates the relative safety of tests performed under ideal circumstances. The unexpected degree of exertion which even modest exercise testing may inflict on some unfit or diseased subjects, however, dictates that wherever there is the possibility of cardiac risk, e.g. in the assessment of the middle-aged subject with possible heart or lung symptoms, precautions should be taken. First, warning signs should be obeyed and tests immediately terminated. Secondly, suitable resuscitation equipment and experienced staff must be immediately available in such circumstances.

Indications for immediate cessation of a test include chest pain or the onset of pain in the neck, jaw, back, shoulders or arms. This may indicate angina due to cardiac insufficiency. Sudden irregularities of the pulse may herald more serious cardiac symptoms. Giddiness, faintness, sickness, undue fatigue or breathlessness call for a halt.

For practical purposes, scientists and practitioners who test only young fit subjects for athletic fitness would not expect to face the problems of resuscitation, subject to the important proviso that no subject should be tested when febrile or ill.

If subjects are tested who are free from cardiorespiratory symptoms and who are untrained but wishing to take up exercise, simple step tests or bicycle ergometry would probably be considered justifiable without further precautions, subject to the same proviso of not testing febrile or ill subjects.

Beyond this, and despite the apparently favourable odds quoted above, the performance of maximum effort stress testing or exercise programmes for the rehabilitation of cardiac patients calls for medical supervision and the availability of resuscitation equipment. It might be difficult to justify legally the lack of such equipment and professional experience in the event of a death occurring under such test conditions in patients with risk factors. It is true that a number of North American programmes have been admirably conducted in detail by exercise physiologists, but they are trained in immediate resuscitation techniques and overall responsibility is usually retained by an experienced clinician who is recommended to be physically available to help in cases of collapse. The greater danger of cardiac arrhythmias and collapse occurring immediately after exercise, for instance in the changing room or showers, means that personal supervision and warning devices must be available at this time as well as during the preceding exercises themselves. For this reason, saunas, hot baths or showers which may lead to hypotensive collapse after exertion should be forbidden in this context.

3 Factors limiting performance

Performance should be assessed by comparison of the subject's recorded performances with known standards for the appropriate age and sex groups.

Objective assessments include static and active tests. Static tests involve biopsy, blood tests, grip tests and so on. Active tests start with the simple step test, up and down from a measured height, and progress to more complex tests such as bicycle ergometry and treadmill testing, and special laboratories for events such as swimming or rowing where the performer remains static while the flow of the surrounding water is adjusted to produce a known resistance against the performer's efforts.

Muscles are assessed by exercise test performances, or by direct muscle biopsy examination which identify the individual muscle fibre types, which are inherited (*see* Chapter 5).

The lungs are responsible for gas exchange between the blood and the atmosphere (*see* Chapter 4). Individual lung capacity and functional ability to exchange respiratory gases at the capillary lining of the lung is also largely determined by heredity. It is influenced by altitude and the quality of the athlete's blood. Measurements of respiratory function include: overall measurements of breathing capacity which measure the amount of air which the lungs can exchange in a given time; simple tests of chest expansion, which reflects total breathing capacity; measurements of breathing power by respiratory flow meters; and measurements of the haemoglobin capacity of the blood itself. Deficiency in oxygen-carrying power due to anaemia or blood disease means a lower capacity for oxygen uptake, hence also for muscular performance.

For cardiac function there is a range of tests from simple pulse and blood-pressure measurements through electrocardiography to complex laboratory determinations of cardiac output (*see* Chapter 4).

The body's chemical systems can be measured by analysis of blood and urine components and much research and controversy surrounds the relative usefulness of many tests (*see* Chapter 11).

The central nervous system (*see* Chapter 11) is highly trainable throughout life and motor tests of function, including reflexes and visual and spatial awareness, give some measure of ability. Psychological tests of function such as personality and response patterns to stimuli or situations are available (*see* Chapter 10).

Despite advances in the study of human performance, the average coach will have only his senses, judgement and experience to rely on, together with a stopwatch and tape measure. These, together with a simple knowledge of physiological responses, will be sufficient to take most sportsmen to the limits of their capacity. Despite the hopes and dreams of most sportsmen, the sad and inevitable fact remains that inherited capacity is the main limiting factor in sports performance. The inherited dimensions of the body on the large scale, measured by stature and somatotype, and on the fine scale, measured by muscle fibre type and cellular biochemical capacity, impose the ultimate limits upon performance. The challenge of sport is to bring the player as near to his ultimate limits of biological capacity as possible and to this end sports medicine and science exist to serve the performer.

The Gaussian frequency distribution curve (*Figure 14.1*) applies to all biological functions. A few people have very poor or very good abilities on either side of the average population level in any given physical, mental, chemical or other biological function or capacity. It is, by definition, impossible to exceed one's potential but it is not always easy to define, or even achieve, that level.

The aim of any scientific selection programme for sport is to match the abilities of individuals with the requirements of the particular sports events rather than to allow selection by chance or misguided preference.

Many individuals may have some optimum abilities for sports success but may lack others and thereby fall short of their hopes. For instance, a runner might have outstanding cardiorespiratory and muscular abilities but inappropriate limb leverage for his event and therefore be intrinsically handicapped by comparison with a more advantageously endowed rival.

It is part of the fascination of sport, and particularly of coaching, that, because so much is not yet scientifically explicable and much is unpredictable, there is still great scope for individual ideas and achievements.

Somatotyping is the description of body build according to detailed body measurements related to the three attributes of muscularity (mesomorphy), thinness (ectomorphy) and squatness (endomorphy). Measurements are made of the body dimensions, weight and fat content and tabulated in graphical form on a somatotyping chart. The extreme endomorph is short and fat, the ectomorph tall, thin and relatively unmuscled and the mesomorph is the typical well-muscled and trimly built athletic figure.

Surveys of different sportsmen show that there is a high degree of conformity between performers in the same event, or in the same team-game positions. Thus, middle-distance runners tend to be clustered

halfway between mesomorphy and ectomorphy with the marathon runners nearer ectomorphy and sprinters towards the endomorphic and mesomorphic builds.

Somatotyping is a useful tool in sifting and comparing populations for sport suitability and performance. It may occasionally prove helpful in the detailed assessment of a sportsman of evident talent but uncertain event.

The limits of performance are continually improving as a reflection of the population's increasing living standards and increasing body size. There has been a general increase in stature in most advanced countries in the last century and this would in itself create the possibility of a growth in performance.

Technical innovations, ranging from lightweight alloys for motor vehicles or bicycles to aerodynamically designed javelins or flexible fibreglass poles for vaulting to synthetic tracks and other sport surfaces, constantly push the sportsman to new levels of performance. They create a corresponding need for technical mastery of new events and implements which may both raise standards and diminish the overall number of participants in some of the highly technical events.

Other reasons for improvement in athletic standards are the increase in the number of people taking up sport because of social advances and the increase in leisure time made available by technology. This broadens the base of the pyramid of participation and in turn pushes up the top standards by increasing competition.

Thus, coaching and selection methods become important in developing athletic talent. Fitness and training increase the body's ability to withstand mental and physical stress. The body must be conditioned to overcome fatigue, to learn and improve new skills and to acquire new strengths and co-ordination. The coach is seeking sportsmen with aptitude and looks to society to create general opportunities in which he can develop their talents through long-term structured training programmes aimed at both the strengths and weaknesses of the individual sportsmen. The coach has to supply incentive and inspiration as well as technical knowledge because the athlete is rarely capable of the maturity or objectivity required for comprehensive self-assessment, especially in events in which self-observation of technique is impossible. The understanding and respect between coach and athlete must be complete; it is general knowledge that many coaches are technically sound but very few are really inspirational for more than a few athletes.

The monotony of long training programmes can be broken up by frequent changes of approach. The law of diminishing returns often brings sportsmen to an apparent halt in a training programme when increasing effort is not rewarded by improved performance. At these times a switch of training, say from cycling to weight-training or flexibility work, will often bring about dramatic improvement.

Why train? The general effects of training are to condition the body and mind to resist fatigue and to develop the maximum potential of muscle strength, heart, lung and muscle endurance, motor skills and co-ordination, and the general physical and mental experience and judgement necessary for success.

4 Cardiovascular and respiratory systems

It is simplest to look at the heart, the lungs and the rest of the body as three interrelated systems which change in response to exercise or illness. Changes affecting any one system lead to compensatory changes in the others.

The heart is a tough, muscular pump which receives used blood from the rest of the body and pumps it from its right side, where it is received from the body, to the lungs. The lungs allow exchange of the carbon dioxide end product of the body's metabolism with oxygen, from the atmosphere, which is transported in the blood from the lungs to the left side of the heart, then to the rest of the body.

The heart

The heart consists of four muscular chambers. Two atria receive the blood, the right atrium from the veins of the body, the left from the lungs. The atria pump blood through one-way valves (right, tricuspid; left, mitral) into the more powerful ventricles. The right ventricle then forces the blood through the pulmonary valve to the lungs. The left ventricle ejects its load through the aortic valve into the main artery of the body, the aorta, which eventually branches to reach all parts of the body.

Cardiac muscle has an intrinsic contractile rhythm of its own and the experimentally denervated heart continues to beat. In some heart diseases the atria and ventricles beat at different rates and the ventricles' own spontaneous rate is about 40 beats/min. For efficient functioning, however, the heart is under the control of the autonomic nervous system (Chapter 11) and thus under the largely involuntary control of sympathetic and parasympathetic mechanisms.

Heart function

The normal adult has a resting heart rate, easily felt over the left chest or the peripheral arterial pulse points as the pulse rate, of about 72 beats/min. With each heartbeat, the left ventricle ejects about 70 ml of blood. The total cardiac output in a normal resting person is the number of heartbeats multiplied by the amount pumped out per beat or

$$CO = PR \times SV$$
$$\text{Cardiac Output} = \text{Pulse Rate} \times \text{Stroke Volume}$$

The blood pressure is a measure of the force with which the blood is ejected from the heart and travels through the main arteries; it is traditionally recorded in millimetres of mercury (mm Hg). Measurement is taken by constricting the brachial artery in the upper arm with an inflatable cuff and, as the cuff is slowly deflated and the pressure falls, listening for characteristic sounds over the same artery at the elbow with a stethoscope.

Heart valves and failure

Heart valves, especially the mitral and aortic valves, are affected by rheumatic fever. The effect is to increase the workload required by the left ventricle to maintain output. If the aortic valve is narrowed (stenosis), the ventricle has to beat harder to squeeze out sufficient blood. If the same valve is too loose (incompetence), the ventricle must force out both the appropriate stroke volume per pulse plus the amount added by leakage because the valve does not shut off the ventricle from the column of blood in the aorta. To a certain extent, the heart muscle responds by hypertrophy, or thickening, as in athletic training. Depending on the severity of the valvular disease, cardiac function may be maintained for many years without failure. When the point of maximum hypertrophy has been reached, the ventricle cannot stretch further or beat harder and increasing load causes cardiac failure. The heart can no longer keep pace with the general circulatory requirements and fluid accumulates in the peripheral tissues together with salt, causing weight gain and swelling of the body (oedema or dropsy).

At this point there is a choice of drug therapy. Digitalis reinforces the power of contraction of the heart muscles; the diuretic drugs eliminate the surplus salt and water; and the beta-blockers slow the pulse and limit the cardiac response to exercise thus effectively lowering the stress on the heart muscles. It is clear, however, that from the point of view of exercise, a heart which has come to the end of its range of compensation cannot be loaded further with athletic stress until the abnormality is corrected. Both the young person with rheumatic-valvular disease or the veteran with aortic stenosis will have considerable limitation of activity but, given satisfactory medical control, may well be capable of modest sporting exertion. The former may take to walking but not running and the latter not pursue anything more active than playing bowls – but this must be a matter for individual medical consideration.

Myocarditis

Heart muscle may be inflamed in myocarditis. It is now known that myocarditis is a common accompaniment of many viral illnesses, including influenza and glandular fever. There are two stages. In acute myocarditis, inflammation may cause sudden death on exertion at any age. Later chronic myocarditis is one of the causes of cardiomyopathy which can also be fatal. Warning symptoms of progressive exercise intolerance include breathlessness and tiredness.

Acute myocarditis almost invariably settles very rapidly after a viral illness has run its course but active sport during the illness should be expressly forbidden. The myocarditis associated with rheumatic fever is usually associated with sufficient general illness to cause the subject not to wish for sporting exertion.

Blood pressure

The standard adult blood pressure is given as 120/80 (i.e. 120 mm Hg systolic/80 mm Hg diastolic). The blood pressure varies continuously according to activity and emotion. There is a progressive elevation with age and a proportion of the population develops an abnormally high blood pressure which does not reliably settle with rest. The upper, or systolic, reading is a more volatile measure and is responsive to physical or emotional stress. The diastolic, or lower, reading is the more important in terms of long-term effects, for instance chronic mechanical stress on the heart leading to failure.

Hypertension

There is no disease of low blood pressure in athletic practice, although the blood pressure falls in association with fainting. Hypertension is one of the cardiac risk factors (see Chapter 1). On a population scale, studies have shown that routine screening of the population followed by very long-term treatment of symptomless hypertension will lower the rate of coronary thrombosis and stroke. Controversy surrounds many of the surveys and their implications: final answers are awaited. It has been known for years, from Life Assurance data, that the higher the blood pressure, the higher the associated morbidity (illness) and mortality. It is therefore reasonable to expect that reduction of high blood pressure is desirable at all ages. There are no symptoms due to hypertension alone.

Hypertension causes its problems in two main ways. First, by increasing the workload of the left ventricle, it causes changes leading to heart failure. Secondly, by its sustained effect on the larger arteries, it is associated with progressive arterial degeneration. Peripherally, the major hazard is stroke illness, caused by arterial haemorrhage or thrombosis in the brain. In the heart, the combination of poor muscle and arterial supply leads to increasing attrition of the heart muscle itself, left ventricular heart failure and coronary thrombosis.

There are many effective drugs for hypertension, most of them compatible with moderate sporting exercise once a satisfactory level of control has been achieved. It should be remembered that isometric exercises cause a rapid and severe increase in both systolic and diastolic blood pressure and sudden lifting or straining should be avoided. Intermittent exercising does not raise the diastolic pressure so greatly, although the systolic level may rise. Strong emotion causes severe rises in blood pressure as well as pulse rate.

The causes of hypertension are not all clear. It is not known why only some individuals become hypertensive. Family history is a significant factor and it is likely that diet plays a role. For instance, primitive populations have low or normal blood pressures but respond to increasing 'civilization' with progressive hypertension. One possible factor in diet and lifestyle is salt. Civilized man takes far more salt in his diet than is necessary physiologically. There may thus develop a gradual build-up of surplus salt which attracts fluids to maintain the body's standard osmotic pressure and hence a progressive loading of the body's fluid volume which acts as a hypertensive mechanism. The corroboration of this idea is that a salt-free diet tends to lower blood pressure. Diuretics are widely used in the control of hypertension and these act by causing excretion of excess fluid and salts.

Pulse rate

The pulse rate is controlled by nervous and chemical factors which act on the heart muscles. The sympathetic part of the autonomic nervous system raises the pulse rate, the parasympathetic lowers it.

Sympathetic factors include the catecholamines, adrenaline and noradrenaline, secreted by the body in states of arousal, fear and aggression, as well as chemical analogues including the sympathomimetic agents such as ephedrine or isoprenaline (*see* Chapter 12). Diseases such as thyrotoxicosis and some rare tumours which secrete hormones also raise the sympathetic drive and pulse rate.

The parasympathetic slowing mechanism of the pulse is through the action of the vagus nerve. At the cellular level parasympathetic function is transmitted by the release of acetylcholine. Inhibition of this drug by cholinergic drugs such as atropine reverses the vagal slowing of the heart. Few diseases slow the heart but myxoedema or thyroid deficiency slows up all bodily functions, including the pulse.

Training increases parasympathetic tone and slows the pulse of athletes (bradycardia of training).

Pulse

The pulse may be regular or irregular. In fact, the pulse is never perfectly regular for long because of the natural 'sinus arrhythmia' associated with respiration. The pulse accelerates slightly during inspiration, with a corresponding slowing during expiration. This is normal and very obvious in the slow pulse of the fit athlete.

Extrasystoles are occasional extra beats due to stimuli which arise outside the electrical conducting mechanism which spreads from the atria through a conducting bundle to the ventricles. The extra beat arises before the ventricle is fully ready for it and is therefore followed by a compensatory pause during which the ventricles are refractory to the stimulus of the next correct beat. They thus have time to overfill and the next contraction may be forceful enough to be felt as a thump or palpitation. Extrasystoles are harmless and may be caused by excessive tea, coffee or alcohol, smoking, stress or organic heart disease (and sometimes the drugs used in treating it). In the athlete, a trial avoidance of stimulant drinks should be tried and reassurance given. These extrasystoles always disappear during the onset of exercise.

Atrial fibrillation causes a very irregular pulse and is due to a disease-induced disorganization of the normal conduction mechanism in the heart. The atria beat incompletely and rapidly. Although only a proportion of the atrial beats get through the AV (atrioventricular) bundle to the ventricles, they contract more rapidly than usual. As atrial fibrillation is related to disease, medical investigation and control is required. The outlook in terms of permissible exercise depends upon the disease, which must be individually assessed by the physician.

Paroxysmal tachycardia consists of occasional attacks of very rapid heartbeats. There are two main types of tachycardia, classified by the origin of the electrical stimulus in the atria or the ventricles.

The commonest is paroxysmal atrial tachycardia. This is usually harmless, not associated with disease and often caused by smoking, alcohol, irritant foods, tea or coffee, as well as anxiety. The pulse rate averages about 180 beats/min and is completely regular. In contrast, the normal tachycardia of strenuous exercise may reach 180 beats/min, but usually decelerates rapidly on stopping exercise and may show sinus arrhythmia (see above). Paroxysmal tachycardia, by definition, usually switches off as spontaneously as it switches on. If spontaneous reversion does not occur, various ways of stimulating the vagus nerve may be tried, for instance: massaging the carotid sinus in the neck near the angle of the jaw; rebreathing expired air from a plastic bag; prolonged breath-holding; trying the Valsalva manoeuvre of breathing out hard against closure of the glottis; or by

direct stimulation of the back of the throat. If these simple measures fail, drug or electrical conversion is possible.

The tachycardias may cause faintness because the heart rate is too rapid to allow efficient maintenance of the blood pressure required to keep the brain adequately supplied with oxygenated blood.

Ventricular tachycardia, caused by rapid uncontrolled ventricular contractions, is life-threatening. It is usually due to heart disease but can be due to other causes including, rarely, effort. Electrical conversion is indicated; in emergency, a blow to the chest may cause the rhythm to revert.

The ECG

The ECG (electrocardiograph) measures the electrical potential difference between different parts of the heart as seen from electrode pick-up points over the chest, trunk or limbs. Its three-dimensional electrical picture of the heart gives a fairly accurate picture of the state of health or disease and is particularly useful in elucidating cardiac rhythm.

Peripheral resistance

The peripheral resistance is an important factor influencing cardiac output and blood pressure. If the peripheral resistance is increased, either by a disease's causing an obstruction to free circulation, or by more temporary vasoconstriction which causes a tight-valve effect for the circulating arterial blood, then the left ventricle is forced to work harder to maintain stroke volume, and the blood pressure rises. The opposite occurs if peripheral resistance is lowered, for instance, by vasodilation associated with exercise, warmth, alcohol or drugs. One of the long-term effects of exercise is to lower the peripheral resistance by opening up a more efficient capillary circulation in the muscle bed and this lowers the blood pressure, although it is relatively ineffective compared with some drugs.

Cardiovascular response to training

At rest, the average adult has a cardiac output of oxygenated blood of about 5 litres per minute (5ℓ/min) of which the muscles throughout the body consume about 15 per cent – roughly 800 ml in an average-sized man. At maximal exercise in the most highly trained subjects the cardiac output leaps to over 40 ℓ/min with the muscle share approaching 90 per cent. In order to meet this enormous increase in demand for oxygenated blood, major adaptations occur in the heart with important supporting changes in the lungs, blood and skin.

The heart has to increase its output in response to exercise and both pulse and stroke volume increase. As exercise begins, nervous and mechanical factors act. The increasing venous return from the pumping muscles acts directly on the heart muscle, forcing it to stretch into bigger contractions in response to the bigger mechanical workload, and to increase the force of contraction, blood pressure and stroke volume. At the same time, the sympathetic nervous drive to the heart is increased, causing the heart rate to rise. The stress of impending exercise plays a part in this mechanism through the release of sympathetic hormones.

Training increases the efficiency of the cardiac response to exercise and, as would be expected, trained subjects perform all work more efficiently and with less distress than untrained subjects.

In moderate exercise, the trained subject increases his cardiac output by increasing his stroke volume with a relatively small increase in heart rate. The untrained subject raises the heart rate considerably more than stroke volume. Pulse rate correlates well with the degree of oxygen uptake, exercise intensity and its degree of perception. Thus, greater distress is felt by the fast-pulsed, untrained subject than his trained colleague at the same moderate workload.

With graduated training, the heart is progressively conditioned into greater efficiency at rest as well as during exercise. In the autonomic nervous system, the balance swings towards the parasympathetic dominance of vagus nerve tone which slows the heart rate. Most cardiovascular responses to training are best seen in endurance athletes, for example long-distance cyclists, runners or swimmers. These athletes gradually descend to resting pulse rates as low as 40 or fewer beats/min. As the resting pulse rate drops, the exercising heart rate for a given workload falls; the same training sessions become easier and new targets become possible.

'Athlete's heart'

While the pulse falls, the stroke volume increases and the continued effects of hard cardiac workloads cause structural changes in the heart itself. These may be of two kinds. In chronic endurance or stamina training, the ventricles gradually enlarge to give the characteristic condition of 'athlete's heart'. In the early days of X-ray assessment, many athletes, by virtue of their enlarged hearts, were thought to be suffering from cardiac disease. It is now known that 'athlete's heart' is a physiological adaptation to training stress and consists of a gradual enlargement of the chambers of the heart but not a corresponding thickening of the walls of the ventricles. Thus, a well-conditioned heart is now beating more slowly with greater force to eject a larger volume of blood in its stroke volume to achieve the same resting effect as the faster, smaller heart before training began. There may be an increase in heart volume approaching 30 per cent but this is healthy and in sharp contrast to the cardiac enlargement found in disease.

The heart itself needs more fuel during exercise to service its own requirements and this is brought about by the chemical stimulus of anoxia, or oxygen lack, and metabolites within the heart itself so that there is a four- to fivefold increase in the rate of perfusion of the heart muscle with blood from the coronary vessels.

This is part of the general drastic redistribution of blood flow in response to exercise. The top priorities are the heart itself, the brain, and the muscles which are being used. The skin has increased needs as temperature rises and the lungs continue to oxygenate the much increased blood flow. In contrast to the left ventricle, the blood pressure in the pulmonary circulation is low and, in health, offers no comparable peripheral resistance to flow. Pulmonary hypertension is always pathological.

Where does this extra blood flow come from? At rest, the viscera, including the intestines, liver, spleen, kidneys and body fat, are relatively well supplied with, and effectively act as a shunt for, some of the blood. In the switch to exercise, their flow is drastically cut from about two-thirds of the cardiac output to 2 or 3 per cent. This causes postponement of some functions, like food digestion, until the end of exercise. For example, the kidneys undergo a relatively drastic shut-down from a perfusion of 1200 ml/min to 200–300 ml/min. The brain, however, preserves its perfusion intact throughout exercise, at least until the extreme stages of exhaustion. *Table 4.1* illustrates the drastic shunt of blood from viscera to functioning muscles between the extremes of rest and exercise. Symptomatically, gastro-intestinal symptoms (e.g. indigestion) and reduced urinary output illustrate the effectiveness of this shunt.

The second type of cardiac response to a hard training load is seen in power training as opposed to endurance training. Repeated heavy loading, for example isometric training, causes a muscular

Table 4.1. Circulatory response to exercise (all figures approximate)

	Rest	Maximal exercise
Cardiac output (100 per cent)	5 ℓ/min	40 ℓ/min
of which		
Muscles	15 per cent	90 per cent
Heart	5 per cent	2–3 per cent
Viscera	60 per cent	5 per cent

thickening of the ventricular wall but not the overall dilatation characteristic of 'athlete's heart' with its increased ventricular cavity volume. Thus, the fully trained power athlete does not share the endurance athlete's main benefit of stamina.

The endurance-event athlete has cardiorespiratory benefits without the risk of sudden sustained peaks of blood pressure common to power training. Power-event athletes are conditioned to their stresses but may also have the disadvantages of greater body weight and fat content because of their way of training and eating. Both power and endurance athletes revert to normal population levels of unfitness and obesity if they stop training. *Table 4.2* summarizes some aspects of the cardiac response to work and shows how increase in cardiac output goes hand in hand with increase in oxygen

Table 4.2. Some cardiac responses to exercise

	Resting adult	'Fit trained adult' at maximal exercise	Elite runner at maximal exercise
Cardiac output (CO)	5 ℓ/min	25 ℓ/min	42 ℓ/min
Heart rate	72/min	180/min	228/min
Stroke volume	70 ml	140 ml	212 ml
Maximum O₂ uptake ($\dot{V}O_{2max}$)	3.5 ml/kg/min (1 MET)	45 ml/kg/min (12 MET)	85 ml/kg/min (24 MET)
Blood pressure (BP)	120 mm Hg (systolic)	180 mm Hg (systolic)	200+ mm Hg (systolic)

uptake by the muscles at maximum workload. The figures for elite runners are maximum values quoted by different sources and do not occur necessarily in the same subject. They are the end products of inherited capacity plus severe training and would not be attainable with training alone.

The 'MET' is the popular American unit denoting a workload equivalent to the resting metabolic rate, equivalent to an uptake of 3.5 ml/kg/min of oxygen (i.e. 3.5 ml of oxygen per minute are taken up for each kg of total body weight, at rest). Many aerobic training programmes use the MET as a simple measure of activity; for instance, basic activity has a rate of 1 MET, moderate exercise with a pulse of about 100 beats/min, approximately 4 MET, and jogging with a pulse of about 140 beats/min, approximately 8 MET.

As the athlete's heart slows and enlarges in response to endurance exercise, a greater functional reserve is developed. *Table 4.3* shows how this relates to potential performance. By lowering the basal heart rate and raising its maximum capacity, performance is gained at both lower and upper ranges of workload. Figures given for maximum performance in elite athletes are often technically difficult to obtain but serve as fair approximations of potential capacity and performance.

ECG changes in exercise

The normal ECG (electrocardiograph) has a 'P' wave showing the potential difference generated by the passage of the contraction through the atria. This P wave is followed (*Figure 4.1*) by the 'QRS' complex of the ventricular contraction. Following contraction, the 'T' wave corresponds to electrical recovery in the ventricles.

The classic 12-lead ECG consists of bipolar and unipolar connecting leads. Bipolar leads show the potential difference between two widely separated points: lead I, left arm and right arm; lead II, left leg and right arm; lead III, left leg and left arm.

Unipolar leads are arranged so that the limb leads are neutral and a simple exploring electrode is used to gain a more selective view of the heart from different electrical viewpoints. By convention, these are usually further adjusted so as to augment electrically these readings to give leads aVR, aVL and aVF from, respectively, the right arm, left arm and left leg, together with the chest leads V1 to V6.

It is not necessary to take the full 12-lead ECG for most purposes and a continuous reading of lead II usually gives a clear indication of rhythm throughout an experiment.

As exercise begins, the pulse accelerates and the simplest response is an increasing frequency of the ECG complexes which can be easily measured from

Table 4.3. Differences in trained, untrained and elite athletes at maximum exercise

	Untrained	Trained	Elite
Heart rate (beats/min)	72 (rest) 180 (max.)	60 (rest) 190 (max.)	40 (rest) 220 (max.)
Difference (beats/min)	108	130	180
Stroke volume (ml)	70	130	210
Cardiac output (ml/min)	5040	24 700	46 200*

* Theoretical value only, see remarks above; usually 40 000–42 000 ml/min

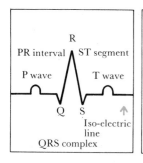

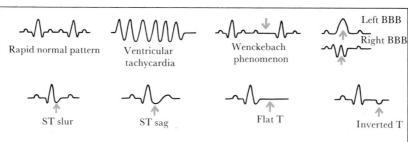

Figure 4.1 (left)
Normal electrocardiograph
(ECG) tracing
Figure 4.2 (right)
Some variations in ECG
tracings (*see* text)

the squared paper used. More sophisticated apparatus with oscilloscope display and measuring devices allows for automatic display, measurement and recording of data.

In more severe exercise, characteristic changes appear. Unfortunately, some of these are similar to those found in disease and the inexperienced interpreter may mistakenly exclude sportsmen from participation.

In apparently fit athletes there may be significant changes in cardiac rhythm and in ECG waveforms (*see Figure 4.2*). Changes include tachycardia, marked sinus arrhythmia or more complex arrhythmias. For instance, supraventricular tachycardia, with or without some degree of heart block, ventricular ectopic beats and, very rarely, ventricular tachycardia may occur in bursts on exertion or during recovery.

Various degrees of conduction block may be seen, including the Wenckebach phenomenon of an increasing PR interval over three or four beats leading up to a missed pulse or QRS contraction. Some degree of right bundle branch block may occur physiologically but left bundle branch block should be regarded as an indication for specialist cardiological assessment.

During intensive exercise the ST segment may become slurred or depressed. While this is often taken as an indication of myocardial ischaemia, there is usually no clinical evidence of this in athletic subjects. P and T wave variations are common in trained subjects, particularly T wave flattening and

inversion. ST segment and T wave changes often revert to 'normal' on exercise, in contrast to the changes of ischaemic heart disease.

These ECG changes may occur during exercise but are most likely to occur during the immediate recovery period. There are well-documented studies in the medical literature of the relation of ECG changes to increasing exercise loads and also of their reversion to normal after cessation of training.

While a wide variation of ECG changes related to exercise might therefore be permissible as 'normal' in the athletically fit, ECG tracings must always be related to clinical symptoms. As a general rule, simple waveform changes affecting P and T waves and marginal changes of the ST segment can probably be disregarded, but paroxysmal disturbances, particularly of bizarre configurations and those suggestive of ventricular tachycardia, must always be referred for expert cardiological assessment. The fact that many 'normal' athletes have very 'abnormal' ECGs must not be extrapolated to the suggestion that athletes are endowed with cardiac immortality. Under severe stress, ventricular arrhythmias may occur and cause myocardial infarction or death, even in the 'very fit'.

The blood

Blood consists of cells and plasma. The cellular element includes red (erythrocytes) and white cells (leucocytes). Platelets, derived from larger cells in the bone marrow, are responsible for clotting. Plasma is the fluid in which the red cells circulate and also contains all the other chemical and cellular elements of the blood. The serum is the watery exudate remaining after red cells and clotting components have been removed. The white cells combat infection and are responsible for antibody responses. They also initiate tissue healing and repair processes after injury.

Erythrocytes

Erythrocytes are formed in the bone marrow and have an average life of 120 days. They contain the pigment haemoglobin, a complex compound of protein and iron, which binds the circulating oxygen and carbon dioxide to transport them between lungs and tissues. As the cells age, they liberate their stored iron which is then taken up by the bone marrow for further red cell production.

The number of erythrocytes is normally constant. Under the stimulus of oxygen lack, the kidneys secrete the hormone erythropoietin which stimulates the marrow to produce further red cells. This mechanism is the basis of altitude adaptation.

Healthy red cell production needs a mixed diet. The absence of Vitamin C causes scurvy, with anaemia and poor wound healing. Iron is necessary but the binding of iron into the protein pigment haemoglobin is so efficient that extra iron is usually unnecessary given a normal mixed diet. Only about 1 mg of iron is excreted daily and a daily average of a further 1 mg covers menstrual blood loss. Pregnancy and lactation use further iron. The total body iron amounts to about 5 g in the adult – two-thirds of this is in the erythrocytes, the rest is stored in the reticuloendothelial system in the liver, spleen and bone marrow. In normal health the iron store is full and surplus intake is excreted.

Erythrocyte formation also needs Vitamin B_{12} and folic acid, which is taken as folates in the diet, for example in vegetables. In practice, folic acid deficiency is unusual in health, although it may occur in pregnancy. Folic acid supplements are therefore unnecessary, provided the diet is adequate.

Much mystique surrounds Vitamin B_{12}, the deficiency of which causes pernicious anaemia. As this is a rare condition which occurs spontaneously or after gastric surgery and is rarely seen before middle age, it is clear that Vitamin B_{12} supplements are totally unnecessary in normal health. So great is the body's ability to take up Vitamin B_{12} that, without disease being present, there is virtually no chance that B_{12} deficiency will occur except on vegan (extreme vegetarian) diets. Replacement of Vitamin B_{12} involves regular injections for life as oral preparations are not well absorbed.

Normal values of blood components

The healthy adult male has about 14–15 g of haemoglobin per 100 ml of blood and the female 12–14 g/100 ml. The value varies considerably between individuals and in general through life, levels in infants and children being higher. There is no overall standard fixed figure for the 'normal haemoglobin' level. Many coaches erroneously believe that there are certain fixed values which must be attained and, if at all possible, exceeded by whatever means, including gross supplementation with iron and Vitamin B_{12}. This belief has no medical or scientific foundation whatever and should be strongly discouraged.

The red cell count in normal blood is about 4–5 million/mm^3 and the white cell count between 5000 and 10 000/mm^3. In disease, changes occur in total white cell count (WBC) and also in the proportions of constituent cells (differential WBC).

The standard blood tests routinely performed are as follows (with normal values):

- Haemoglobin (Hb) $\begin{cases} 14–15\,\text{g}/100\,\text{ml (male)} \\ 12–14\,\text{g}/100\,\text{ml (female)} \end{cases}$
- Red blood cell count (RBC)   4–5 million/mm^3

- White blood cell count (WBC) 5–10 thousand/mm^3
- Differential WBC (*see* text above)
- Erythrocyte sediment-ation rate (ESR) up to 15 mm in 1 hour (Westergren method)
- Packed cell volume (PCV), haematocrit 45 per cent
- Red cell dimensions and haemoglobin content (MCH, MCHC and MCV)

The ESR (erythrocyte sedimentation rate) is a useful indicator of inflammatory and other disease conditions. A small blood sample is diluted with anticoagulant citrate and set up in a calibrated tube. The rate at which the red cells fall to leave clear plasma is read off after 1 hour.

The PCV (packed cell volume) or haematocrit gives an indication of the volume of red cells relative to plasma and is prepared by spinning down a sample so that the heavier cells collect at one end of the tube.

Blood oxygen transport

Respiratory gases are carried in the blood by attachment to the complex protein haemoglobin in the erythrocytes. As blood flows through the lung capillaries, the red cells absorb fresh oxygen (O_2) avidly in exchange for the waste product carbon dioxide (CO_2) and are pumped back to the muscles. As a result of muscle metabolism, the arterial blood becomes desaturated of its O_2 and this is replaced by CO_2, one of the end products of tissue metabolism. Now dissolved in the blood, this CO_2 returns to the lungs via the right side of the heart for elimination as expired CO_2 gas in the breath and is replaced in the new cycle by fresh atmospheric O_2.

The blood's efficiency in transporting O_2 depends on the amount of haemoglobin to which the O_2 can be attached. Each erythrocyte carries haemoglobin which consists of an iron-bearing pigment, haem, attached to the protein globin. O_2 attaches to the haem. In anaemia, the amount of haemoglobin is reduced and there is therefore reduced oxygen-carrying capacity. The anaemic athlete is easily breathless and tired as his blood is not carrying enough O_2 for the exercise requirement.

Conversely, if the amount of haemoglobin is increased, there is an enhanced oxygen-carrying capacity. Can this be achieved in the athlete?

Excessive haemoglobin exists in certain diseases but these can be disregarded in the athletic context. Stimulus to the formation of extra red cells is given by anoxia, or tissue oxygen lack. This occurs at altitude (*see* Chapter 5) and by the conditioning stresses of hard training.

An increase in the number of red cells is beneficial even if there is a corresponding increase in plasma volume and one problem in the trained athlete is interpretation of blood measurements in the presence of training-induced changes in haemoglobin or red cell content. If plasma volume also increases, Hb and RBC may be relatively constant but there is a greater absolute oxygen-carrying capacity. Chronic endurance training may bring about a possible 40 per cent increase, both in blood volume and total or circulating haemoglobin.

Blood doping

'Blood doping' is another way of increasing the athlete's haemoglobin. Some blood is withdrawn from an athlete and stored to be reinfused later. Meanwhile, the loss of this blood stimulates the bone marrow to form more red cells so that the athlete's blood has returned fully to normal in about 3 weeks. He is then given back his own red cells (and haemoglobin) with a consequent boost to oxygen-carrying capacity proportional to the volume of blood retransfused. Several studies have been published with conflicting results in actual response gained from this procedure. The following points are relevant. First, in all blood transfusion procedures there are inevitable risks including infection, transfusion reaction owing to confusion of specimens, and reaction to the anticoagulants used. These should all be eliminated by good practice however. Secondly, and more practically, the frozen stored red cells deteriorate so that they may be relatively inefficient by the time of their retransfusion, thus the whole procedure may be a waste of time. Thirdly, retransfusion of whole blood may embarrass the circulation at a crucial time in a competition, or replacement of the oxygen-carrying part as 'packed cells' may cause an increase in viscosity of the athlete's circulating bloodstream. Thus, in order to be effective in the enhancement of performance, it would have to be certain that, not only were there no technical mistakes but that, in the given subject under study, the red cells would remain sound, the extra O_2 transport would actually be available and the benefit gained would exceed any possible inefficiency incurred by increased blood viscosity which would slow the circulation.

In summary, while this method is theoretically attractive, its practice must be extremely difficult to regulate safely and efficiently under all the stresses of athletic competition and, in view of all the provisos outlined, it is unlikely to become widespread.

Heat loss

As part of the circulatory shunt already discussed, there may be a 50-fold increase in circulation to the skin at maximum heat loads. Muscle work produces heat which has to be dissipated despite the body's ability to accommodate a considerable degree of hyperthermia, or overheating. Core temperatures of up to 106°F (41°C) have been recorded in long-distance runners; these values are associated with heatstroke and death in untrained subjects. Skin perfusion may reach 3–4 ℓ/min and heat loss may occur by conduction, convection and radiation, and particularly by evaporation of sweat which can be secreted at a rate of up to 2 ℓ/hour.

Lungs

Breathing is a complex mixture of voluntary and involuntary actions. During inspiration, the chest expands due to action of the intercostal muscles and, possibly, the accessory muscles of respiration at the top of the chest. The diaphragm is lowered and the lungs attain their maximum volume. The process is reversed during expiration. As atmospheric air flows in and out of the lungs, gaseous interchange occurs in the capillary bed where the pulmonary capillaries meet the very thin alveolar lining of the lungs. O_2 is extracted from the inspired air and replaced by CO_2.

Breathing is under the overall control of the medullary respiratory centre in the brain as well as mechanical factors which influence the elastic recoil of the lungs and chest wall. The rate and depth of breathing are highly sensitive to changes in O_2 and CO_2 levels in both blood and air. Both temperature and the degree of acidity or alkalinity (pH) in the region of the nervous receptors affect their sensitivity to the gas levels. While breathing requires minimal effort at rest, at exercise considerable work is performed simply to move the chest wall and, for this reason, increasing effort brings the accessory muscles of respiration into play. These are the neck muscles, the sternomastoids and scaleni, together with the intercostal and abdominal muscles which play a more active part by raising intra-abdominal pressure and forcing the diaphragm up to aid expiration. The work of respiration is increased in certain lung diseases, particularly bronchitis, emphysema and asthma, where great effort may be required to force air out through the constricted airways.

Measurements of breathing

Figure 4.3 summarizes respiratory function. Total lung capacity (TLC) is the maximum capacity of the lungs which is roughly 6 ℓ in male adults. Only about 10 per cent of this large capacity is required during quiet breathing at rest where the tidal volume (TV) is only

about 500 ml of air. This requirement increases
gradually with exercise, however, until a maximum
level of inspiration and expiration is reached which
represents the vital capacity (VC). This capacity is
between 3 and 5 ℓ in adults, with levels in males being
some 50 per cent greater than those in females. The
VC is the tidal volume at maximum breathing effort.
Even at this maximal level, however, there remains a
residual volume (RV) of 1–1.5 ℓ. The dead space is
the volume of the air passages from nose to alveoli
which are not available for gas interchange in each
breath. Thus, of the resting tidal volume of 500 ml,
some 150 ml represents an average dead space,
leaving about 350 ml of the original 500 ml available
for respiratory gas exchange.

The maximum breathing capacity (MBC) or
maximum ventilation volume (MVV) measures the
rate of breathing. The breathing measured at any
time is a reflection of all the respiratory functions –
lungs, muscles, chest wall and nervous and chemical
control. An average male has an MBC of about
125 ℓ/min in a normal atmosphere.

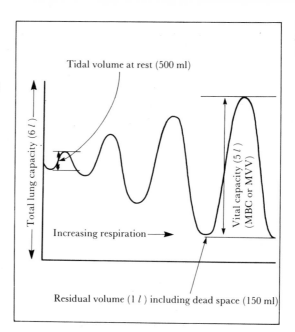

Figure 4.3
Some respiratory measures
(*see* text)

Alveolar gaseous exchange

Efficient exchange of O_2 and CO_2 in the lungs
depends on appropriate supplies of air and blood
reaching the alveoli and the efficiency of the alveolar
membrane itself. The alveoli are ventilated by the
amount of the tidal volume which is left after the dead
space has been filled. Diseases which increase the
dead space, e.g. emphysema, detract from respiratory
efficiency. At the alveolar interface, the ventilation:
perfusion (V:P) ratio must be appropriate, in other
words, the right amount of inspired air must tally
with the optimum amount of blood. If all the air went
to the top of the lungs and all the blood to the bottom,
no effective gaseous interchange could occur. There is
considerable regional variation in blood flow to
different parts of the lungs both during disease,
including asthma, bronchitis and emphysema, and in
normal health. Effective shunting mechanisms exist
which influence the regional flow through the

different parts of the lungs. In full health, the athlete
may take an efficient V:P ratio for granted but, in
respiratory disease, inefficient V:P will further limit
exercise tolerance, which partly explains why the
asthmatic athlete cannot perform efficiently during an
attack.

Alveolar diffusion capacity

The alveolar diffusion capacity is a measure of the
efficiency of gaseous interchange and this capacity is
impaired when there is pathological interference with
the lung lining. This condition is caused by diseases
such as pulmonary fibrosis or emphysema both of
which slow down the rate of exchange which in turn
leads to breathlessness and underoxygenation of the
blood. In contrast, CO_2 does not accumulate in the
blood because it diffuses some 20 times faster than
O_2, so that the primary problem is the level of O_2 in
the blood and not the level of CO_2. Diffusion defects
cause breathlessness in asthma, bronchitis and those

viral inflammations which affect the alveolar membrane. There is, however, variation in individual diffusion capacity which is essentially an untrainable function. Hence, at normal atmospheric pressure the athlete cannot absorb more O_2 because the blood is already fully saturated through efficient diffusion and respiration. Intensive training will teach muscles to cope with some relative anoxia and also the production of metabolites but will not teach alveoli to take up more O_2.

Breath-holding and overbreathing

Some sportsmen try to improve performance by overbreathing before a sprint, especially in swimming. The idea is that if CO_2 can be removed from the bloodstream, a few seconds respite may be gained from the urge to breathe, and thus performance may be enhanced by delaying the need to breathe. It may also be thought that removal of the CO_2 increases the O_2 level beneficially. What, in fact, does happen?

First, the unprepared subject, after a full inspiration, can easily hold his breath for about a minute. At the end of this time, the falling O_2 and rising CO_2 levels in the bloodstream compel him to breathe again. Next, if he simply overbreathes, as quickly and as deeply as possible, he does indeed wash out CO_2 to lower the alveolar CO_2 concentration by 50 per cent or more with a corresponding increase in O_2 concentration of about 50 per cent. At the end of overbreathing, there is a period of compensation beginning with non-breathing. This is due to the lack of sufficient CO_2 to stimulate breath-taking and not because there is enough oxygen in the lungs. Over the next few minutes, the surplus oxygen is absorbed and CO_2 is exchanged. Eventually, a severe shortage of O_2 produces a stimulus to further respiration while the blood CO_2 level is still low or nearly back to the normal level at which it will also stimulate breathing. Respiration then resumes its normal pattern.

If overbreathing and breath-holding are combined,

breath-holding time may easily be doubled. This, however, doubles the time during which O_2 can be absorbed before the CO_2 level comes up to breathing-stimulus levels. There may thus be a discrepancy between the two breathing stimuli of CO_2 excess and O_2 lack. As both stimuli need to interact, there is a risk that the underwater swimmer who has overbreathed before breath-holding may become severely anoxic and faint under water. This practice is therefore extremely dangerous. Breath-holding can be even more prolonged after overbreathing with O_2 but this would in any case create practical difficulties in competition.

Interesting experiments involving the rectal infusion of O_2 into swimmers did not lead to improved performance, either through buoyancy or through mucosal O_2 uptake!

Blood oxygen uptake

The total surface of the alveolar membrane is about the size of a tennis court. During exercise the circulation rate is so great that contact time between blood and alveolar membrane is no more than a third of a second. This suffices for the haemoglobin to become at least 97 per cent fully saturated, however.

Arterial blood acquires an O_2 content of 19 ml/100 ml at a pressure of 100 mm Hg with a further small amount in simple solution in the plasma. The corresponding CO_2 content is 48 ml/100 ml at 40 mm Hg pressure. At rest, the tissues take up O_2, exchanging it for CO_2, so that the desaturation of O_2 leaves venous blood containing only about 14 ml/100 ml O_2 at a pressure of 40 mm Hg while the CO_2 rises to 52 ml/100 ml at 46 mm Hg pressure in the venous blood returning to the lungs. On exercise, total O_2 desaturation can occur in the active muscles, although the final venous blood reaching the lungs contains O_2 remaining from the non-muscular tissues.

The O_2 dissociation curve, which relates the degree of O_2 saturation of the haemoglobin to the atmospheric pressure of O_2 (*Figure 4.4*) shows the rapid rate at which the blood takes up O_2. This is influenced by the amount of available haemoglobin as well as by atmospheric pressure. Binding of haemoglobin, for instance by carbon monoxide (CO) as a result of smoking, limits the residual haemoglobin available for O_2 and CO_2 transport. For instance, 10 cigarettes or a large cigar may bind 10 per cent of the circulating haemoglobin so that the athlete is substantially impaired in terms of oxygen carriage. Bearing in mind that in severe exercise the muscles can use almost 100 per cent of the oxygen supply, if these muscles are offered only 90 per cent of this amount in a smoker, it is obvious that maximum performance is not possible. This is so even though it is true that exercise is one of the factors which promote the restoration of carbon monoxide-bound haemoglobin to normal oxyhaemoglobin (HbCO to HbO_2).

Asthma

Ten per cent of the population may suffer some degree of bronchial spasm induced by exercise. This discovery obviously introduces a totally new dimension into the subject of asthma. Apart from known asthmatics with a tendency to exercise-induced asthma (EIA), EIA may be the only asthmatic manifestation in otherwise completely normal subjects. A proportion of the population has been found to be latently asthmatic or allergic and there may be a strong family history of these conditions.

A common complaint is that an athlete, after some years of comfortable exertion, realizes that at a certain level of intensity he simply cannot get a satisfactory chestful of air and his performance declines. A practical difficulty is that symptoms may be so specific as to be extremely difficult to demonstrate and treat. For instance, EIA may be caused by specific pollens and be highly seasonal; may be induced by air pollution including chemicals or photochemical smog; or related to ambient air temperature; for example, it may be precipitated by

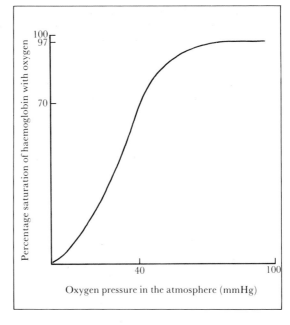

Figure 4.4
Oxygen dissociation curve

Percentage saturation of haemoglobin with oxygen

Oxygen pressure in the atmosphere (mmHg)

cold air breathing only. Stress, also, is often a potent precipitant of symptoms. Various atmospheric conditions, including humidity, play a part, with swimming producing fewer attacks in vulnerable subjects than dry-land exercising, and running causing more problems than cycling. The reasons for this are not clear and have been shown not to relate simply to the degree of atmospheric humidity.

The presence of EIA can be demonstrated by listening to the chest, which shows the expiratory wheeze, or by peak flow meter changes. Such meters measure the rate of flow of exhaled air on a simple dial. Normally, 80 per cent of the total forced expiratory volume (FEV) is exhaled in the first second (i.e. $FEV_1 = 80$ per cent of FEV). In EIA the obstruction of the airways resists this forced exhalation and FEV_1 falls drastically.

Characteristically, EIA comes on after a few minutes of continuous exercise or within a few minutes of stopping. The intensity of exercise is not clearly related to attacks and there is considerable variation from time to time in individuals as well as between different individuals, factors which make management of EIA specific to the individual sufferer.

The attack then lasts for 10–15 min and gradually eases as normal breathing returns. This is reflected in gradual reversion of the FEV_1 to normal. It is sometimes possible for exercise to be continued through a mild attack of EIA which does not recur because of a refractory period during which bronchial spasm cannot occur after the acute attack. Some athletes find it possible to induce their predicted EIA in the pre-race warm-up, knowing that actual competition, perhaps half an hour later, is guaranteed to be free from bronchspasm.

Why should the asthmatic stress himself with exercise? The general benefits of exercise apply no less to asthmatic than to non-asthmatic subjects. There is, therefore, considerable reason for asthmatics to benefit from regular exercise. Secondly, many asthmatics are of high athletic ability which, in itself, gives them the desire to continue at high level. Thirdly, the ubiquity of EIA has brought a new impetus to the general management of asthma which encourages the asthmatic to look for much better control of his condition than heretofore and opens up new vistas of enjoyable sports participation in a way that was previously impossible.

Drug management of asthma

Common and effective antiasthmatic drugs such as adrenaline, ephedrine, isoprenaline and other sympathomimetic drugs are expressly forbidden by international doping regulations. Drugs are now available, however, which will control most competing asthmatics without risk of disqualification. For instance, salbutamol (Ventolin) and terbutaline (Bricanyl, Brethine) are sympathomimetic drugs but, because of their highly selective beta-2 bronchodilating action, are permitted for Olympic usage. The forbidden sympathomimetic drugs have wider sympathetic activity than these two drugs and

their possible stimulant effect upon performance is the reason for prohibition (*see* Chapters 12 and 13).

While salbutamol and terbutaline act by local action on the constricted airways, a prophylactic drug is available in sodium cromoglycate (Intal). This works in a different way and inhibits the allergically induced release of the histamine which actually triggers the bronchial constriction. Because it works prophylactically, it obviously has to be taken in advance of competition. At present, it must be taken in a locally acting form, e.g. by spray, powder, or by a spin-haler which releases the standard dose of powder directly into the airways.

For the general prevention of asthma during exercise, a combination of drugs may be highly effective. Salbutamol or cromoglycate may be necessary as basic medication or can be substituted for other effective but athletically prohibited maintenance therapy. Either salbutamol or cromoglycate can be taken about half an hour before the beginning of exercise. Aerosol or puff delivery to the airways is quicker and more reliable than oral administration.

Because the general management of asthmatics is often complex and variable, it is essential that the asthmatic competitor be fully assessed and the prescribed drugs brought into line with permitted sports practice, well before the crisis of a major competition with the danger of disqualification because of doping.

Cardiorespiratory symptoms

Fatigue

The commonest causes of fatigue in the athlete are overtraining and anaemia. Overtraining states include loss of enthusiasm for, and impaired recovery from, hard exercise. More common is simple fatigue due to overambitious training schedules and recognition of this should be obvious to the experienced coach. Failure to increase training on a gradual scale is probably the commonest reason for undue fatigue. It rarely pays to undertake a drastic increase in training or competitive load.

Occasionally, training leads to iron deficiency anaemia and the female athlete is commonly iron-deficient. Other general illnesses can causes anaemias.

Glandular fever is a common viral illness in the athletic age group and is sometimes the cause of slight anaemia. Fatigue and depression following a 'flu-like illness raises the possibility of glandular fever. It may impair athletic performance for 6 months, or longer in some cases. The basis of this fatigue and breathlessness is a combination of myocarditis, anaemia and general viral toxaemia which affects the reticuloendothelial system and may be reflected in abnormal levels of immunoglobulins in the blood.

Any illness increases fatigue and it is important that adequate time is given for full convalescence, including a graduated return to full training loads. Depression may be a cause of fatigue in athletes. This may be part of the overtraining state or a disorder in its own right, commonly associated with anxiety.

Breathlessness

This may be due to anxiety, anaemia or lung disease of any type. Anxiety often causes hyperventilation, or overbreathing, leading to tingling of the lips, hands and feet. Cardiac causes include valvular disease, myocarditis, cardiomyopathy, ischaemia and hypertension. It is important to recognize that relatively young athletes, although highly successful, may still be victims of rheumatic carditis which may reach the stage of decompensation and heart failure. Important symptoms include a history of rheumatic heart disease and breathlessness at rest or when lying flat at night. An athlete with decompensated rheumatic heart disease cannot be fit for high-level training again because the cardiac limits have been reached.

On the other hand, the symptom-free presence of cardiac murmurs due to rheumatic valvular disease is not necessarily a contraindication to any degree of effort. This is because the heart is compensating adequately. Nevertheless, it is impossible to give a definite prognosis in such cases, from both the long-term medical and the athletic viewpoints. The patient and his parent or coach should be realistically aware of the situation and know that unaccustomed breathlessness or fatigue will need further medical assessment. Mild degrees of treated cardiac failure may be compatible with some exercise under medical guidance.

Palpitations

This means undue awareness of normal pulse, or awareness of abnormal pulse. Anxiety, tension and exertion all make the normal subject aware of his pulse (*see* above).

Giddiness and dizziness

Anxiety, or vasovagal attacks of fainting may produce giddiness or dizziness. Anaemia has to be fairly severe before giddiness occurs but symptoms on sudden change of posture are common.

Giddiness or fainting habitually related to particular positions, or changes of position, is rare but may be due to extremely serious cardiac disorders, including the presence of a tumour, and needs urgent specialist investigation. This is one of the few conditions where an absolute prohibition of training is required on the story alone, pending full diagnosis.

Giddiness or collapse after exertion

In the vast majority of cases a simple faint at the end of hard effort is caused by the athlete's having suddenly stopped leg movement and with it the active muscle pump mechanism. This allows blood suddenly to pool in the legs, due to vasodilation, with a consequent sharp drop in blood pressure and cerebral circulation. It is a distressing but self-correcting event because falling to the horizontal position reverses the cause.

Very rarely, collapse at the finish of competition has the more serious significance of being due to heart disease and if there is doubt in the interpretation of the athlete's account of the symptoms a medical check is necessary.

Some athletes tend to exert themselves to a point of considerable gastrointestinal distress with retching, vomiting or abdominal cramps. There is no particular reason for this or, usually, any serious cause. It is partly due to the acute circulatory shifts which occur during strenuous exercise, to which some subjects may be more vulnerable symptomatically than others. In general, such symptoms relate to relative unfitness and tend to improve with continued training.

Chest pain

The most serious cause of chest pain, particularly in older subjects on general exercise or jogging programmes, is angina, or cardiac pain related to effort. This is characteristically a tight, heavy or gripping pain felt in the middle of the chest and radiating to either, or both, shoulders and arms, to the jaw or through to the back.

Such pain calls for prompt cessation of exercise and full investigation. Unfortunately, differential diagnosis of chest pain may sometimes be extremely difficult. This is because classic angina may be associated with a totally normal ECG at rest and on exertion. On the other hand, some of the ECG changes found in active athletes may cause diagnostic confusion, particularly to less-experienced observers. Furthermore, patients vary considerably in their ability to express symptoms which are of themselves difficult to put into words or pin down anatomically. The commonest causes of confusion in diagnosis are indigestion, particularly oesophagitis and hiatus hernia pain; chest-wall musculoskeletal pain; and the so-called Effort Syndrome.

Indigestion usually becomes apparent when the subject admits to food-related symptoms at rest, or relief with positional change or antacids.

Chest-wall pain tends to relate to movement such as change of position, rather than the general effect of, for example, sustained jogging. It is fairly common for chest pain to be due to pectoral muscle strains from overenthusiastic weight-training, press-up exercises, throwing or swimming by unfit sportsmen. All these efforts may cause minor strains of the muscles and fibrous tissue and of the many small joints which make up the thorax and shoulder girdle. Nevertheless, a careful clinical history and detailed examination should usually make a positive and clear diagnosis of mechanical pain without the need for cardiac investigation.

The Effort Syndrome is an obscure condition mimicking angina with left pectoral pain which may radiate to the shoulder and arm. This has been blamed on neurosis because it has often been found in fit but reluctant performers, such as military recruits.

Other possible causes of chest pain may include diaphragmatic irritation, shoulder capsulitis or a referred pain from spinal osteoarthrosis in older subjects. Medical treatment of all these conditions is along conventional lines, the most important factor from the sportsman's point of view being the clear elimination of angina as a diagnosis.

Subject to the physician's assessment in each case, angina does not necessarily disqualify from sport. Prophylactic use of cardiac vasodilators, such as trinitrin, may allow comfortable participation in the gentler sporting pursuits such as walking, golf or bowls but, as strong emotion can exacerbate angina and cause coronary thrombosis, the older sportsman is well advised to modify both his attitude and levels of physical participation in sport.

Coughing blood (haemoptysis)

Haemoptysis may be due to disease or simply to an irritation of the airways in some susceptible subjects. The latter is particularly likely in winter when the harsh inspiration of cold air may cause bronchial irritation and congestion leading to a small haemoptysis. The condition is unimportant but may be alarming.

Nose-bleeding or dental haemorrhage may cause haemoptysis when blood runs down the back of the nose and throat and is coughed up. Again, this of itself may not be serious but the cause should certainly be found and treated.

More important causes of haemoptysis include tuberculosis and bronchiectasis. Cough associated with malaise and haemoptysis, especially in Asian populations in whom tuberculosis is common, needs full investigation. Vigorous exercise is forbidden during active tuberculosis but is allowed once the disease is fully controlled by drugs – treatment which may be necessary for a year or more.

Bronchiectasis is a form of lung scarring following a severe chest infection, usually in childhood. An otherwise fit person may suffer recurrent attacks of cough during which some blood may be produced. Occasionally an alarming amount may be coughed up but usually small amounts tinge the purulent sputum. Initial medical management is important to exclude tuberculosis but it is not usually necessary to stop sport.

Vomiting blood (haematemesis)

Major haemorrhage with vomiting is usually due to peptic ulceration. Aspirin, other anti-inflammatory drugs and steroids may cause bleeding and ulceration, especially if combined with alcohol.

Violent retching can lead to the production of a small amount of blood, however, usually flecking some mucus. This is the Mallory–Weiss syndrome due to mechanical irritation by straining of the blood vessels which line the lower oesophagus. It is of no pathological significance but the athletic subject producing these symptoms should be considered against the above remarks on post-exercise distress.

5 Muscle and training adaptations

Training improves efficiency by conditioning the body to the stresses imposed by progressively heavier workloads, and the whole body shares in these adaptations. The cardiovascular and respiratory responses are outlined in Chapter 4.

Muscle

The crucial step in exercise is the conversion of energy, by muscles, from the chemical to the mechanical form. This brings about muscle contraction which can be energized through different chemical pathways. These reflect different muscle structures and functions, fuels and waste products. An overall synopsis is shown in *Figure 5.1*.

Initiation of contraction

Voluntary movements are initiated in the cerebral cortex and impulses are transmitted down the spinal cord and along the peripheral motor nerves to the muscles. There is a continuous flow of sensory impulses relaying information back from the joints and muscles about position and movement, as well as pain. Muscle tone is monitored and controlled by spinal reflexes through which alpha motor fibres respond to changes indicated by sensory nerves supplying stretch-sensitive muscle spindles. This tone-controlling mechanism is partly overruled by the voluntary impulses from the brain when active movements start.

The peripheral nerves split up into fine branches which supply the muscle fibres as a motor unit. Some motor units have a very rich innervation, others receive fewer nerve endings, but all the muscle fibres supplied by a particular nerve fibre are of the same functional type (fast or slow reacting, *see* below).

The impulses transmitted along the nerve ultimately affect the electrical potential of the muscle cell membrane. The membrane is first depolarized by acetylcholine secreted at the nerve ending and then has to be repolarized, through the metabolism of acetylcholine by cholinesterase, before a further impulse can be transmitted.

Muscle structure

Muscles are built up of bundles of individual fibres together with connective tissue, collagen and elastin, and a rich supply of blood vessels, lymphatics and nerves. The fibres themselves contain smaller bundles of fibrils containing the individual contractile filaments of actin and myosin.

Voluntary muscle has a characteristic banded appearance under the microscope; involuntary (or smooth) muscle lacks this. Staining techniques distinguish between different types of muscle fibre, notably fast or slow, and show the changes which occur in muscle damage, disease or wasting through disuse. Specimens of muscle are easily obtained by biopsy (needle sampling) under local anaesthetic; such samples are then prepared for chemical and microscopic examination.

Figure 5.1
Synopsis of muscle function

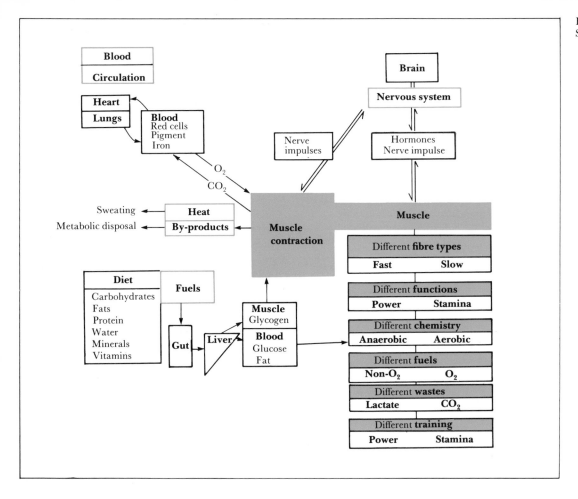

Muscle contraction

Nerve stimulation triggers the changes which liberate the stored chemical energy of ATP (adenosine triphosphate) in the muscle fibre. This change releases chemical bindings between the actin tubes and myosin rods to allow them to interdigitate, or slide together, thus producing the actual contraction. Relaxation reverses the movement which is partly limited by fatigability of the chemical processes, i.e.

the local supplies of chemicals run out. Training increases the size and chemical efficiency of the cellular fibres as well as their blood supply.

Muscle chemistry (*see Figure 5.2*)

The energy for muscle contraction is supplied by the conversion of ATP to ADP (adenosine diphosphate). This instant mechanism can only last a few seconds and, in order to keep exercising, the muscle must

Figure 5.2
Energy pathways in the
muscle cell

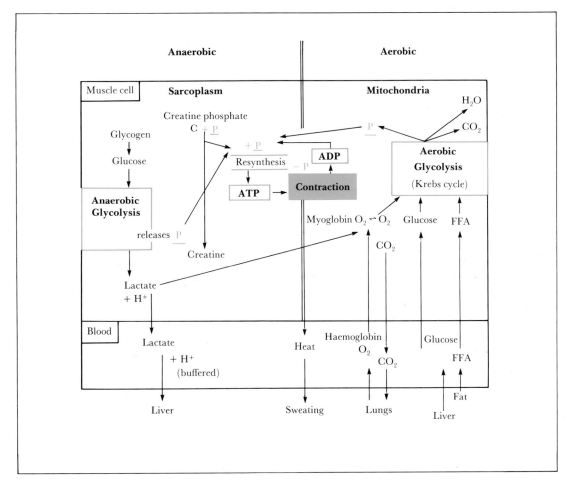

recycle the ADP back to ATP for further high-energy phosphate radicals to become available for contraction. This resynthesis is achieved by using the energy from the main fuels – carbohydrate and fat – which are oxidized to carbon dioxide (CO_2) and water or metabolized to lactate in the process.

If the muscle contracts suddenly there are three sources of energy available within the cell. First, pre-existing ATP itself breaks down. Secondly, as ATP breaks down to ADP, creatine phosphate (CP)

gives up its phosphate to restore ADP to ATP. As there is only a small amount of ATP and CP in the cell, this can only last perhaps 5 seconds. Thirdly, the small supply of oxygen (O_2) attached to the muscle pigment myoglobin in each cell may initiate aerobic glycolysis but is insufficient to last more than a few seconds. Thereafter ATP replacement energy must come from fuel breakdown, with or without using O_2. These mechanisms occur before O_2 and glucose are used and do not therefore generate the waste product lactate. Hence they are called 'alactate' mechanisms and form the 'non-lactic' part of the subsequent O_2 debt to be repaid in recovery.

Maximum contraction needs immediately available energy and the first contractions exceed the ability of the O_2-fuelled ATP replacement mechanisms to keep up with demand. Hence, for the short-term maximum efforts of the sprinter, energy is obtained by non-O_2-dependent sources. However, these are strictly limited in duration (about 30 seconds) and the energy stocks used can only be replenished eventually with the help of O_2. Thus there are two main ways of fuelling the muscle – with or without O_2. Aerobic metabolism uses O_2; anaerobic (literally 'non-air using') metabolism does not. The sprinter depends on anaerobic metabolism but builds up an energy debt which can only be repaid with O_2 later by aerobic metabolism, the process which also fuels longer, slower exercise.

Muscle cells possess a permeable cell membrane, a nucleus containing genetic material and a matrix – the sarcoplasm – in which anaerobic processes occur and in which are suspended numerous bodies, the mitochondria, in which the aerobic pathways are found. Oxygen, which diffuses from blood haemoglobin to attach to muscle myoglobin, is freely available within the cell; so too are ATP and glucose (derived from blood glucose or pre-stored muscle glycogen in the cell). Thus all the components needed for contraction are freely available.

Alactic anaerobic mechanisms initially provide energy for contraction. ATP is resynthesized using phosphate released mainly from creatine phosphate (by the enzyme creatine kinase) and to a lesser degree generated by aerobic glycolysis using the oxygen from myoglobin already inside the cell (*see Figure 5.2*).

Continued maximum exercise draws on the immediate conversion of stored muscle glycogen through glucose in the process of anaerobic glycolysis (literally 'sugar breakdown') to generate phosphate and lactate. The phosphate's energy goes to resynthesize ATP from ADP while the lactate accumulates. If there is no oxygen available, lactate accumulation is the main limiting factor in exercise. The sprinter becomes fatigued, his muscles cramped and sore and he has to stop. Anaerobic processes are quicker and more powerful than aerobic processes, but more quickly fatiguing because of lactate production associated with increasing acidosis.

If O_2 is available and the pace drops sufficiently to reduce lactate production to a level at which it can be both tolerated and partly metabolized, then lactate joins the mitochondrial pathway of aerobic glycolysis and is converted with the help of O_2 to CO_2 and water (H_2O), with the restoration of further phosphate to replenish ATP stores.

During steady-state exercise, aerobic glycolysis operates using O_2 to generate energy through the breakdown of glucose and fat to CO_2 and H_2O. This is the typical 'jogging' or 'cruising' state where movement can continue indefinitely but at a level well below maximum capacity. The greater the effort, the more the muscle changes from fat to carbohydrate metabolism.

There is a conflict, however, between endurance and speed (or power) in sport at a high percentage of maximum effort. Some degree of O_2 debt is inevitable even in the longest races; extra stamina is crucial in the longer sprints between 300 metres and the mile. The sprinter can operate anaerobically for short races – the 100-metre and 200-metre races can be run without a breath as far as energy is concerned. For the 400 metres a fine balance must be found between anaerobic and aerobic work. If he keeps sprinting flat out, the runner will 'die' in the last 100 metres because of the lactate build-up and excessive level of O_2 debt. If, on the other hand, he cruises too soon, or too slowly, he may not be able to incur his maximum tolerable O_2 debt before the finish and hence loses time or place in the competition. In practice it seems most difficult to accelerate from a state of increasing fatigue and most recent 400-metre, 800-metre and 1500-metre records have been set by runners able to start fast and then cruise fast at a high proportion of both maximum effort and tolerable O_2 debt, with relatively less last-phase acceleration than is usually found in top competitive races where overall time is usually sacrificed to tactical expediency, and victory usually won by the runner capable of the most drastic change of pace towards the end. Only rarely do record and competitive interests coincide. This raises the question of selective training of the different chemical processes and will be further discussed below.

Fuels for exercise (*see Figure 5.3*)

Most exercise is fuelled by carbohydrate which is stored as glycogen in the liver and muscle. Some is in free circulation in the blood and tissues as glucose, the most important function of which is nourishment of the nervous system. Protein is not a direct fuel for exercise; tissue or dietary protein is converted in the liver to glycogen before it is available for use in exercise.

Fats provide a large store of energy. Dietary fats are converted in the liver to free fatty acids (FFA) which are circulated and stored in the body's adipose tissue.

The average male has about 15 per cent of his body weight as fat, the average female 25 per cent, but these levels fall drastically with training to about 5–10 per cent for males and 15–20 per cent for females. Nevertheless, the fat stores represent a theoretical energy supply for 100–200 hours of hard work. In contrast, the glycogen store is good only for a couple of hours – witness the 2-hour 'barrier' in marathon running where the muscle glycogen becomes depleted.

How does the muscle 'choose' its fuels? Initially, the alactic anaerobic mechanisms are the instantly available sources of energy. Thereafter, the lactate anaerobic metabolism is quick and powerful but totally dependent on carbohydrate and limited by its end product of lactate which not only causes symptoms of fatigue but at a certain level chemically inhibits glucose metabolism.

Thus aerobic metabolism is the key to sustained effort. The mitochondria can use glucose, lactate and FFA for aerobic glycolysis in the presence of sufficient O_2. Initially carbohydrate is the most efficient and quickly available fuel but the small reserve compared with fat limits its use in endurance events. Hence the muscle switches progressively to fat metabolism in longer events.

If a runner sets out to run indefinitely, he uses glycogen for a couple of hours of hard effort but then as he changes over to fat his energy output drops. He may feel worse and his pace slows, often dramatically. He has lost the power-rich carbohydrate source of his speed (*see Figure 5.4*).

The effects of training for long-distance running, however, include an earlier switch to fat metabolism. This may be enhanced by long slow distance ('LSD') type running programmes. The athlete learns to use fat (FFA) almost immediately while sparing carbohydrate to a degree which allows longer maintenance of speed and reduces fatigue levels. Caffeine enhances FFA release and use. It is probable that women may have a more effective fat-burning metabolism than men which may benefit them in marathon events. Thus the use of FFA spares

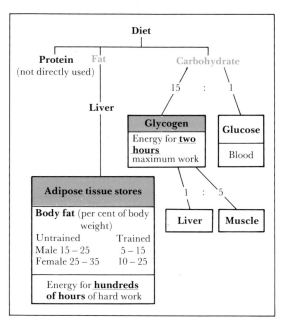

Figure 5.3
Fuels for exercise

39

glycogen and, in steady-state exercise, glycolysis and lactate formation are curtailed.

Only high-carbohydrate diets are effective in increasing performance. By increasing the glycogen stores, more 'power' fuel is available. The marathon 'carbohydrate loading' diet achieves a doubling or more of muscle glycogen levels in the week before a race. Best results follow a hard run, or harder training over a day or more, one week before the target day. If a carbohydrate-free diet is followed for about 3 days, the muscle's avidity for glycogen is enhanced and a switch to a very heavy carbohydrate diet will cause the cells to overcompensate in the next few days.

This diet does not suit all runners, particularly not those with very low 'fast' muscle fibre percentages. For no clear reason, it may be effective only on some occasions and may not work if repeated too often, perhaps 4–5 times a season. Many prefer simply to train harder the week before rather than to exhaust themselves. Others simply load their diets with extra carbohydrate during the week before a race. These variable responses indicate the need for each person to experiment with this method well before any key competition.

Any diet which is low in carbohydrate (including the first phase of the loading diet) may leave the athlete feeling weak, fatigued and miserable. Hard training should not be undertaken. Muscle glycogen can be depleted in one day of starvation. Other effects of carbohydrate deprivation include lowering of the blood glucose level (hypoglycaemia) which causes hunger, irritation, fatigue and inco-ordination of central nervous system function.

Muscle cell types

Individual muscle fibres can be classified according to their anatomical, chemical and functional characteristics into different types. There are slower- and faster-reacting fibres, called, respectively, slow twitch (ST, or Type I) and fast twitch (FT, or Type II) fibres, with division of Type II into IIa and IIb variants, and also intermediate fibres.

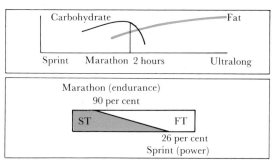

Figure 5.4 (top) Fuels for exercise

Figure 5.5 (bottom) Muscle fibre proportion related to event

The FS/ST proportion may vary in different muscles as well as between individual people and it is clear that this is due to inheritance. There is no evidence that substantial change of fibre type or proportions can be induced by training, except in the limited circumstances described below. It is also possible that not all fibres are equally fast or slow, thus the FT fibres of the champion sprinter may be 'faster' than those of a mediocre athlete. Debate continues about fibre classification and function because there is no clear demarcation between types. Fibres vary between two responses to each test or chemical stain, but Type I fibres respond differently compared with those of Type II. A list of FT and ST characteristics is summarized in *Table 5.1*.

As might be expected, the individual's 'fibre mix' can be related to athletic event. Top sprinters possess over 75 per cent of FT fibres in their leg muscles whereas top distance runners have up to 90 per cent ST fibres (*see Figure 5.5*).

Training effects

The aim of training is to maximize physiological adaptation to the demands of that event. The main determinants of response are the type and the intensity of work undertaken. Muscle training can be roughly divided into static or dynamic types, summarized in *Figure 5.6*.

Static exercise ('isometric') represents muscle contraction against a fixed resistance, without

Table 5.1. Differences between FT and ST muscle fibres

I	Type and characteristics		II	
slow (ST)	'Twitch'		fast (FT)	
red	Muscle colour		white	
smaller	Relative size		larger	
high	myoglobin content	} Aerobic	low	
high	mitochondrial content	} capacity	low	
lower	Anaerobic glycolytic capacity		higher	
slower	Speed of contraction		faster	
less	Enzyme myosin ATPase content		more	
more	Capillary blood supply		fewer	
sparser	Nerve supply		richer	
low	Fatigability		high	
	Training responses:			
+ size increase	Static (power)		+ size increase; ++ especially if high intensity	
+++	Dynamic (endurance)		+ to ++	
			'FTOG'	'FT'
			Type IIa	*Type IIb*
			++	+

movement. Examples are static contraction exercises of the quadriceps muscle, pushing in a rugby scrum or against a fixed object.

In contrast, dynamic exercise ('isotonic') involves muscle work during movement, such as running, swimming, cycling or weight-training with light weights.

In fact, few exercises represent 'pure' static or dynamic work. For instance, isometric efforts usually involve a maximum hold at one point during a range of movement, while isotonic movements imply a maximal loading at initiation of effort, for instance lifting the weight or starting to run, cycle, etc. In order to try to standardize these variables, isokinetic

training has been developed. This applies a constant resistance throughout a planned range of movement. The drawback of this system is that accurate and expensive machinery is required.

Dynamic exercise is expressed as workload per time, most conveniently in such sport-related terms as timed-interval swims or runs, or number of weight-lifting repetitions and weights lifted. Its major effect is to increase endurance or aerobic capacity.

Static exercise is measured as the maximum attainable load initially, then as a percentage of the maximum voluntary contraction (MVC) of the muscle. It is used to enhance muscle power for strength and speed events.

Isokinetic exercise is expressed as a rate of resisted work because the variables include the mechanical resistance, the arc of movement performed and the rate at which movement occurs. Its effects depend on the balance of work and speed applied but early comparative studies showed that isokinetic exercise produced consistently greater gains in power and games movements than isometric or isotonic training.

The complexities of planned training are further increased by the way in which muscle fibres are progressively recruited to a task. In endurance exercises ST fibres are used at low intensity. As effort increases, FT fibres are recruited. If maximum effort is achieved, all the FT fibres are active even to a point where only FT fibres are working. In very intensive dynamic exercise, such as flat-out sprinting, the work becomes virtually static rather than dynamic and dependent on anaerobic instead of aerobic mechanisms (*see Figure 5.7*).

Below about 20 per cent of maximum voluntary contraction (MVC) the contraction is held by ST fibres working aerobically. Hence training effects of low-grade exercise of any type can only be directed towards improved endurance. At about 20 per cent of MVC, however, FT fibres take over for two reasons. First the increasing workload calls for the greater power of the FT fibres. Secondly, the increasing intramuscular pressure of sustained contraction blocks the blood supply. This stops the O_2 supply and

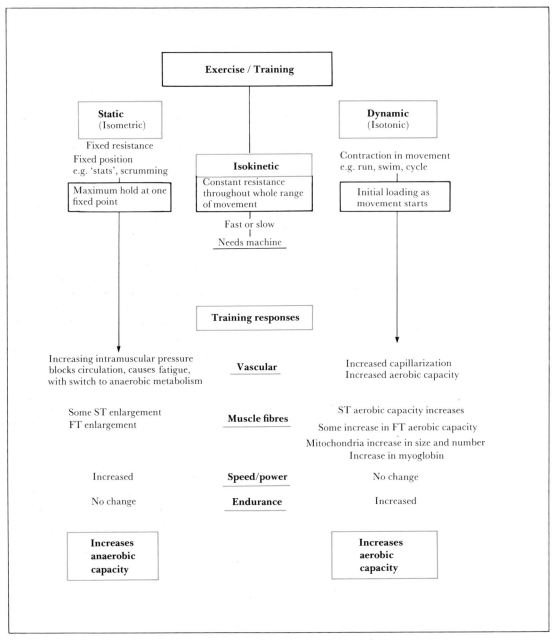

Figure 5.6
Summary of training
responses

forces the cell into using anaerobic energy. Hence, in order to train for power, training must stress the muscle to well over 20 per cent of its MVC, otherwise no strength will be gained (*see Figure 5.8*).

Both FT and ST fibres enlarge with power training such as static exercising or maximum power work. The ST fibre cannot, however, be made faster. In contrast, both ST and FT fibres may develop extra endurance in response to dynamic training. Thus the sprinter has a chance of maintaining his pace for longer.

This change is related to the subdivision of Type II/FT fibres. Some fibres, Type IIb, have minimal endurance response but others, Type IIa, or FTOG, fibres, have more scope for acquiring extra endurance through increased oxidative capacity. In sustained exercise, Type IIa (FTOG) fibres are brought in because of their aerobic power and Type IIb FT fibres are used only in the final anaerobic phase.

Nevertheless, fibre proportions are inherited and training response is likely to depend on the inherited chemical capacity of the muscle cells more than on any type or intensity of training. Bearing in mind the mixed FT/ST nature of each muscle, training should always be sufficiently planned and varied to provide adequate stimulus to each type of fibre. Training response is specific to the type of training and the site trained.

Specific training changes

Training responses of the heart and lungs are described in Chapter 4.

Training brings about changes in the blood supply to the muscle cells through increased capillary development and changes in the size and chemical functions of the specific cells trained. Further changes, for instance enzyme induction in the muscles or liver, help to increase the tolerable workload by more efficient release of fuels or removal of waste products.

Muscle changes Both ST and FT fibres are trainable. Both can increase in size and work capacity. ST fibres do not gain strength but FT fibres can gain strength and endurance. Static training increases the size and amount of contractile protein in FT fibres. Specific training intensities for each function are outlined above, with stamina/aerobic effects predominant below about a quarter of maximum workload and power/anaerobic effects predominant thereafter. Prolonged but low-grade endurance work is needed to boost the aerobic capacity of the FT fibres. This increases the size of the cell and the size and number of mitochondria within it.

It is not likely, under normal circumstances, that there are increases in the number of muscle fibres or their innervation, though some branching of muscle fibres may occur.

Capillaries Blood supply to muscle is increased by aerobic work. New capillaries open up to supply the harder-working, enlarging muscle. Experiments suggest that certain electrical stimuli applied to whole muscle through the nerve supplying it can increase oxidative/aerobic capacity of both ST and FT fibres by inducing increased capillarization in addition to chemical changes in the fibres. Some speed or power may be lost but more endurance is gained. These experimental methods remain outside the practical sphere at present but suggest future lines of research and training.

Figure 5.7 (top)
ST/FT fibre work during endurance race

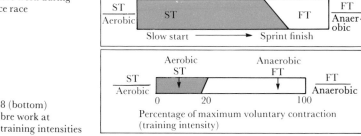

Figure 5.8 (bottom)
ST/FT fibre work at different training intensities

Cell chemistry and specific training The final effect of training lies in enhancement of the cell's chemical efficiency. During energy-yielding processes, one compound (e.g. glucose) is converted to energy plus breakdown products (e.g. lactate, CO_2, H_2O). These processes are accelerated and regulated by enzymes, or organic catalysts, which are complex substances present in small amounts. All such systems become more efficient with use and enzymes can be 'induced' by practice to become more effective.

Similar enzyme changes may improve the energy transfer systems within muscle, between muscle, blood and liver (where overall metabolic control is achieved), and from stores such as muscle glycogen or adipose tissue for the liberation and transportation of fuels.

Chemical efficiency can be estimated by staining tissue samples and measuring the amount of specific stains taken up by different cells and enzyme systems. The same cells can be stained in different ways to give an overall profile of their different chemical capacities; for instance, the enzyme succinate dehydrogenase reflects mitochondrial metabolism. The aim of training is to relate the workload to the specific chemical function which is to be enhanced.

Anaerobic training The alactic phase involves instant anaerobic energy production in short bursts before going on to induce lactate production from glycolysis. This implies the ability to 'surge' for a few seconds, hoping to drive a less capable opponent into lactate production and oxygen debt. Recovery can occur during the cruising phase between surges if oxygen debt is avoided. A logical way of improving alactic capacity is to train in short bursts of a few seconds' flat-out effort with ample rest between bursts. For example, a runner might sprint for 15 seconds flat out, rest for 4 or 5 min and repeat this 10 times, thus learning to recharge his creatine energy pathways. The rest period is required to ensure full 'recharging' of the creatine system.

The next phase of anaerobic training conditions the mechanisms that dispose of the lactate which builds up rapidly to cause fatigue. The body disposes of lactate in three main ways. First, lactic acid is buffered in the tissues. Some individuals or races are able to tolerate very much higher levels than others, sometimes because of their conditioning by a high-lactate diet. Secondly, lactate is neutralized in the liver and kidneys along normal metabolic pathways. Thirdly, lactate can be used in muscle metabolism as one of the energy sources in aerobic glycolysis, to be converted finally to water (H_2O) and CO_2 (*Figure 5.2* and *Table 5.2*).

To train these lactate disposal systems, intensive intermittent exercise should be performed to stress the athlete's lactate tolerance which lies at about 40 seconds of maximum effort. Therefore, maximum effort repetitions should be done for up to about 1 minute, to be followed by several minutes' rest for 'recharging'. A few seconds' worth of instant energy can be supplied by the O_2 which is bound to the myoglobin in the muscle cells, although this will subsequently have to be replaced, along with any other O_2 debt, through the haemoglobin-bound O_2 in the blood. Intensive training increases the haemoglobin and myoglobin levels and these increases might benefit the athlete's instant energy, or surging ability.

Aerobic training In contrast to the short bursts of anaerobic energy available from fuels within the cells, aerobic work depends on the sustained supply of O_2. The cardiorespiratory aspects of this are described in Chapter 4; capillary blood supply to the muscles may be increased by 25–50 per cent through endurance training.

Because the muscles switch increasingly to anaerobic mechanisms as work intensity increases, it is important that endurance training should remain within the aerobic range, i.e. at clearly submaximal work levels.

The three main types of endurance training involve sustained pace (tempo) exercise, rigid alterations of fast and slow work (intervals) or a less rigid

Table 5.2. Summary of metabolic training methods (*see also Figure 5.2*)

Anaerobic (speed, surge, strength, sprinting)

    Alactic (instant surge)

        Creatine phosphate + ADP $\xrightarrow{\text{creatine kinase}}$ creatine + ATP

            gives: a few seconds' 'surge'

            train by: flat-out efforts 15 s, rests 4–5 min

        Myoglobin (instant, but *see* text)

            uses O_2 already in cell

            gives: a few seconds' 'instant energy'

            train by: intensive efforts, (altitude ?)

    Lactic (sustained sprint/power)

        Glycogen $\xrightarrow{\text{anaerobic glycolysis}}$ lactate

            gives: about 40 seconds' 'sprint'

            train by: flat-out efforts 60 s, rests 4–5 min

            might be increased by: enzyme induction (high-lactate diet) to increase
                                  acid/base buffering

Aerobic (prolonged submaximal events, cruising speed)

    Glycogen

    Fat $\quad\xrightarrow[\ O_2\ ]{\text{aerobic glycolysis}}$ $H_2O + CO_2$

    Lactate

        gives: endurance (glycogen – 2 hours; fat – days)

        train by: intermittent or sustained submaximal efforts

---

racing pace, e.g. about 75–85 per cent of $\dot{V}O_{2\,max}$ for middle-/long-distance training. The disadvantage of such a regimen ('running a mile to train for a mile') is that, apart from boredom, the athlete stereotypes himself and misses important benefits of other training, such as the ability to change pace comfortably.

Such running would train carbohydrate-based aerobic pathways at fairly fast running speeds. Steady-pace training at faster speeds leads to earlier fatigue and the need for frequent rest. It might also train the anaerobic mechanisms as a fast-paced run approached its end.

Interval training is a development of this technique to its logical conclusion. Fast or hard efforts are deliberately interspersed with slow or rest periods. Each component is timed and this offers an entirely controlled and deliberately planned form of training.

Longer-distance fast runs with shortish rests are, in effect, the interrupted tempo running described above. At the opposite end of the scale, interval running of near-maximal intensity with short rests combines speed with stamina training and this type of interval training is highly effective in speeding up recovery from effort and in increasing rapidly the athlete's workload. It is extremely demanding both physically and mentally on the athlete, however, and ample rest and variety are essential to avoid breakdown.

Repetition training is similar in principle to interval training but the emphasis is on the intensive efforts, with a more generous time allowed for recovery than in the strict interval regime.

Long slow distance ('LSD') training is now widely used by joggers and longer-distance runners. Here the emphasis is on long-sustained low-intensity effort. Biochemically, this type of exercise enhances fat metabolism, with its promise of weight control for the obese jogger, and is virtually entirely aerobic. An important advantage is that its lower intensity puts less strain on the locomotor system and therefore minimizes the stiffness, soreness, fatigue and soft-tissue injury so frequently associated with higher

alternation of different speeds within a long continuous effort (fartlek, or speed play). Each method has its different advantages and all should be used by the athlete to vary the routine of training to avoid boredom as well as to increase his physiological flexibility. The same principles apply to all sports; any movements can be used including, for example, running, swimming, cycling and rowing.

Traditionally, tempo-type training consists of running a given distance at a fairly constant pace. This improves aerobic function but may have different effects at different speeds. At the different proportions of maximum oxygen uptake ($\dot{V}O_{2\,max}$), the athlete may build up stamina if he approaches his intensity exercise. It is, therefore, the training method of choice for the older athlete, the jogger or the casual sportsman. Its disadvantage is obvious – no speed or power training – but it is probably underused by younger competitive athletes who might gain in stamina and capillarization from a regular long slow outing as a refreshing break from the intensity of interval training. The training of the fat metabolism may also help the longer-distance racer to use fat more efficiently as a fuel in his competition, thus preserving carbohydrates and averting the painful switch to fat which has to occur when carbohydrate runs out, e.g. 'the wall' in marathon running.

Fartlek or speed play, consists of running at frequently changing pace so that a single outing can include all speeds of running. Ideally carried out over varying terrain, it is an effective way of increasing enjoyment or avoiding routines and its training results depend entirely on the actual workloads performed, which may vary greatly from run to run.

Other aids to training

The principle of carbohydrate loading is described above. Large amounts of sugar should not be eaten shortly before endurance events because the insulin reaction may cause a sudden fall in blood sugar level (hypoglycaemia) and insulin also inhibits the release of free fatty acids, thus further embarrassing fuel supplies.

Fat release for fuel in exercise can be enhanced by taking caffeine, e.g. drinking coffee, about 1 hour before endurance exercise. A serious disadvantage of this may be the cardiac stimulant effect of caffeine in some individuals. This can raise the resting pulse and effectively pre-empt some of the heart's exercise capacity. Therefore such a technique should be tried in practice before any competitions and not persevered with if the response is unsatisfactory – or if symptoms such as palpitations occur. A small coffee may be a help, a large one a hindrance!

Recently proposed doping regulation changes banning caffeine should be checked in international competition, though most experienced clinicians doubt if such a ban would be either realistic or enforceable in practice because of the universality of caffeine consumption in normal diets.

Nervous stimulation through the sympathetic nervous system may induce the reduction of ATP to ADP. This is a (more or less) controlled fear reaction and its benefit to the athlete depends on its correct control. Overstimulation hinders – witness the lacklustre performance of the nervous sportsman. Controlled anxiety is an important factor in athletic success (*see* Chapters 10 and 14).

Electrical stimulation may have useful physiological results but remains for the most part an experimental procedure. First, electrical stimulation can improve the capillarization of voluntary muscle by increasing the aerobic capacity of FT fibres and/or, possibly, by partial conversion of some fibres from fast to slow. The new stamina may be gained at the cost of power loss. Secondly, electrically introduced isometric contractions may increase maximum voluntary contraction by up to 30 per cent. It is possible, though inconvenient experimentally, to stimulate muscles during technique learning so as to boost actual patterned athletic movement. Thirdly, electrically induced muscle contraction may help players in competition or heavy training, perhaps by the enhanced relaxation induced following full contraction, which has probably become impeded by increasing fatigue or cramp.

Monitoring of training (*see* Chapter 2)

Nobody consciously wants to be a 'Training Champion' and the acid test of any training programme is its competitive outcome.

Nevertheless, physiological monitoring may be of practical help to athlete and coach. It may include gross and micro-anatomy, biomechanical analysis and physiological and biochemical studies. Unfortunately, many sportsmen feel that test programmes are indispensable to their progress. In fact, resources are very limited and skilled scientists more so. As so much remains unknown about human performance it is essential that it is studied as intensively as possible in all classes of athletes. Few top sportsmen care to be experimental subjects, however, and most coaches lack the physiological knowledge to put the results of any tests into useful practice – or, worse, get irrelevant tests done.

Because of the cost and complexity of exercise testing, more research papers are now correlating the results of elaborate tests with basic measurements, e.g. pulse rate, so that the coach can, with confidence, make and use his own scientific observations. Nevertheless, the athlete and his coach who 'only want immediate information and help' and resent experimentation, must realize that scientists can only acquire the ability to give this help as a result of experimental and practical experiences. Mutual understanding between coach and scientist is therefore imperative.

The exercising body can be monitored in almost any activity on the ground or in the water. Laboratory studies tend, purely for convenience, to concentrate on bicycle ergometers and treadmills but it has been shown that the nearer the activity to the sportsman's chosen event, the more meaningful the test results. Also, tests tend to be biased in favour of particular attributes. For instance, distance runners usually score unduly well compared with field-event athletes, yet the shot put champion with a 'poor' O_2 uptake cannot be regarded as 'unfit' for his own event – rather, the test is irrelevant to the event.

Pulse rates, electrocardiographs (ECGs) and O_2 uptake are readily measurable by direct and indirect methods. Automated gas analysers now make it easy to gain immediate print-outs of respired gases. Blood tests can monitor haemoglobin levels, for anaemia, haematocrit and metabolic products such as lactate, but are an unpleasant experience for the subject and not applicable at competitions. Even less welcome are muscle biopsies!

For the vast majority of sportsmen, the tape, the stopwatch and pulse-meter are the essential monitoring equipment, the readings to be recorded faithfully with details of training loads and competitive results as well as subjective phenomena. From a well-kept diary it is usually possible to give sound practical advice to the sportsman, provided that the adviser has sufficient personal knowledge and experience.

Factors limiting performance

Anaerobic exercise is self-limiting. The duration of effort is related to both training and the degree of exertion. Because the intracellular fuel supply is very small each phase is limited as described above – the creatine and myoglobin mechanisms to a few seconds each and anaerobic glycolysis to only about 40 seconds. These are trainable to some extent as outlined earlier.

The precise mechanism of exhaustion is uncertain. It is not simply lactate excess but is probably due to cellular consequences of this with alteration of the cell membrane permeability which allows minerals, especially phosphate, to escape.

Aerobic exercise is more subtly limited by many different factors. It is always difficult to assess endurance performance because of such variables as ambient temperature, track variation, wind resistance, altitude and competition. Nevertheless, it is common experience that the individual's 'form' may vary inexplicably from day to day.

This may be due to psychological factors (see Chapter 10) but physiological fluctuations which underlie performance variations have also been shown in work capacity from day to day. The classic explanations of biorhythm theory, with its three variable parameters set from the moment of birth, have been comprehensively debunked by statistical analysis. Man is a highly variable animal and the natural rhythms are far more complex and interrelated than simple theories would permit.

Performance limits can be considered from the cell outwards. Within the cell, the exhaustion of available creatine phosphate and glycogen may supervene towards the end of the aerobic event when greater effort forces the athlete from his controlled O_2-fed movements into a hectic sprint finish, recruiting FT fibres into an almost static anaerobic contraction. Pace control is the key factor so that such a sprint finish is well timed, or that cruising pace is within tolerable limits of O_2 uptake. Some individuals, however, will be able to 'surge' in mid-race and then continue more slowly while aerobically metabolizing their sudden flush of lactate, while others will be 'burnt off' because they cannot eliminate, but only accumulate, this lactate until they are forced to slow to the place at which they both compensate chemically and lose the race. Training can improve lactate handling – blood lactate monitoring shows a sudden rise in lactate concentration as the effort forces the switch from aerobic to anaerobic. The trained athlete gets to a much higher percentage of his maximum O_2 uptake before switching (around 80 per cent compared with the untrained 30 per cent). The athlete must clearly identify his individual physiological capacity, then train and race to it, not waste too much effort trying to train the untrainable. For instance, if the distance runner cannot sprint he must aim to race to his maximum cruising capacity, not hold back and thus allow the fastest sprint finisher to relax earlier in the race.

Lactate build-up, cellular phosphate leakage, changes in cell membrane permeability and exhaustion of fuels stop the cell exercising. Neuromuscular exhaustion, with possible acetylcholine depletion, impairs the nerve impulses stimulating the muscle to contract. Further up the nervous system, hypoglycaemia, or glucose depletion, causes nervous exhaustion – witness the breakdown of skilled movement in the tired player. Psychological factors are discussed in Chapter 10: nervous tension is exhausting work at the cellular level too!

While the body's carbohydrate store can fuel 2 hours or more of very hard effort (compared with a week or more of fat energy) use of this energy can be helped or hindered. Carbohydrate loading can increase muscle glycogen stores threefold, but if sugar is taken shortly before (within a couple of hours of)

endurance work, the resulting insulin secretion inhibits both the use of sugar for exercise and also the release of free fatty acids (FFA), so that the subject feels weak, tired and unable to work hard. Caffeine taken before exercise may enhance FFA release and increase endurance capacity.

Within the muscle, vascular and pressure changes impair performance and may cause symptoms overlapping with frank injury. While lower levels of aerobic exercise stimulate the capillary circulation, the more intensive the effort, the more completely the blood supply within the muscle is blocked off during contraction. This may lead to swelling within the muscle and symptoms of cramp and, rarely, to severe pain and gangrene. Examples are the compartment syndrome in the runner's leg (see Chapters 25 and 28) and forearm pain in oarsmen. Changes in training, technique and equipment may relieve these symptoms; medical treatment is discussed in the relevant chapters. Variations in tissue hydration may underlie cramp-like symptoms which may cause difficulty in differentiating between a muscle tear and old scar, metabolic cramp or stitch, vascular insufficiency, or pressure symptoms leading to compartment syndromes.

Biomechanical factors are important in fatigue. The more mechanically efficient the movements, the less wasteful they are of energy and the less likely they are to cause the injuries. Examples include correctness of swimming style and bowling or throwing movements. Light footwear reduces energy consumption, although it may cause injury through giving insufficient protection. Disordered gait, for instance overpronation, may accelerate fatigue by causing local pain or increased intramuscular tension.

Cardiorespiratory limits are discussed in Chapter 4. Dehydration accelerates exhaustion; by lowering the cardiac output and increasing the pulse rate it effectively pre-empts some cardiac work capacity, thus lowering the limit of possible effort. Caffeine, e.g. in coffee, has a similar pre-emptive effect on cardiac work capacity. High altitude limits aerobic performance (*see* below) because there is less available O_2.

Ambient temperature may be an important limiting factor. While the advantage of warmth is reflected in the initial increase of 10–15 per cent in metabolic efficiency per 1 °C rise in body temperature, justifying a 'warm-up' for short events, a long-lasting effort in hot surroundings may lead to heat exhaustion with body-core temperatures over 41 °C (106 °F). The athlete's success suddenly depends no longer on getting warm but on losing heat (*see* below).

Illness is a potent but usually evident cause of limited performance and may cause a threat to life (*see* especially Chapter 11). It is unclear why athletic performance should be impaired for such variable periods after illnesses in some subjects and not others. Convalescence is never speeded up by hard training; staleness may be caused by training during and soon after illness. Fluctuations in the body's immunity mechanisms have been shown in relation to different sporting efforts and individual variations in immune responses may play a part in impaired performance.

Overtraining/overuse states: staleness

A major problem for the serious sportsman is survival of extreme mental and physical stress. Aspects of this are discussed in Chapters 10 and 14. Staleness, or loss of form, is perhaps the commonest cause of performance failure and should be recognized and avoided by the competent coach. It is important that hard training is interspersed with rest periods. Athletes vary greatly in their exercise capacity – some can only manage maximum effort training occasionally, others more frequently – yet competitive results may be the same.

The stress of forcing the athlete to train too hard ensures that all cellular, physiological and biomechanical mechanisms are always at full stretch. There is then no safety margin and breakdown is always imminent. The irony is that many feel that the absence of pain indicates insufficiently hard training,

but the next step up causes the pain of overuse injury which then prevents more work. All the factors outlined above as limiting factors are present in overtraining. Clinically the symptoms include a sharp loss of appetite for, and recovery from, hard work and competition; a rising pulse rate at rest as parasympathetic tone is overwhelmed by the adrenergic signs of stress; and mental and physical symptoms such as loss of appetite and weight, insomnia, loss of concentration, overanxiety and aches and pains, strongly resembling the clinical picture of depression with anxiety.

Acclimatization

Circadian rhythm and travel

The bodily functions of all animals exhibit diurnal rhythms related to a cycle of daylight and darkness. These rhythms are not all identical and need time to adapt to changes brought about by travel to new time zones. Sleeping–waking rhythm, body temperature, basal pulse, hormonal and organ activity rhythm all adapt differently. Mood fluctuates diurnally and there are personality differences between 'morning' and 'night' people in their adaptation to new time zones (the latter doing so more quickly): 28 per cent of people find exceptional difficulty in adaptation.

As a rough guide, an average adaptation, or entrainment, of 1 hour/day gives an idea of the overall adjustment time needed and an appropriate number of days should ideally be allowed for local acclimatization after travel to distant venues. This is not always feasible however, and the athlete can prepare for travel by changing his home training time to conform to competitive requirements before his departure. For instance, an athlete training regularly at 5 pm would train an hour a day earlier for 3 days before a 3-hour time zone crossing eastwards, or later for westward travel, so that his body could adjust to the new competition time before departure. **Exercise** helps adaptation. Sedative drugs probably hinder rather than help by altering the natural sleep rhythm and response to fatigue. Initial benefit can be gained by sedation in transit, however, followed by a prolonged sleep on arrival then full exposure to the new environment with its 'clock stimuli' which prompt the body's rhythm adjustments.

Circadian disruption can cause general symptoms – insomnia, fatigue, loss of appetite and indigestion, bowel and bladder changes, and time disorientation. Menstrual rhythm can be altered with periods being induced or delayed, although the cycle returns to normal if travel stimulus is prolonged (e.g. aircrew). Mood changes may be dramatic and biochemical response to drugs can be altered remarkably, e.g. some drugs may take twice as long to be metabolized so that regular medication should be reviewed. Especially important is diabetic care with altered response to insulin superimposed on altered metabolism and diet. Circadian resynchronization is helped by exercise and by keeping sleep deficit minimal. Adaptation improves with practice but becomes more difficult with increasing age.

Exercise in the heat

Because the body is not completely efficient, only about a quarter of the energy of the exercising muscles is converted to movement; the remainder is converted into heat. The longer exercise continues, the more important becomes effective dissemination of this metabolic heat which would otherwise lead to overheating, or hyperthermia. Initially, a 'warm-up' raises body-core temperature by 2–3 °C, during which the metabolic efficiency of muscle action increases by 10 per cent or more per 1 °C. After this, efficiency declines and at core temperatures over 41 °C (105 °F) heat injury is liable to occur in the untrained. The body adapts well to heat; trained athletes may compete without ill effects at core temperatures up to 42 °C (107 °F).

Heat is produced by contracting muscles (400–1000 Calories/hour (Cal/hour) (1.67–4.18 megajoules/hour; MJ/hour) according to the intensity of exercise). The body may also gain heat directly from the environment, e.g. on clear sunny days by solar radiation (up to 150 Cal/hour (627.6 kJ/hour)).

Heat is lost mainly through the evaporation of sweat (up to 2 ℓ/hour). Smaller amounts may be dissipated to the surrounding atmosphere by convection, depending on ambient temperature, wind speed and clothing. Theoretically sweat evaporates to cool off some 500 Cal/ℓ (2.092 MJ/ℓ) (up to 1000 Cal/hour (4.184 MJ/hour)) so hyperthermia might not occur. In practice, a variable proportion of sweat is not evaporated, being lost as fallen drops, or held in clothing – from where it might evaporate later. Any clothing, especially of restrictive waterproofing type, hinders sweat evaporation and may create serious hazards, for instance many deaths were caused by hyperthermia in American football before the hazards of clothing, especially of synthetic fibres, were recognized. Poor adjustment to heat may cause 'prickly heat' (see page 104).

Heat loss is impeded in the obese, where body fat insulates the heat in the body's core. Dehydration is dangerous because the body reduces the store of water available to become sweat. Dehydration levels of over 5 per cent of body weight lower strength and stamina. For example, a 10 stone (140 lb, 64 kg) man would be significantly impaired during an event in which he lost 5 per cent body weight, or 7 lb (3.2 kg) representing a water loss of over 3 ℓ or 5½ pints.

Illness, especially febrile, may dangerously impair temperature control and is inconsistent with safe exercise (see Chapter 11). Certain drugs also impair sweating and have caused death in competitions (see Chapters 12 and 13).

Unacclimatized and unfit subjects cannot cope well in heat. Acclimatization is enhanced in trained people – the sweating/heat loss function is made more efficient by the regular heat challenges of training even in cool climates. It takes 4–8 days for most athletes to make the necessary adjustments to heat by which efficient sweating starts at a lower body temperature. Regular exercise speeds this up, but two warnings are necessary. Exercise in the heat uses more glycogen than normal and gradual depletion of muscle stores may insidiously undermine performance. Chronic dehydration also impairs performance. Below the more dramatic sweat losses mentioned above, a water loss of 3 per cent of body weight causes a pulse rate increase of 20 beats/min, thus effectively increasing cardiac workload for a given task and hastening fatigue. The body can gradually increase its plasma volume by 10 per cent by renal compensatory mechanisms if the daily training loss is fully made up each day. Thus the athlete who goes to a hot climate should train more lightly than usual in the heat, drink more than enough to compensate sweat loss and make sure that his carbohydrate intake is full. Water loss can be roughly monitored by twice-daily weighing or by urine output. Dark coloured, concentrated urine indicates dehydration – therefore one should drink until frequent pale urination occurs.

Heat illness

This is a spectrum of symptoms starting with discomfort, and progressing as core temperature rises to cramps, fatigue, confusion and finally to delirium and coma as sweating may finally cease.

The essential preventive measures are education and recognition. The ill and unfit should not be exposed to likely dangers, plentiful fluids should be available and used, clothing should permit heat loss, sufficient first aiders should be present to recognize the early confusion and staggering of those near collapse, and emergency resuscitation facilities should be near at hand.

Prevention of heat illness The athlete should start his event fully hydrated and with energy and mineral stores replenished from previous exercise demands.

Water is the main substance required for sustained submaximal exercise, e.g. a marathon run. It has been shown that water can, with practice, be drunk at the rate of 150 ml/15 min for several hours during long-distance running. Thus, perhaps two-thirds of

the continuing fluid loss can be compensated in action. This will both provide water for continuing an effective sweat rate and defer the fatigue due to dehydration.

Mineral loss occurs in the sweat. Salt may be lost at a rate of up to 1.5 g NaCl/hour. This, in relation to the body stores and the average content of 3–5 g NaCl per meal is a trivial amount and well made up by liberal salting of the diet. Similar considerations apply to magnesium and other trace elements.

It is unnecessary, and possibly dangerous, to add sugars or minerals to water during events of marathon type and duration. At this intensity of continuous exercise, water is freely and rapidly absorbed from the bowel. Concentrated solutions are not absorbed and their osmotic strength attracts water into the bowel from the already dehydrated tissues. Thus the metabolic situation is worsened and the symptoms of bloating, nausea, griping or diarrhoea can only hinder the athlete's progress. The maximum concentration recommended for additives to water is only 2.5 per cent glucose, a totally insufficient energy supply in a marathon. The dangers of miscalculation and wrong dilution of energy/mineral drinks and powders should also be remembered.

Intermittent events, of course, provide a metabolic pause for refreshment of glucose, minerals and fluid and the aim should always be to try to maintain the fullest possible hydration and chemical balance, in the heat as in temperate climates.

The American College of Sports Medicine issued, in 1975, a major policy statement on the prevention of heat injuries during distance running which included two important recommendations. First, distance races (over 10 miles or 16 km) should not be conducted when the wet bulb globe temperature (WBGT) exceeds 28 °C (82.4 °F). The WBGT measures temperature by a damp-cloth-enclosed thermometer within a black globe, thus taking account of radiation and humidity as well as ordinary (dry) ambient temperature. Secondly, where seasonal temperature often exceeds 27 °C (80 °F), distance races should be conducted before 9 am or after 4 pm to reduce the impact of radiant heat on the athlete.

Not all athletes adjust equally well to climatic changes and there are situations where all participants are at risk. It is the responsibility of the event organizers to minimize such risk by intelligent planning and detailed arrangements. Above all, the possibility of hyperthermia or overheating must be remembered in cool climates. The overclothed dehydrated sportsman can be at risk in the same event in which an underclothed exhausted participant is drastically cooled into hypothermia by a strong wind.

Exercise in the cold

Body chilling occurs if surroundings are colder than the body. If severe exposure occurs to water, snow or wind, body temperature falls to hypothermic levels at which clumsiness, mental confusion and coma may occur.

Particular dangers attach to water immersion (the majority of recreational deaths in Great Britain are due to exposure and/or drowning) or wind cooling of the inadequately clothed body. Even cross-country hiking can kill the unwary who cannot walk fast enough to produce enough heat to counteract climatic cooling and slip into hypothermic confusion. A number of long-distance running deaths have been due to hypothermia – the underclad runner drops his pace and a cool wind lowers his core temperature. This may occur even if the weather is cool rather than freezing. A strong wind cools more drastically than a light breeze.

The sportsman can acclimatize to some extent with cold-weather practice. Suitable clothing is important as is the need to dress up immediately a trial or game is over in order to prevent cooling at peak body temperatures. In particularly cold climates more cumbersome clothing may be necessary, including gloves, ear muffs and masks which prevent gasping of icy air. Even a solitary case of frostbite of the penis has been reported in an underclothed winter jogger!

Exercise at altitude

With increasing altitude the air becomes thinner. Its component gases are present in the same proportions as at sea level, but the pressure is lower. The thinner air gives less resistance to people or objects and sprinting, jumping and throwing records are remarkable in medium-altitude competition (e.g. Mexico City, altitude 7500 ft (2300 m)). The disadvantage at this level is increased solar radiation because of thinner air, which causes easier sunburn and accelerates hyperthermia in endurance events. The cooler drier air also increases evaporative loss, especially from the respiratory tract, leading to respiratory symptoms as well as dehydration which in turn impairs performance (*see* Heat, above).

The main consequences of sport at altitude stem from the lower availability of oxygen (O_2) in the air. Lower O_2 pressure in the inspired air gives a lower O_2 pressure in the lung alveoli (*see* Chapter 4) and this in turn leads to less O_2 saturation of the arterial blood. For instance, the pressure of O_2 in the air is 150 mm Hg at sea level and the blood haemoglobin is 96 per cent saturated, while at 7500 ft (2300 m), the figures are approximately 110 mm Hg and 90 per cent, respectively. As aerobic work capacity depends on O_2 supply, it falls. Between sea level and about 5000 ft (1500 m) there is little significant fall in maximal oxygen uptake ($\dot{V}O_{2_{max}}$) but thereafter $\dot{V}O_{2_{max}}$ falls by about 10 per cent per 1000 m height gain. In the Mexico Olympics, track races were faster than sea-level records up to the 800 metres, in which event the world record was equalled, and progressively slower at longer distances.

People born and resident at altitude have a built-in advantage over low-level dwellers. Gradual, albeit partial, adaptation is possible, however; a minimum recommended exposure being about 3 weeks. Some athletes do not adapt well. Adaptations are maintained for about 2 weeks back at sea level, so that intermittent altitude exposure may be undertaken.

The physiological changes compensate for the lower O_2 availability at altitude. The immediate changes affect breathing and pulse rate. In order to try and inhale the same volume of O_2, pulmonary ventilation is increased. The carotid bodies monitor blood gas concentration and trigger the brain's respiratory centre to increase the depth and rate of breathing. Simultaneously, the heart increases its output by up to a third by raising the pulse rate and stroke volume.

The effect of increased respiration is to wash out more carbon dioxide (CO_2) than usual, thus causing respiratory alkalosis. This may cause periodic, or irregular, breathing and add to sleeping difficulty. Insomnia may further add to fatigue and impair both training and recovery. Other symptoms include irritability, headache, dry throat, gastrointestinal upsets and visual disturbances and giddiness.

With more time, further compensations occur. The blood rapidly concentrates itself, raising the haematocrit, or proportion of red cells, from 45 to 50 per cent by a reduction in plasma volume. A natural block then stops further concentration because, despite further increase in oxygen-carrying capacity, the blood's viscosity increases and this increased stickiness tends to slow the circulation, thus cancelling out the benefit of the O_2 increase.

As this change occurs, cardiac output and stroke volume fall and the pulse drops. By these changes the initial drop in the blood's O_2 carriage is partly made up but nothing can compensate for the basic lack of sufficient atmospheric O_2 pressure fully to saturate each red blood cell, so aerobic capacity and $\dot{V}O_{2_{max}}$ must remain impaired.

The longer-term altitude adaptations include the production of more new red cells so that there is an absolute increase in the blood's oxygen-carrying capacity rather than the temporary shorter-term concentration effect. Muscle enzymes adapt to altitude stress and myoglobin concentration increases.

Mountain Sickness may occur at fairly low altitude. The older person is at greater risk of illness than the young fit athlete. It is particularly important that older less fit people coming to mountains for holidays take time to adapt. Unaccustomed exercise stress may precipitate cardiac symptoms. The more serious high-altitude pulmonary oedema may rarely affect people at a moderate altitude, but is more usually a complication of rapid exposure to much higher altitudes, 4000 m or more.

With the possible exception of myoglobin increases, careful and repeated studies have shown no advantage of altitude training on subsequent sea-level performance, despite widely accepted myths. The commonest misconceptions have followed remarkable improvements in groups of unfit athletes. While all athletes must train for altitude competition, the highly trained athlete has little to gain but a holiday effect. A notable disadvantage of altitude training is the 'locomotor detraining' effect whereby the athlete, despite fully stressing his heart and lungs at altitude, cannot, because of the O_2 limitation, equally stress his muscles which therefore lose some work capacity. While this is rapidly recovered on return to sea level, the time scale is uncertain and variable and the runner may feel particularly heavy-legged for some time after his descent. Blood doping is discussed on page 26.

6 The female athlete

Physical characteristics

Some of the physical differences between the sexes have a direct influence on athletic performance. These form an inherited biological limit to comparative sports performances. The Gaussian frequency-distribution curve of physical characteristics reflects this limitation in both sexes (*see Figure 6.1*).

The relative rate of improvement of female performance in many sports, for example, swimming and marathon running, has led to suggestions that women will in future be able to beat men in any sport. An explanation is that, for any biological characteristic amenable to training, and even sports performance itself, the distribution curves for females approach those for males (*see Figure 6.2*). The rate of approach and the possibility of equality depend on the particular aspect being studied. At the same time, more intensive training for both sexes ensures that the leaders are drawing further away from the norms and the most highly trained females are coming further up the male ranking lists. It is likely that in many events there will be times when a woman happens to have a better physical capacity than men for some events and will therefore win competitions (*Figure 6.3*).

Final sexual equality sought by the Women's Lib. movement seems to imply that both distribution curves are identical with complete overlap, something not yet foreseeable in Darwinian terms, as illustrated by some of the physical characteristics now considered.

The characteristic skeletal shapes of the sexes differ. The female frame includes a broader, more tilted pelvis suitable for childbearing and this necessarily calls for a different angulation of the femur compared with the slimmer-hipped male. Such an angle, in its more extreme form, is positively disadvantageous to athletic performance. Also, the lower centre of gravity associated with the female build may be unhelpful in jumping events. Bone strength and density favour the male but this does not mean that men are automatically 'stronger'. Bone strength reflects the muscular, tendinous and gravitational demands made upon it during movement. The female's musculoskeletal system is fully efficient as a closed system and direct comparisons between sexes must take account of body weight as well as muscular strength acting on the bones. For example, there is no greater incidence of stress fractures in females than males on equivalent training.

The fat content of the body varies widely between individuals. The average male level is around 15 per cent of body weight, falling as low as 4 or 5 per cent in highly trained subjects. This compares with an average of about 25 per cent for females, again subject to training. Female breast size influences the total proportion of fat and the presence of large breasts may cause serious inconvenience in some events.

The lean body mass is lower in females than in males and various studies suggest that absolute strength in the female is roughly 60 per cent of maximum male strength. This has, however, been shown to vary with individual build and between the different limbs, the differences being greater in the arms than the legs. While much of muscular strength and lean body mass is amenable to training in both sexes, male strength must be partly ascribed to the active influence of the male hormone testosterone, which has anabolic or muscle-building effects. The adrenal glands of both sexes produce this in small amounts and the testicles produce the majority of the testosterone in males. In normal health, the female's naturally occurring amount of testosterone is not enough to provide as much muscle strength as in males and taking male hormone has serious adverse virilizing effects on the female.

Although oxygen (O_2) uptake is different in the sexes, there is no significant distinction between boys and girls until the age of about 10 years. After that age, girls tend to level off in maximum O_2 uptake capacity while boys continue steadily through their adolescent growth phase to reach, on average, a level some 20 per cent ahead of the female. Again, these group differences are difficult to assess in individuals. In functional terms, the O_2 uptake capacity must be related both to cardiac efficiency and to the amount and efficiency of the muscles which are to consume the O_2. If due allowance is made for the female excess of fat, then the sex difference narrows. The point is, however, that surplus fat has to be oxygenated and carried which, in terms of many sporting activities, will be disadvantageous. If a female of suitable body type becomes highly trained to the point of shedding most of her body fat, she will approach the ideal male athletic shape and performance. The dramatic improvement in female marathon running times shows how closely the sexes can be matched in an event more dependent on physiological function than on body bulk or strength.

There are four possible advantages for the female in sport. First, female capacity for coping with heat loss in sustained exercise may be more efficient. Women sweat less than men and are fatter but do not suffer the expected degree of hyperthermia, or overheating, which limits performance. This mechanism is unclear

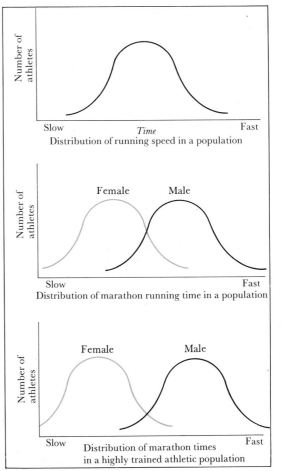

Figure 6.1 (top)
The frequency-distribution curve plots measures of a function against its frequency, i.e. running time against the number of people able to run at each speed. This type of distribution curve applies to all natural phenomena.

Figure 6.2 (centre)
Plotting, say, marathon speed against male and female populations, a range exists for each sex but there is clearly considerable overlap, i.e. fast women beat slow men.

Figure 6.3 (bottom)
Taking this further to selected populations of trained athletes (i.e. at the fast extreme of the original curve of Figure 6.9), two features become clear. First, the leaders have already diverged greatly from their 'norms' and secondly, there is more overlap, with the fastest women able to beat most men, i.e. occasionally winning mixed races.

and currently the subject of study.

Secondly, the greater proportion of body fat proves an advantage in events where buoyancy and insulation are important, for example in long-distance swimming at which women have long excelled.

Thirdly, in the marathon-type events, women may have a more efficient fat-burning metabolism which has considerable advantages in sustained performance. Paradoxically, however, if we are searching for our perfect running female, equal to her male rival, is she not trying to shed her fat to approach the male levels of O_2 uptake efficiency per gram of lean muscle?

Fourthly, body flexibility of the female is influenced by the hormone oestrogen. Her flexibility is greater than that of the male with obvious advantage in events such as gymnastics. On the other hand, increased laxity in major joints is disadvantageous and studies have indicated both a higher incidence of knee injury and a poorer degree of recovery from joint operations in females compared with males.

Menstrual cycle

There is no evidence that the rate of growth or age of onset of menstruation is influenced by normal sports activities. Severe overtraining may, however, delay maturation. Menstruation starts at an average age of about 13 in Britain with a wide range from 10 to 17 or older. This age of commencement, the menarche, varies around the globe and is influenced by racial and economic factors. Menstruation, which can be influenced by anatomical and physiological abnormalities, is under the control of hormones. The hypothalamus (*see Figure 6.4*) is the brain's hormone-regulating organ and controls the pituitary gland. This in turn releases hormones (FSH and LH) which have a cyclical influence on the ovaries. The ovaries themselves release the hormones oestrogen and progesterone in varying amounts throughout the menstrual cycle. The relative proportions of these hormones dictate the timing of the cellular changes in the uterus which, if pregnancy has not occurred, lead to the cyclical shedding of the lining as the menstrual flow. Menstrual periods vary greatly in duration, the average duration of loss being 4 days in each 28-day cycle, the norm varying from 2 to 10 days every 3–6 or more weeks.

The menstrual cycle is sensitively regulated by the inherent rhythmicity of the hypothalamus, the circulating levels of hormones, and direct cerebral stimulation of the hypothalamus by emotion or illness. It can thus be influenced by shock, stress such as exams, heavy training or competition, or by strong emotion. There is no consistent pattern of change; virtually any possibility is known.

Administration of hormones changes the menstrual cycle. For instance, the taking of female sex hormones increases the levels circulating in the bloodstream and this causes the pituitary gland to respond by sending out less of its own messenger hormones. Thus, control is by a sensitive feedback mechanism. As with all hormones, giving some may maintain overall levels while suppressing the body's own self-regulating output. This effect is usually quickly reversible but may not always be so. For instance, taking the female contraceptive pill suppresses ovulation and menstruation, which normally occurs as a response to ovulation, is suppressed as long as the pill is taken continuously. Once the pill is stopped, a period ensues which is not a true menstrual period but a withdrawal bleed in response to the cessation of

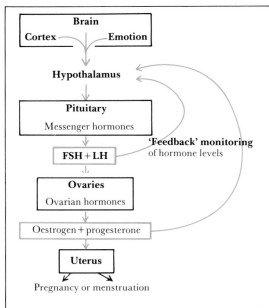

Figure 6.4
Menstrual control by hypothalamus, pituitary and ovarian hormones. Circulating amounts of hormones are monitored in the pituitary 'feedback' system. Ratios (FSH/LH: ovarian hormones) are constant within limits and altered by addition of extra male or female hormone. This is the basis of dope control tests for extra male testosterone given to males or females. (The male ratio, messenger: testosterone, is also limited normally; extra testosterone inhibits the messengers by 'feedback' control.)

hormone therapy, i.e. the pill. Use of the contraceptive pill in female athletes may be beneficial if the individual is inconvenienced by the cyclical changes. The pill may be taken continuously throughout the competitive season, if a suitable preparation is free from side effects. There is no clear evidence about the effect of the menstrual cycle on athletic performance however. Numerous studies have given conflicting results and the mere fact that competition occurs during a menstrual period does not necessarily mean a poor performance. In fact, many women find the opposite – increased well-being and performance around the time of the period.

An emotionally induced change in the menstrual cycle may occur in female communities, for example, in schools, where there is a tendency towards mass synchronization of periods.

Premenstrual syndrome

The premenstrual syndrome consists of bodily and emotional changes which occur at certain phases of the menstrual cycle. This is usually the few days leading into a period but a similar state may occur briefly in mid-cycle when ovulation occurs and the hormone ratios change. Physical symptoms include salt and fluid retention causing weight gains of up to 3 or 4 kg with feelings of fullness, bloatedness and congestion of epithelium including that of the nose, sinuses and vagina. Mental symptoms include anxiety, irritability, lethargy and depression. Occasionally, pain in joints and even swelling may occur at these times without other evidence of arthritis. Symptoms are self-limiting and usually subside quickly once the period starts.

In women suffering from this syndrome there are also mental symptoms which influence concentration and accident-proneness. Physical illness is also more frequent. Specific sports skills may be impaired by slight unsteadiness, minor changes in visual acuity or increased liability to asthma at this time. The increased body weight which occurs in some women

clearly increases the workload imposed by some events and this, of course, has to be undertaken at a time of possible mental and physical malaise.

Nevertheless, studies of menstrual effects on physical performance show no consistent pattern. The apparent advantage enjoyed by sportswomen and physical education students may be due to self-selection of these groups. It is unlikely that a grossly disadvantaged girl will find herself as athletically motivated as her fitter sister.

This syndrome can be treated in three main ways. For those troubled by weight fluctuation, diuretics during the few days of anticipated weight gain each month are a simple and highly effective treatment. In more severe cases, diuretics are insufficient because they simply remove surplus salt and water but do not rebalance the hormones causing the problem, hence the other mental and physical effects outlined above may persist. Secondly, temporary treatment may be offered with progesterone. This counteracts the hormonal imbalance and involves the use of suppositories for the latter half of the cycle. Thirdly, long-term correction is available with the various female hormone or contraceptive pills which superimpose a new hormonal profile and inhibit the changes precipitated by ovulation.

Dysmenorrhoea

Dysmenorrhoea is the abdominal discomfort associated with the onset of menstruation. This can be extremely severe and totally preclude athletic training or competition for one or more days in each month. It is not clear whether exercise itself is an effective preventive or therapeutic measure. The same arguments about the self-selection of sporting populations applies in the studies quoted in the literature which usually favour the sportswoman.

Mild cases respond to simple aspirin. Antispasmodic tablets may be prescribed and act by relaxing the involuntary smooth muscles of the viscera in general. Prostaglandin-inhibiting anti-inflammatory drugs can be extremely effective, e.g. indomethacin (Indocid), ibuprofen (Brufen), mefenamic acid (Ponstan), and have become the standard treatment. In resistant cases, specific hormone therapy is effective in the form of short-term oestrogens or, on a longer-term basis, the contraceptive pill.

Amenorrhoea

Amenorrhoea, or cessation of periods, is well recognized as a response to stress, illness, malnutrition or hard physical work such as athletic training.

The reasons for this cessation are not entirely clear. Studies point to similarities between athletically induced amenorrhoea and the anorexia syndrome. It is possible that the triggering mechanism in some individuals is the rate of marked weight loss associated with training. In other individuals, the severity of training workload may be the key determinant. It is usually promptly reversible by easing the training load. There is no evidence of subsequent infertility.

Menstrual adjustment

Long-term menstrual adjustment involving the cyclical use of contraceptive pills should be carefully and responsibly planned in advance of the season's competitive requirements. Time must be allowed for suitable preparations to be tried and for the athlete to come to terms with her new hormonal environment. As trial of any therapy of necessity needs at least one month, the time to get ready for next season is after the end of this one!

Short-term menstrual postponement is possible with progesterone or progestogens but the latter may not prevent adverse premenstrual symptoms. A practical problem often posed is that of an athlete who wants to postpone a period at very short notice, for example, one day.

Unless there is good evidence of serious menstrual symptoms, such as spasmodic dysmenorrhoea which

would normally prove crippling at this time, it may well be better to have the normal period than to embark on hasty hormonal suppression regimens which may themselves present new adverse side effects. Indeed, as evidence for this, many women athletes have produced career bests on a first day of menstruation, only to improve on them in the next round of competition during the same period.

Pregnancy

There is evidence that physically active women have easier pregnancies and childbirth than those who are unfit. The quoted rate of Caesarian section delivery for athletic women is only half that in other women. There is no evidence that athletic activity either causes abortions (spontaneous miscarriages) or harms the developing baby. Olympic medals have been won by pregnant women and it is safe, in the absence of any medical or obstetric contraindications, to continue exercise up to childbirth. Commonsense, as well as the increasing physical limitation of the growing foetus, will dictate the limits of exercise which is both pleasurable and desirable for each mother. The increasing cardiovascular stress of pregnancy, which reaches its maximum at around the thirtieth week, acts as a sure deterrent to overambition.

The foetus is extremely safe from external blows and this means that women in contact sports such as lacrosse and hockey may safely play as long as they wish to do so.

There are, however, certain contraindications to physical activity during pregnancy, especially in the later months. These stem from the hormone-induced softening of the ligaments, particularly of the low back and pelvis, in preparation for childbirth. This renders them more liable to overstrain by such activities as weight-lifting or jumping.

The same limitation applies for several months after delivery as the ligaments take this time to return to their normal stiffness. Moderate exercise helps prompt recovery from childbirth and should be encouraged. To minimize the risk of injury, heavy straining such as weight-training or jumping should be delayed, certainly for at least 3 months and, according to many, 6 months after delivery.

Lactation is a contraindication to strenuous training for two reasons. First, the breasts are larger and more vulnerable to injury and discomfort. Secondly, the nutritional demands on the mother of lactation may pre-empt satisfactory fulfilment of her own dietary requirements during this phase.

The late results of pregnancy on sports performance can only be described as excellent in many cases, some of them quite outstanding at Olympic level. The reason for this is unclear. The change from a younger less mature woman to a more mature and strongly motivated one may play a major part. There is also the suspicion that 9 months of continuous progressive cardiorespiratory stress coupled with a sophisticated form of weight-training plays a part!

Anaemia

General aspects of anaemia in sport are discussed in Chapter 11. Specific aspects of anaemia concern the pregnant athlete. The tendency towards iron deficiency, together with the increase in the volume of plasma which dilutes the red cells and gives an apparent anaemia in the later part of pregnancy, should fall within the normal medical care of pregnancy.

There are two reasons why the female athlete is likely to become iron-deficient and need occasional blood tests and supplementary iron to remedy this. First, many women take a diet deficient in iron in their attempts to maintain slimness. The athletic woman should remember that a full diet plus full physical activity is far more likely to maintain both health and beauty!

Secondly, the menstrual loss may be incompletely compensated by the dietary intake of iron. Many

woman habitually lapse into iron deficiency and anaemia throughout the childbearing age and remain there unless supplementary iron is taken. In virtually all circumstances, simple iron pills are sufficient. The cheapest and among the most effective is ferrous sulphate in a dose of 200–600 mg (1–3 tablets) taken daily with food. Once the anaemia is corrected, there is, in many women, no point in continuing to take iron supplements as the body's iron stores are complete. Some women clearly do need a small regular and permanent iron supplement throughout their reproductive years however. This should be undertaken with medical direction and based on occasional blood checks.

As with male athletes, the apparent anaemia of heavy training should not be misleading. Some athletes in chronic endurance events develop an expansion of their plasma volume which, by diluting the quite adequate number of red cells present, gives a low haemoglobin value and haematocrit. There is, however, no functional deficiency of iron, the stores are complete and there is therefore no response to therapeutic iron supplements.

'The sex tests', chromosome testing

At present, female athletes are alone subjected to chromosomal tests of their gender. It has never been clear why, in their urge to eliminate non-females from women's competition, the various international regulating committees have declined to ensure equally fair treatment for honest males. A grotesque side effect of the sex testing of individual athletes is that, should a person be found who does not fit exactly certain narrowly prescribed criteria for femininity, they are effectively disenfranchised from competition for life. They are not, by being denied femininity, declared male. There should be little doubt that, in the fairly near future, either the arbitrary testing of females will cease in response to civil rights legislation or that the equally thorough testing of male competitors will begin.

All human beings consist of cells which contain nuclei. In each nucleus are chromosomes which regulate the development and characteristics of the individual. These are assembled in 23 pairs, one pair of which constitutes the so-called sex chromosomes. By convention, these are designated as X or Y chromosomes and the female has two X chromosomes in addition to the 22 pairs of non-sex chromosomes. The male has one X and one Y chromosome. The female is, by convention, designated as having a 46XX chromosomal pattern, the male 46XY.

During reproduction, a male cell divides into two sperms, each containing 23 chromosomes, of which one has an X, the other a Y chromosome, i.e. 23X and 23Y. In contrast, the female produces two ova of 23X constitution. At fertilization, the laws of chance operate to combine these cells to give a theoretically equal number of 46XX and 46XY, i.e. boy and girl, offspring.

Occasional mishaps occur, however, in which either the sex chromosomes or the non-sex (autosomal) chromosomes divide and combine in the wrong way to give abnormal numbers and XY configurations. To add to the confusion, various mixtures of mistakes may occur, sometimes combined with the normal and occasionally with one chromosome missing to give mixed-up or 'mosaic' patterns. Many of these genetic errors give rise to characteristically different people. Many abnormalities are inconsistent with life itself and are aborted or die in infancy. Others lead to bizarre deformities not consistent with a normal life and athletic performance. Some persist as apparently normal people throughout life however.

The chromosomal make-up determines the individual's sex, hormonal function and genital structure. In some instances, however, particularly of 'mosaicism', mixtures of sexual characteristics may occur to create considerable doubt as to the true assignation of the individual to either the male or female gender.

A further complication is that sexuality is determined also by hormonal secretion. Abnormal glands, for example, the male testis in an apparent female, will dictate further abnormal formations. Rare diseases occur in which overproduction of hormones of the 'wrong' sex occur. The commonest types of these rarities are tumours of the adrenal gland which secrete male hormone in females who thus suffer gross virilization which suggests masculinity. On the other hand, secretion of female hormone by the testis in an otherwise normal male will inhibit his masculine development (testicular feminization), as will failure of the testis to respond to male hormones, leaving in each case an apparent female with male chromosomes.

Most of these abnormalities are excessively rare and many of them quite inconsistent with athletic performance. Despite all the sex tests so far carried out, there is no published incidence of chromosomal abnormality so that it remains impossible to judge the true justification of sex testing of females alone.

In the rare instances of trans-sexualism where a person of totally male or female character chooses to change the apparent sex by combined hormonal and surgical interference, there is an obvious and easy detection of genetic sex. It seems unlikely that transvestitism, where a genetically normal person dresses in the clothes of the opposite sex, would create any serious problems as a male transvestite is hardly likely to invoke the characteristic male urge for competition in his new female guise.

Happily, the original sex test imposed upon women of parading their breasts and genitalia before a panel of judges has given way to more scientific and objective methods of chromosome analysis. A few cells are painlessly scraped, by buccal smear, from the mouth lining inside the cheek and specially stained so that chromosomes can be microscopically counted and the presence of the so-called Barr body determined. An alternative is the use of a few cells in a hair follicle, simply obtained by extracting a hair. The presence or absence of Barr bodies gives a quick and reliable method of determining femininity. Barr bodies are only formed by the second (or third or fourth) X chromosome present and therefore do not occur in a male cell. They appear as dark-staining bodies in the nuclei and occur in up to 50 per cent of the female cells. Thus, the absence of any Barr bodies suggests a male cell, the presence of one per cell suggests a normal female and a mixed pattern or the presence of multiple Barr bodies draws attention to more generalized chromosomal abnormalities calling for further investigation. A full chromosome count would then be indicated to map out the exact abnormality present and this is combined with a clinical assessment of the body form, including genitalia, to ensure that a full classification of the individual is made.

7 Age

General effects of ageing

Age brings a gradual decline in muscular strength and cardiorespiratory fitness. The maximum oxygen uptake at age 60 is between only 70 and 80 per cent of that at age 20. Blood pressure also rises with age and pulse rate falls. The tendency to become less active with age leads to increasing obesity. Sedentary habits combine with these physical limitations to leave many relatively young people 'unfit to train'.

There are two important facts concerning age and fitness. First, the age-related decline in strength and cardiorespiratory fitness can be considerably slowed by regular physical activity. Secondly, training can improve these functions at literally any age in life. There are many examples of 80- and 90-year-old athletes and even a centenarian is on record. It is medically and physiologically realistic for patients to train in their sixties and seventies as part of rehabilitation programmes, as well as for fun.

Skills decline with age and neglect but they tend to return relatively quickly once practice is resumed.

Life-long sports

The traditional pattern of sport is that in youth competitive games are pursued intensively and then, for the majority, there is a fairly sudden cessation of all recreational activity. This break is often at the school leaving age when many leave both school and sport for ever. The reasons for this non-participation are not certain and have been the subject of intensive speculation. Some causes may be obvious, for example, work and social responsibilities may make it difficult for individuals to continue in the same games.

Many feel that, with the increasing fragmentation of organized school games and physical education, the school leaver will often be only too keen to abandon overdisciplined compulsory events. The eventual abandonment of school sport and P.E., for instance, coupled with changes in social policy which bring together all the sport and recreation in a community setting outside the more limited institutions in an area, might have considerable advantages for both the individual and society.

The most important concept to be considered is that of introducing to young people during their years of competitive sport one or more recreational pursuits which will be suitable in later life. Thus, it might be sensible to combine, say, field games, cricket and swimming with cycling, hiking or rock climbing. In the long term, the ideal sports for fitness involve regular rhythmic contractions of the large muscle groups. Activities such as jogging, walking, cycling or swimming are highly beneficial in this respect, even if not pursued on a competitive basis. Because youthful participation in these four activities is, in fact, often extremely competitive, it is easy to create in the individual a feeling of reluctance to continue because of failure to meet competitive targets. This is often expressed in such terms as 'I am not going to go on running as a hack'.

If the ideal of a gradual change in recreational pattern with age is accepted, the individual's need for competition must also be remembered. The end point of sporting competition should be to wean the individual off the need for it. Some people, however, have the natural advantage, or disadvantage according to one's philosophical view, of needing competitive stimuli throughout life. This may be concentrated into the competitive energies of work balanced with relaxing non-competitive sport and recreation or, instead, it may bring the individual to a state of permanent competitiveness both at work and play. This type of character, the so-called 'type A', has a sevenfold increased risk of heart attacks compared with the 'type B' colleague who is more relaxed and less competitive.

Childhood

In early life, emphasis is given to the development of normal perception, posture and gait. It is important to avoid bad footwear and to encourage a generally active way of life. Childhood laziness causes the development of extra fat storage cells which in later life lead to obesity. One of the simplest ways of avoiding fat adults is to keep children thin and to counter the age-old myth that a fat child is a healthy one.

School age

The decline of physical education in the school curriculum is regrettable. This decline may be a reflection of a general improvement in the health of the community which thus needs less remedial gymnastic work in schools. The school child needs, however, to continue learning those basic motor skills started in infancy and to add stamina, then strength. Stamina is developed by aerobic endurance training programmes such as long-duration running, swimming or cycling and, provided that overtraining

does not put excessive strain on the musculoskeletal system, these activities can be introduced gradually between the ages of 5 and 10 years. Most children will prefer the hurly-burly and fun of games rather than boring repetition but the danger of overuse injuries must be remembered, particularly in events where there is surface or implement resistance, for example, long-distance running or weight-lifting. Team skills should be introduced at this stage and also, optimistically, a sense of perspective towards both games and fitness and their relative importance to the individual and society.

Middle age

This is the age of voluntary decline. The two most important facts are that most of the decline in fitness between the ages of 20 and 50 is preventable by the motivated individual and that most of the dangers of middle-aged sport are foreseeable. The sense of perspective gained in the school years should by now be providing a realistic horizon for the middle-aged exerciser, particularly in the more strenuous competitive games.

Older age

There is not much evidence to link games with longevity. The evidence suggests marginal statistical advantages slightly in favour of sportsmen but at the individual level there is no guarantee of a long life for the active sportsman. It is clear, however, that the general quality and enjoyment of life can be improved by a modicum of physical and mental fitness which can easily be obtained by very low levels of regular exercise, even though longevity may be largely due to chance and individual genetic endowment. Those who choose to participate in physical activity tend to adopt habits generally favourable to health which tend to reduce cardiac risk factors. For instance, the athlete will probably not become excessively overweight or want to impair his respiratory capacity by smoking.

In view of the active participation of many veterans, as well as the demonstrable trainability of subjects of all ages, the amount of exercise for an individual is a matter of his or her own choice. In general, medical guidance is 'Do what you like and can within the limits of stressful symptoms'.

8 Disability

Exercise and medical rehabilitation

Routine exercises in the rehabilitation of medical disabilities are boring for all but the obsessional. The need to make the necessary tasks acceptable and even enjoyable has led to the increasing use of games in medical rehabilitation. In the gymnasium, the medicine ball allows limb and trunk strength and postural control to develop. Planned swimming can replace repetitive land exercise. In finer neurological disability, games such as quoits, chess or draughts with outsize pieces of variable weight can, by replacing boredom with the concept of games or even competition, encourage longer and keener participation.

One of the advantages of an Athletes' Clinic in a general medical rehabilitation department is that the mixture of ages and motivations usually acts as a general stimulant to both patient and remedial staff. A little adjustment of environment can work wonders. Boring leg exercises become a focus for keen competition on a bicycle ergometer where it is possible to monitor speed or power output against oneself or one's fellow patients. Rowing machines, treadmills or games with throwing or kicking all help to stimulate interest. The simplest resource required to make an exercise programme more stimulating is imagination on the part of the remedial therapist. Given that, there are no limits!

Sport for the disabled

Interest in sport for the disabled began after the First World War and there are now international movements available for virtually all categories of disability. There are two prerequisites. First, the choice of sport or recreation must be appropriate and realistic for the individual. Secondly, the classification of participating and competitive groups must be equally realistic.

There is continuing debate about the degree of integration with non-disabled sport which is desirable or achievable. Schools of opinion favour both open and closed competition for the disabled and a third school advocates stronger emphasis on non-competitive participation in sport and recreation rather than competition.

Two fundamental precepts are 'rehabilitation begins with realism' and 'the individual is all-important'.

It is true that modern science may make possible the successful achievement of, for instance, archery for a one-armed legless archer. This requires so much exceptional support in financial and engineering terms, however, that it is hardly likely to be a realistic goal for all amputees. The individual is, even more than his able-bodied colleague, torn by the conflict between his ambitious ideals and his actual constraints. It is simply realistic, not defeatist, to take careful note of local facilities and their availability to the individual in the choice of sport and recreation. It is also important to take into account the requirement for attendants. For instance, the epileptic may safely swim but a safe occupation becomes hazardous when he swims out to sea alone in cold water, rather than staying with his watching attendant in a warm indoor pool.

Paraplegics blazed the trail for the disabled and there are now organized sports available in many countries for amputees, the mentally handicapped, cerebral palsy patients, the polio-disabled, spina bifida patients, muscular dystrophy patients, the visually handicapped, the deaf, and more. Some of the games available include wheelchair races and ball games, archery, shooting, cycling, swimming, including water ski-ing, canoeing and rowing, table tennis and outdoor walking and climbing.

Because of the need for skilled guidance and expertise, the disabled patient is strongly advised to seek help through one of the organizations appropriate to his disability, e.g. British Sports Association for the Disabled at Stoke Mandeville Stadium, Harvey Road, Aylesbury, Bucks.

It is crucial that the benefits of sports participation should not be destroyed by the demoralization of failure. To those familiar with the consequences of failure in highly competitive non-handicapped sport, there appears to be no reason why 'normal' competitive attitudes in the disabled should not lead to a similar problem of failure and thus provide for the majority of competitive disabled sportsmen the bitterness of sporting failure as well as of the underlying handicap. It is most important to remember the individual's personal attitude to his disability and to life in general as well as to sport and competition. Individual preference may dictate, for instance, non-competitive horse-riding or outdoor hiking and it would be wrong to try and force such a person into competitive swimming. Nevertheless,

many will accept the role of sports such as wheelchair racing and swimming as part of the rehabilitation programme, *en route* to their personal choice of recreation and much depends on considerate explanation and the motivation of suitable rehabilitation programmes.

The disabled player can improve his physiological functions in exactly the same way as the able-bodied athlete doing similar training. For instance, exercise in the wheelchair or swimming pool can bring about improvements in oxygen uptake, pulse rate and blood lipid level.

Disabled sportsmen have completed the marathon in wheelchairs and may on favourable courses exploit gradients to outspeed able-bodied runners. About 30–50 per cent more work must be done by a wheelchair occupant to cover ground, however, because he must move the dead weight of the chair with its frictional resistance in addition to his own body mass.

Access

Access must be made possible to all appropriate facilities. The British Sports Council has given a lead in this respect by trying to ensure that grant aiding of capital facilities is dependent upon provision being made for disabled access. This must go hand in hand with full and appropriate safety measures being built in to sports facilities. In principle, this should be no different for the disabled or able-bodied. In architectural terms, the same amenities which would make sports facilities available to the disabled would also enhance public safety and access. Imagination, rather than money, is usually the limiting factor as the cost of planned access is cheaper than subsequent building modifications.

9 Diet

The athlete's diet remains as controversial as in the past when the Greeks prepared themselves on a special diet of dried figs or in the nineteenth century when it was customary to prepare for cross-country races with steak and wine. There is continuing conflict between physiologists, physicians and coaches. A cycle exists whereby physiologists find that there is little or nothing to commend new dietary fads; physicians therefore take this to mean that no special diet is required for sport, but coaches feel certain that they know best and reject all the scientific evidence in favour of yet more fads.

There are probably several reasons for these conflicts. Most foods are interchangeable within the body as sources of energy because of human biochemical efficiency and under almost all normal circumstances, appetite and thirst take care of demand as natural regulators. Strictly controlled scientific experiments of diet and athletic performance are difficult to set up. Repeated attempts to assess the importance of certain dietary substances show no significant positive or negative effects on performance, whatever the strength of conviction displayed by individual athletes and their coaches about certain substances from Vitamin B_{12} injections to pollen extracts.

Many claims by coaches are based on basic misunderstandings of scientific fact. For instance, the fact that Vitamin C is involved in certain metabolic cycles is extrapolated to mean that massive supplementation will make muscle exercise much more efficient; or the apparent anaemia of the endurance athlete is misinterpreted as meaning that iron supplementation is necessary and will lead to an increase in haemoglobin in all circumstances. These two fallacies, together with statements that Vitamin C is a virus killer and that Vitamin B_{12} enhances performance in explosive events – but, because of its stimulant effect, should not be given in the evening – have all appeared in coaching literature.

Much of this logic is based on evidence from Eastern Europe. Because certain countries with successful sporting achievements use certain diets, it is said that they must be 'right' and ahead of Western scientific competence, but no allowance is made for the many other variables in athletic training, including the widespread use of anabolic steroids which might invalidate many dietary considerations. On the other hand, the medical and scientific professions are certainly guilty of gross underestimation of the athlete's nutritional demands. Almost all dietary advice is based on the sedentary or moderately active person and few doctors understand that a competitor's metabolic demands may show a three- or fourfold increase over that of the sedentary subject. Other misunderstandings concern the special needs of competitors in certain events, as for example, in hot climates or prolonged endurance events where there is clearly need for special dietary planning.

Much misunderstanding between scientists and athletes may simply be due to the difference between the sedentary and the highly active subject's overall energy requirements. Dietary constituents, including minerals and vitamins, may be expressed in absolute terms, for example, the minimum amount required for daily existence or, more importantly for the athlete, may best be expressed in terms of requirement per 1000 Calories (4.18 MJ) of food consumed. Comparison of recommendations from a wide range of sources suggests that the appropriate multiplication upwards of basic sedentary man's requirements would be very near many of the suggestions put forward as ideal levels for the active athlete. Indeed, consideration of this logic might save a great deal of expense and disappointment for the athlete whose coach would do well to ponder why there is so little scientific evidence to support athletic dietary faddism in an age when nutritional and biochemical research has clearly elucidated so much of man's metabolism.

Western populations overeat and official scientific recommendations from the United Kingdom, the United States and Scandinavia have all, in recent years, advocated dietary reductions. Most scientific reviews of the sportsman's diet suggest that a mixed one provides all the basic needs for the athlete, but that particular events may call for specific modifications. It is assumed that an athlete's basic requirements for iron and Vitamin C are fulfilled from ordinary fresh food sources. The greater Calorie requirements of the athlete should, then, be met by an appropriate increase in intake of a mixed diet which will provide the necessary vitamins and trace elements *pro rata*. There are, however, some important variations to be considered in certain events.

Energy expenditure

Basic metabolic requirements of the average adult body run at about 1500 Cal/day. The Calorie (Cal) is the traditional unit used to measure heat and energy exchange. It represents 1000 calories and is sometimes called a kilocalorie. The recent metrication of scientific measurements is gradually replacing Calories with joules; 1 Cal = 1000 cal = 1 kcal = 4.184 kilojoules (kJ). Although quantity of food can be stated by weight it is useful to consider energy intake and expenditure in the same Calorie units. The energy value of a food is expressed as the Calories yielded by combustion of a standard amount, e.g. Cal/g.

The UK Recommended Daily Amount of energy for sedentary young men is 2500 Cal (10.46 MJ); for women it is 2100 Cal (8.79 MJ); 3000 Cal (12.55 MJ) is recommended for moderately active young men (aged 18–34). Heavy workers and athletes naturally expend a variable amount of energy over and above these basic levels. It is useful to look at workrates of certain activities and consider their energy consequences. Thus running fairly hard, say at 5-minute-mile pace, burns 25 Cal/min (104.6 kJ/min), or about 125 Cal/mile (523 kJ/min). If a sedentary person went straight out without warm-up and ran 1 mile in 5 minutes and resumed his sedentary activity, then his basic daily requirement would be 2500 + 125 = 2625 Cal/day (10.46 + 0.52 = 10.98 MJ/day).

By comparison, a highly trained distance runner might maintain 5-minute-mile pace for an hour, in which case he would burn up 25 Cal/min × 60 = 1500 Cal/hour (104.6 kJ/min × 60 = 6.276 MJ/hour) and his daily requirement would be 4000 Cal (16.74 MJ). *Tables 9.1* and *9.2* illustrate some energy expenditure rates.

Table 9.1. Energy expenditure in different activities

Activity	Energy expenditure	
	(Cal/day)	(MJ/day)
Basal living	1500	6.28
Sedentary worker	2500	10.46
Athlete	3000–5000	12.55–20.92
24-hour cycle race	10 000	41.84

Table 9.2. Energy costs and pulse rates

Activity	Pulse (beats/min)	Energy cost per minute (Cal)	(kJ)	Energy cost in one hour (Cal)	(MJ)
Rest	up to 70	1–2	4.18–8.37	60–120	0.25–0.50
Easy walk	70–100	3–5	12.55–20.92	180–300	0.75–1.26
Jog	100–140	5–10	20.92–41.84	300–600	1.26–2.51
Run/cycle/swim	120–200	5–20	20.92–83.68	300–1200	1.26–5.02
5-minute miling	180–200	25	104.60	1500	6.28

Components of diet

A full diet consists of carbohydrates, protein, fats, vitamins, minerals and water. For good health, the total input must match the energy expenditure and a correct proportion of the various components must be present. It is possible to contrive a diet consisting, for instance, entirely of carbohydrate energy sources plus fluid, vitamins and minerals. This intake might be satisfactory for a short time, depending on the subject's activities, but would lead inexorably to wasting and weakness. Because of the body's considerable ability to adjust itself to temporary fluctuations and maintain a constantly stable biochemical internal environment (a process called homeostasis), the pattern of diet over weeks and months rather than hours and days, should be considered.

Carbohydrates

Carbohydrates are molecules containing carbon, hydrogen and oxygen, with the hydrogen and oxygen being combined in a ratio of 2:1, as in water. The simplest carbohydrates are called 'sugars', while 'starches' are more complex. Carbohydrate-rich foods include grains, fruit and vegetables, as well as refined sugars and starches.

In the body, carbohydrates are metabolized to glycogen and glucose which are the basic exercise fuels and glucose is finally burnt to carbon dioxide (CO_2) and water (H_2O).

Proteins

Proteins are nitrogen-containing organic compounds from such sources as meat, fish, eggs or cheese. Proteins are necessary for the formation and maintenance of body tissues. Body-building, or anabolism, is the process of building up proteinacious tissues, e.g. muscle, through natural growth or training in a way which incorporates more nitrogen into the new tissues. In contrast, catabolism is the process of wasting or tissue breakdown, due to disease, injury or relative starvation, of the same tissues. In this case, tissue breakdown yields nitrogen which is excreted in the urine in the form of urea and creatinine.

Despite the bizarre protein gluttony of many athletes, surplus protein is not stored as muscle. The nitrogen is removed and excreted in the urine and the remainder is used as a source of energy or stored as glycogen or fat. As with carbohydrate, there is no positive harm in eating protein in excess of daily requirements although an eventual weight gain from excessive total calorie intake is inevitable.

Fats

Fats of animal or plant origin are complex compounds of carbon, hydrogen and oxygen but without the water content of carbohydrates. Their structure contains carbon chains which may be saturated or unsaturated in their chemical bonding with oxygen and hydrogen. The more saturated a fat, the more tightly bound is its chemical structure. Saturated fats are mostly associated with animal tissues, unsaturated fats with plants, e.g. vegetable oils. Excessive intake of saturated fats, in contrast to unsaturated fats, is one of the risk factors associated with arterial and coronary heart disease and has a tendency to raise the blood fat levels.

Cholesterol is a complex fatty compound whose basic structure of interlocked carbon rings is common to all the body's naturally occurring male and female hormones, as well as their derivatives which include the anabolic steroids.

Vitamins

Vitamins are natural compounds which are necessary in small amounts for efficient metabolism. Most of them act as part of the body's enzyme systems which catalyse or regulate the body's biochemical actions. Because vitamins play well-defined and limited roles in the body's chemistry, they are required in defined amounts which can be related to body size or the level of bodily activity and dietary intake. There is no consistent or reliable scientific evidence that excess of any vitamin promotes health or fitness once the basic requirements have been satisfied. Most of the vitamins cannot be made by the body so they must be included in the diet. Deficiencies lead to characteristic diseases.

Minerals

The most important mineral requirements are those for salt (NaCl) and potassium (K) because the body's osmotic pressure is largely managed by the balance of these key elements, together with protein molecules.

Other elements required in relatively large amounts include calcium (Ca) and iron (Fe). There are numerous others required in smaller amounts such as manganese (Mn), magnesium (Mg) and zinc (Zn). Their importance is better established for some than for others. For instance, magnesium deficiency may occur due to prolonged diarrhoea or diuretic therapy and causes neuromuscular disturbance including tremor and convulsions. Calcium deficiency, usually combined with Vitamin D deficiency, leads to the serious bone diseases rickets or osteomalacia. Zinc deficiency impairs wound healing,

however normal zinc levels and requirements are not clearly established.

Dietary balance

Carbohydrates

Most authorities suggest that the proportions of carbohydrates, protein and fat should be in the ratio of roughly 6:1:1.3. It is suggested that carbohydrate should provide some 60 per cent of calorie requirements, of which most should be in the form of complex carbohydrates, e.g. grain and vegetables and fruit, with restriction of refined sugars to no more than about 15 per cent of the total carbohydrate.

Protein

Protein intakes are recommended to make up some 10 per cent of the total energy needs. Actual intakes are usually about 12 per cent of calories. The basic requirement for the average person, including a generous safety margin, is about 1 g/kg of body weight (1 g/kg BW). The training demands of the athlete which include the regular chemical servicing of a greater and more active muscle bulk, would be fully met by this intake, i.e. 12 per cent protein out of some 4000 Cal (16.74 MJ) total daily intake. Negative calcium balance has been shown in men on intakes of 2 g/kg BW daily, so that selective protein overeating may induce bone weakening. Nevertheless, while many authorities regard this as an absolute maximum requirement, others suggest that rather lower intakes are perfectly adequate.

Fats

A recommended intake of fats from all sources would provide some 30 per cent of the total calorie requirement with vegetable fats constituting two-thirds of the intake. Cholesterol intake should be regulated: one authority recommends no more than

300 mg daily for the average 70 kg man (one egg provides about 250 mg cholesterol) but there is so much individual variation in fat metabolism and energy levels that some scepticism should be maintained. The more exercise the subject takes, the more efficiently can he handle all forms of diet. Inactivity is associated with dietary excess and biochemical disadvantages.

Energy value of foods

Carbohydrates, protein and fats all yield different amounts of fuel during metabolism. For instance, 1 g of carbohydrate yields about 4 Cal (16.74 kJ); 1 g of protein also yields about 4 Cal (16.74 kJ) but 1 g of fat gives about 9 Cal (37.66 kJ). Thus, fat appears to be a most efficient fuel but in athletic pursuits, as shown in Chapter 5, it is not the immediately available fuel of choice under most normal circumstances except in longer-duration aerobic exercise. Thus, a large store of body fat is not so much a useful supply of energy as an increasing liability in terms of dead weight which has to be carried around at great expense in terms of energy.

Basic dietary deficiencies

Students often live on college-cooked diets in which both overall calorie content, as well as balance, may be deficient. Furthermore, overcooking diminishes vitamin content. Thus, there may be overall nutritional deficiency in athletes who are students and besides a lack of quantity, specific additions of Vitamin C may be required through fresh fruit and vegetables.

Many younger women are unduly figure-conscious despite trying to maintain athletic training. Anaemia is discussed further in Chapter 4 but, in addition to undereating and poor institutional diets, iron deficiency due to heavy menstrual loss is common and supplementary iron pills may be essential.

Relative undernutrition may occur in athletes from poor home backgrounds and will affect training in events demanding very high energy output, e.g. athletic field events, swimming or cycling. Because this is likely to be a problem of general nutrition, rather than simply a deficiency in one or two items, a general policy on diet should be planned by the coaches in conjunction with governing bodies, the individuals and their families involved. It is notable that many sponsorship schemes for sportsmen in recent years have been specifically involved with nutritional support of individuals or squads.

Malnutrition is rife in the developing countries. Also, intestinal infestation by parasites is endemic and this is an additional cause of iron-deficiency anaemia. Here specific treatment is required and iron supplements may be unnecessary if this can be achieved. Probably the leading causes of athletic non-achievement in the world at large are poverty, malnutrition and anaemia. Those working to establish sport in the poorer countries must realize that public health measures will do more to improve the basic level of fitness of many populations than sports training schemes alone.

Salt (NaCl)

The estimated daily need for salt is about 0.5 g. Under circumstances of heavy sweating and hot climates, this may rise to between 3 and 5 g. The present estimated daily intake in the Western world is between 5 and 10 g however, so that, under average circumstances, it is clear that no supplementary salt is required for sportsmen. Indeed, there is evidence linking sustained overconsumption of salt with the development of high blood pressure and official recommendations for salt intake are set at a target of only 3 g daily, which, however, still leaves the average citizen to excrete most of his daily intake.

In good health, the kidneys are extremely efficient at conserving necessary salt and excreting clear surpluses. If excessive salt is eaten, however, then it has, by osmotic attraction, to hold an appropriate amount of fluid within the body to maintain a concentration equivalent to that of the blood so that the two liquids are isotonic. Thus, if the athlete drinks 1 ℓ of pure water, by far the greater part of this is passed as urine within 4 hours. If, instead, he drinks 1 ℓ of a saline solution isotonic with his body fluids, it takes most of the next day to rid the body of surplus salt and water.

Specific indications do exist for salt supplementation. Assuming normally balanced nutrition, the indications are confined to circumstances of profuse sweating, indoors or outdoors. Indoors, in prolonged competition in such events as judo or fencing, in which thick or ill-ventilated clothing is worn, it is possible that some extra salt may occasionally be required. Liberal salting of the normal diet should be more than adequate in providing an extra 5–10 g/day however.

For sustained outdoor performance, such as heavy manual labour, hard training, or marathon running, some extra salt may be required in hot weather. In most events, however, it cannot be absorbed during participation and prior 'stocking-up' may be indicated to avoid salt deficiency from profuse sweating. For instance, under such circumstances, sweat loss may amount to 1.5 ℓ/hour, i.e. 3.75 ℓ in a 2½ hour marathon run. With a sodium concentration of up to 2.2 g/ℓ in sweat, up to at least 8.25 g of sodium could be lost during that period. As one of the effects of training and acclimatization is to reduce the salt content of sweat, the more experienced athlete should suffer minimal distress from this cause. More likely is the tendency to chronic salt depletion among athletes training intensively under hot conditions without adequate salt and fluid replacement day by day. This leads to fatigue, listlessness and cramp. Losses should be made good as soon as possible after the event but drinking large volumes of pure water may precipitate the cramps of salt deficiency by diluting the blood. Overconcentrated salt solutions exacerbate dehydration by osmotic attraction of fluids into the bowel from the tissues. Hence, modest salt replacement, about 0.5 per cent solution, is adequate.

As a rough guide, a big pinch of salt to a mug of liquid is a safe replacement drink. Salt tablets are useful in preparation for high-temperature events.

Saline drinks and tablets may cause nausea or vomiting if taken in excess but enteric coated preparations, e.g. Slow Sodium (Ciba), have proved most effective. In these formulations, the salt is embedded in a wax core which allows the slow release of salt in the small bowel without the sudden gastric concentrations which cause nausea. Slow Sodium contains 600 mg of actual sodium chloride and a recommended prophylactic dosage is between four and eight tablets daily. It should again be emphasized that there is no point in deliberate overdosage because of the fluid-retaining effects which may occur.

Minerals

Calcium (Ca) Calcium salts are the main components of the skeleton. They are absorbed from the gut with the help of Vitamin D but in some diseases this absorption is impaired, e.g. certain forms of diarrhoea. Absorption is also impaired by foods which precipitate calcium and cause its excretion in the stools. These foods include spinach, rhubarb and unrefined cereal grains containing phytic acid. To compensate for this effect, extra calcium is added to commercial flour. A daily calcium intake of 500 mg for adults, 600–700 mg for adolescents, and 1200 mg during pregnancy and lactation is advised. A pint of milk contains about 600 mg of calcium, and vegetables and cereals are other rich sources. Drinking water may provide considerable calcium intake especially in hard-water areas. Efficient calcium metabolism needs the presence of Vitamin D and this vitamin is synthesized by the action of sunshine on the skin.

Iron (Fe) Iron is present in meat and vegetables, and liver, eggs and wholemeal cereals are rich sources. An average mixed diet contains about 4–5 mg per 1000 Cal, or 12–15 mg of iron daily and of this, only about 10 per cent is absorbed – such an amount being more than adequate for males. In women, menstrual loss varies but if the average monthly loss, equivalent to between 25 and 50 mg of iron is not replaced, anaemia develops; the UK Recommended Daily Amount of iron intake for young women is 12 mg. Supplementary iron pills may be necessary to ensure this level.

During childbearing and lactation, an average iron loss of 2 mg daily must be made good. Iron absorption is improved during pregnancy and lactation, however, so the increased requirement will be met for most women, provided that their initial iron stores were adequate.

A possible further source of iron deficiency in prolonged heavy exercise is through the iron content of sweat. An estimated maximum possible loss through day-long sweating is given as about 14 mg of iron and, if this were to be sustained, then a good chance of mild chronic iron deficiency would exist. It is most unlikely that many people would sustain this level of sweat loss, but the theoretical hazards of lesser degrees of sweat loss would be compounded by a diet which is marginal or deficient in iron. Similar theoretical considerations apply to blood loss due to haematuria after exercise, but *see* page 100 for discussion of this condition.

All other minerals are normally found in fully adequate proportions in a mixed diet and no supplementation is required.

Vitamins

Athletic folklore is particularly rich in vitamin mythology. It is important to relate vitamin intake to total diet bearing in mind the two- or threefold increase in fuel requirement and metabolism of the active athlete compared with the sedentary subject.

Vitamin A Vitamin A, from milk, butter, cheese, eggs, liver and fish (particularly fish liver oils), as well as carrots, green vegetables and fruit, plays a vital part in visual acuity with deficiency leading to 'night blindness'. Deficiency also causes deterioration of skin texture. The recommended daily intake of up to 1200 micrograms (μg) for adults is so small compared with the average amount of 150 mg (1 mg = 1000 μg) stored in the adult liver that, in the Western world, dietary deficiency is virtually impossible in the absence of specific disease. Gross deficiency states do exist in the very underdeveloped countries, however, where starvation is widespread.

Vitamin B The 'B' group of vitamins occurs in the highest concentrations in foods such as yeast and liver which are rich in metabolic activity. These vitamins play an important part in the body's enzyme systems. For practical purposes, a well-mixed Western diet of adequate calorie intake automatically contains a fully adequate supply of the Vitamin B complex. The severe deficiency diseases of beriberi (deficiency of thiamin or B_1) and pellagra (niacin deficiency) are rarely seen in the developed countries, although they are common in the Third World.

Of more practical importance in European countries is depression due to pyridoxine (B_6) deficiency associated with taking some oral contraceptives and megaloblastic anaemia due to Vitamin B_{12} or folate deficiencies. Vitamin B_{12} deficiency may be dietary due to a strict vegan diet, but is usually caused by gastrointestinal disease or surgery. Folate deficiency is not uncommon because body stores are low and the richest dietary sources, fresh green vegetables, liver and kidney, are often ignored or their folate content lowered by cooking. Pregnancy and anticonvulsant drugs may also lead to folate deficiency.

Recommended intakes of the Vitamin B complex include: thiamin 0.4 mg, nicotinic acid 6.6 mg and riboflavin 0.44 mg, all per 1000 Cal (4184 kJ) of total dietary intake. Normal adult requirements of pyridoxine (2 mg/day), Vitamin B_{12} (2 μg/day) and folate (0.2–0.4 mg/day) should be scaled-up from these reference levels for a 2500 Cal (10.46 MJ) diet to match the higher calorie diets of the more active athletes.

There is no evidence to warrant the use of injections of Vitamins B_{12} or B_{15} in healthy people under athletic training who enjoy a balanced diet and the absence of disease. The most likely cause of apparent improvements from these treatments is the 'placebo' effect which, in most drug trials, yields a positive response of up to 30 per cent due to suggestion when inert compounds are administered.

Vitamin C Vitamin C (ascorbic acid) is plentiful in fruits, vegetables and liver. The daily requirement is 30 mg (10–15 mg per 1000 Cal (4184 kJ) of diet). Deficiency leads to the disease scurvy and, in lesser degrees, to impairment of tissue healing.

Reference has already been made to the real possibility of Vitamin C deficiency due to overcooking and lack of fresh foodstuffs in institutional diets. The massive overdosage of Vitamin C commonly found in sportsmen is hard to justify however. There is no evidence that huge doses prevent or cure diseases, though many claims have been made for its use in protection against the common cold. Excessive overdosage may cause oxalate kidney stones, a rather more serious problem than a cold.

Vitamin D The D group vitamins work closely with calcium metabolism. These fat-soluble vitamins, are plentiful in fish and liver oils, margarine, milk, butter and eggs. Recommended daily intakes are between 2.5 and 10 μg, a level well exceeded in any reasonable diet. The deficiency disease rickets is rarely seen in the Western world because of the generally satisfactory level of diet and sunshine. It is imperative to realize that gross excess of Vitamin D causes dangerous toxicity with sickness, diarrhoea, renal failure and abnormal deposits of calcium in the body.

Vitamin E Vitamin E has for long been one of the scientific jokes of the athletic scene. Massive consumption of its various forms, including wheat germ oil, have made fortunes for many. In medical terms, however, there is no known deficiency state of vitamin E and, in the words of a standard textbook of medical practice, 'it has no proven therapeutic value'. Attention is again drawn to the 'placebo' effect.

General conclusion

A general review of diet suggests that excessive attention to the minutiae of dietary balance is counterproductive and expensive. There is little evidence that gluttony or the esoteric faddism which is such a common part of the sports scene has other than placebo value. Provided that the individual components of the diet are considered in their overall proportions to each other, as found in a well-mixed Western diet, or in terms of so much constituent per 1000 Cal (4184 kJ) of overall food intake, all should be well.

Specific dieting

Not only is the sportsman's overall diet important but his eating habits must also be considered. Correct preparation for specific events and intelligent timing of dietary intake are important. Endurance events and sustained competitions with intermittent rounds or periods of intense exertion call for specific consideration.

Endurance events – fluids

The key to nutrition for the endurance events is the level of sustained effort. In the marathon race, for instance, it is simply impossible to take in food or useful amounts of mineral in transit due to the high level of energy expenditure and gut inhibition. Because efficient heat loss is essential for safe marathon running, adequate hydration is absolutely vital. Fully adequate salt and water intake must be achieved by drinking fluids up to the start of the race. Unfortunately, international regulations still forbid unrestricted fluid replacement in all longer races, although there is hope of early change in this respect.

A trained runner can drink about 200 ml of fluid at 15-min intervals for most of the marathon but he cannot absorb significant amounts of minerals or sugar. The American College of Sports Medicine recommendation is that fluids in this event should not contain more than 2.5 per cent glucose and many authorities claim that, because the amounts of glucose thus available are so small, pure water is the ideal fluid for use during the actual race.

Carbohydrate loading

The carbohydrate loading diets developed in recent years have allowed the marathon runner to more than double his resting muscle glycogen stores. This can lead to very substantial improvements in endurance as an average muscle contains enough glycogen to fuel between 1 and 2 hours' running. Without rest and preparation for the event, the athlete classically 'hits the wall' which causes him to slow up markedly as he runs out of muscle glycogen somewhere around the 20-mile (30-km) or 2-hour mark when he is still short of the finish.

In principle, hard effort carried out about a week before a marathon will deplete the muscle glycogen stores. Experiments have shown that muscle glycogen levels can then be raised by 2 or 3 days of carbohydrate starvation, with a diet rich in protein and fat only, followed by a switch to an extremely high carbohydrate-only diet for the 3 or 4 days leading up to the race itself. In this way, muscle glycogen content can be trebled. A point to remember is that the chronic training load of most long-distance runners ensures that muscles rarely get to their optimum glycogen levels and, indeed, many such runners may find themselves chronically fatigued in long-distance runs because of low average glycogen levels which then tend to fall even further with subsequent training. Thus, even a couple of days' rest with no dietary modification would be expected to produce a muscle glycogen bonus in many long-distance runners.

Most authorities find that the carbohydrate loading diet has a variable effect on different runners and that, even with those who find it most beneficial, it is not likely to work successfully more than a couple of times a year.

Many experienced runners find that the idea of running to exhaustion, as originally proposed, within a few days of a race, is highly unsatisfactory. They achieve good results simply by stepping up their training over 2 or 3 days about a week before racing and then proceeding to increase their carbohydrate intake for several days before the big race while reducing their training. Hard training must be avoided during carbohydrate-free days when fatigue, irritability and malaise are common.

The coach and athlete must experiment with individual response so that unpredictability is avoided.

Intermittent endurance diets

At the lower level of energy output associated with intermittent events spread over a long time – such as canoeing races with heats, or ultralong-distance sports – there is clearly a need for the intake of actual fuel, most simply in the form of glucose. In sustained events, constant fluid replacement remains essential and salt supplementation becomes more important in the avoidance of cramp.

In training and competition the timing of meals is important. There should be at least 1 hour between eating and training and 1–4 hours before competition. This is a matter for individual experiment. Because of increasing gastric inhibition due to nervousness before competition, only well-timed light nutritious meals, rich in carbohydrate, should be taken. Heavy or rich meals fill the bowel and cause indigestion.

Liquid meals

There are various products available and these are more expensive than normal diets. Some products, e.g. 'Nutrament', provide a balanced diet in a can of flavoured drink. Such an intake is more easily absorbed than solid food and is, therefore, useful for those with tight schedules or insufficient time both for eating and for resting around their extended training schedules or competitions. A comprehensive dietary mix, e.g. 'Complan' powder, can also be made into a drink. A protein-only supplement, e.g. 'Casilan', is not relevant in the immediate sporting context. The limiting factor in intake is the comfortable absorption time of whatever is ingested and this must be worked out by the individual and his coach.

During severe endurance effort, such as marathon running, water is probably the simplest and optimum supplement and this should be drunk on the 'little-and-often' basis. Any attempt to take significant amounts of salt, sugar or other foods leads to gastric stasis, non-absorption and sickness.

Energy drinks

Some energy drinks for example, Dynamo and Hycal, contain high concentrations of glucose solids and are invaluable for use in intermittent events such as field games, pole vault competitions and rowing events. Between heats, regular topping-up is thus possible throughout competition. This is important for two reasons. First, maintenance of blood sugar levels prevents the hypoglycaemic symptoms of fatigue and fall-off in performance. Secondly, the nervous system uses glucose exclusively as its fuel. Low blood sugar levels, even with high tissue glycogen reserves, 'starve' the nervous system and impair skill and concentration.

Sugar supplements given to football teams at half time significantly reduce the rate of error and goals conceded in the last quarter of the game. Glucose is usually regarded as the instant energy sugar but glucose syrup (BPC) may be even better as the sugars are partly hydrolysed into their constituent polymers. Such hydrolysis allows a greater carbohydrate load to be given without the sweetness which many find sickly. Other sugars have been used because glucose is rapidly absorbed from the small bowel and calls

forth prompt secretion of insulin which itself causes secondary hypoglycaemia, or drop in blood sugar. Fructose has been used for this purpose; there is some evidence that it may lead to more sustained output of insulin over a longer period which might even out drastic variations in sugar and insulin levels. Strong concentrations of fructose easily cause diarrhoea, a misfortune discovered by many marathon runners. Other energy drinks, such as Best-1, XL-1, Staminade, in suitable dilutions, supply small concentrations of glucose (5 per cent). Up to this concentration gastric absorption of useful energy and fluid replacement can be achieved. A minimal concentration (0.6 per cent) of salt may accelerate gastric emptying. Greater concentrations cause gastric stasis, hence non-absorption.

Isotonic drinks

Isotonic drinks, for example, Accolade and Gatorade, in contrast to the high-energy drinks, contain a low percentage of carbohydrate, together with electrolytes designed to replace sweat and fluid losses. These are intended as iso-osmotic replacements for plasma fluids and compensate for minerals lost through sweat; they also provide a minimal energy replacement. These drinks replace sweat losses if the effort is low or intermittent enough to allow gastric absorption.

Sweeter replacement fluids are less tolerated than slightly sharper tasting drinks and, for this reason, some citrus flavouring should be used in any home-made drinks. Gastric absorption is most efficient during effort if the replacement drinks are cool and not, as might be anticipated, at body heat. The coolness stimulates peristalsis, or intestinal movement, and absorption.

Dieting and weight loss

Exercise is a very powerful fat-burning mechanism, particularly at the continuous low-grade aerobic level. The metabolic effect of exercise on fat burning (lipolysis) outlasts the duration of exercise itself and blood fat levels are reduced as well as, eventually, body weight. Initially, exercise leads to an increase in appetite and weight as the increasing bulk of trained muscle replaces some fat. Thereafter, exercise leads to weight loss and the appetite falls to less than that required for full caloric restoration of the exercise load.

The most effective slimming diet is a normal calorie-controlled mixed food diet with added exercise. Exercise leads to a higher basal metabolic rate and more efficient 'burning off' of fat than with untrained people. The metabolic benefit of running is more efficient and sustained than the usual equation of 'a slice of cake per 2-mile run' suggests. The steady expenditure of, say, 100 Cal/day (418.4 kJ/day) in the brisk jogging of about a mile would burn about a pound of fat a month.

Some voluntary restriction of excessive food intake such as nibbling between meals is desirable. The key to a change in lifestyle is really to replace automation with feet.

Other diets are less satisfactory. Artificial carbohydrate restriction leads to the ketosis associated with excessive fat burning. People feel tired and uncomfortable on this regimen, as they do on artificially low-protein regimens. A high-protein diet is pointless because excess is inefficient and protein is not a significant primary fuel for exercise. Sugars should be avoided because of the insulin response and their possible relation to vascular disease. Complex carbohydrates, including vegetables and whole grain cereals which are also rich in fibre, are more satisfactory.

10 Mental aspects of sport

Psychology is the scientific study of human behaviour and thought processes; psychiatry is the clinical application of psychology and medicine to the management of mental illnesses. The clinical psychologist is trained in the application in a clinical situation of psychological methods to mental disorders and disturbances of behaviour in patients – usually in close liaison with the physician or psychiatrist.

Psychology

Psychology has developed from earlier philosophical preoccupations with thoughts and mental processes to a more scientific analysis of human behaviour. As a young science, it is beset by much confusion over definitions, language, classifications and methodology. Its development along scientific lines has seen the gradual accumulation of a core of proven facts, experimentally tested and reproducible, as a basis for practice. Scientific approaches may be either empirical, with conclusions being inferred from actual observations, or deductive, with hypotheses being devised which must then be tested and rejected or proven.

At present, in sport, behavioural psychology is predominant. Its methods are based on the practical application of conclusions gained from observed behaviour, its objects are to modify subsequent behaviour in the sporting (or any other) context.

It is important to identify the differing roles of coach, physician and psychologist in the athlete's life. The physician tends to be injury- and disease-orientated, the psychologist perhaps more health-minded and, as a scientist, still rather constrained by the discipline of his scientific approach; the coach alone is free to explore the fullest range of science and nonsense, practical and theoretical, in the manipulation of his pupil's progress. Only if the inherent limits of each party's approaches are seen and accepted, can the logic of the team approach really be understood. The advice offered by each member of a team of advisers to an athlete should be given only after joint consultation. It is unfair to expect the athlete to have to hawk himself around after failure, trying to piece together his jig-saw from the fragmented advice of experts in different fields, few of whom have the vision to see the whole context.

Personality type

All scientific action is based on an ordered classification and man has long been assessed by temperament as well as physique. Modern personality studies have been greatly influenced by Eysenck's work in classifying people into broad personality types. By contrasting minimal and extreme reactions to certain basic characteristics, it is possible to map out some important aspects of behaviour. Eysenck's basic criteria concern stability and social responsiveness – the latter varying from extreme introversion to extreme extroversion.

Similarly, stability can grade down to extreme instability or neuroticism. A convenient graphic expression of these two scales can be made on a simple chart with introversion/extroversion plotted against neuroticism/stability. On such a chart different sports groups can be plotted together as shown in *Figure 10.1* where marathon runners, who tend to be introspective, are compared with more extrovert wrestlers.

It is important to stress that all such groups contain exceptions. Top marathon runners can be extrovert and wrestlers can be torn by introspection. Personality classifications are not, by themselves, indicators of any level of sports achievement but are valuable and comparative tools for study and clinical work.

It follows that no one classification is entirely satisfactory and several questionnaires and inventories are used in psychological practice. These include the widely used MMPI (Minnesota Multiphasic Personality Inventory) and the Cattell 16 PF'(Cattell 16 Personality Factor) tests which plot a wider range of different personality traits in more complex fashion.

On the basis of such classifications, certain opinions may be formed. There are differences between the event groups and between elite and non-elite performers. As an overall trend, however, the most successful sportsmen tend to be stable extroverts. There are, for example, demonstrable personality differences between elite sportsmen and 'club athletes' and between all sportsmen and the non-sporting population. The more neurotic a person, the greater the tendency to drop out of sport.

The intriguing questions arise as to how much of one's personality is determined by inheritance and how much can be changed by environment and conditioning? Can we create an elite athlete, or is he, or she, born with all the qualities required?

Many animal experiments, as well as human twin studies, have shown a basic and unchangeable genetic component in each individual's personality. Furthermore, this stable component has been linked

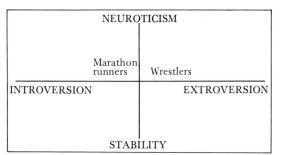

Figure 10.1
Personality assessment chart of introversion/extroversion and neuroticism/stability, with relative positions of marathon and wrestling groups

by some researchers to the basic neurophysiology of the brain and the nervous system. For instance, it is possible that neuroticism is related to the nervous system's excitability, which, in turn, is directly related to the basic chemistry of the brainstem. Extroversion may reflect the relative balance between excitation and inhibition mechanisms of the brain and nervous system. Arousability, a crucial factor in competition, may reflect individual variations in neurophysiological responsiveness to stimuli. The stable extrovert may perform consistently well but suffer chronic underarousal. This makes it difficult to find sufficient uplift for the big occasion. In contrast, the more introverted, or neurotic, performer with pronounced labile arousability may have difficulty in preparation for more minor events as well as optimal arousal for major challenges. Such competitors have a resultant tendency towards brilliant, if erratic, achievement.

Arousal affects the ability to control anxiety. Tests of learning, reaction, pain tolerance, perseverance, fine skill performances and response to stimuli all reflect differences between introvert and extrovert personalities. For instance, extroverts are more tolerant of pain, introverts more adept at finely skilled performance. The effect of personality type and arousal may affect overall capacity to persevere with the sustained and boring training loads necessary in many events. Regardless of the athlete's physical attributes, he must be able to overcome the psychological stresses of the chosen event.

Is personality influenced by sport? There is

evidence that adult sportsmen and sportswomen do not show changes in personality type but there may be some change in young adolescents strongly exposed to specific sports training. This may be in the development of greater extroversion and stability but also, less fortunately, greater dependency. Even so, these changes are in line with the development of the typical profile for sportsmen and do not represent the fundamental changes in personality type.

Learning, training and coaching

Learning experiments have provided models for the study of athletic behaviour. As the individual develops his own personality and range of day-to-day behaviour patterns and responses, influence may be applied in various ways. Pavlov's work on conditioned reflexes showed that an individual can be induced to behave in certain ways by repetitive applications of stimuli linked with rewards or punishments. In athletic terms this would be analogous to a long-jumper landing on thorns if a required distance was not reached – naturally, subtler techniques are more effective.

In human terms there is usually a choice of behaviour available to the individual. Successful choices can be rewarded, for instance, by knowledge and experience gained, comfort of action, freedom from pain or injury, greater distance jumped or more prizes won. Apart from any natural aptitude or inclination, the individual gradually learns by trial and error to do what is most effective.

Teachers and coaches have as their main function the guidance of this development and the presentation of the most appropriate choices of action and reward or punishment to the learner. This applies to sport as it does to other fields of learning. The variables in all cases include the ability and motivation of the learner and the knowledge and skill of the teacher or coach.

The learner's correct choice of action can be influenced by certain well-established techniques. The use of rewards and punishments so prevalent in infancy and school has its analogies in sport, for instance, in successful advancement for those who succeed in mastering skilled techniques or who win races. The coach usually manipulates the psychological punishment/reward system, which may comprise team selection, award of colours, prizes or status or simply personal approval from a stern mentor, to condition the pupil.

New techniques are imprinted into the athlete's behaviour pattern. The establishment of this pattern involves chemical changes in the brain and central nervous system. Repeated efforts to learn skills leave their mark until the new movements become almost automatic but the process needs time. If training proceeds relentlessly, however, the sportsman may get stuck, or stale. A change or rest becomes essential after which it is usually found that there is permanent improvement. The relevance of this mechanism to intermittent or interval training is obvious.

The most essential aspect of learning concerns competitive experience. Whatever the wisdom of the coach and the intensity of preparation it is the athlete alone who faces the actual competition. Only by exposure to competitive stress can responses be refined. At the same time, overexposure to stress leads to staleness and rest periods are essential if performance is to be well maintained throughout a long season.

Learning and coaching are influenced by many individual psychological factors and the different responses of introverts and extroverts have been mentioned. Pain tolerance is also important in sport. External or traumatic pain in contact sport is an obvious factor and the typical stable extrovert shows a higher pain tolerance than the sportsman in non-contact sport who, in turn, surpasses the non-athlete.

Little mention is made in the experimental literature of the intrinsic pain of solo events such as swimming, cycling or longer-distance running. This pain is not simply comparable to externally induced injury and should not be overlooked in general remarks about introspection. Where there is soft-tissue overuse injury present, the solo athlete is often able to overcome the discomfort but it is still unknown whether this pain tolerance, or induced analgesia, has a basis in local circulatory and neurological physiology, or in the brain and central nervous system reflexes or chemistry.

People interpret sensations differently, again with variation between different personality types. Some augment sensory input – 'make the most' of everything – others reduce it ('play it down'). Again, the mechanism is uncertain but contact sport extroverts tend to be sensory reducers for pain. Perception of other environmental factors in the same ways may explain some aspects of competitive variation in form – crowd awareness, sensitivity to climatic conditions and so on. Furthermore, cultural differences in response to pain are well documented and this may be a factor influencing attitudes and responses to different sports.

There is individual variation in self-awareness. Neurotic people have a heightened awareness of their own bodies and minds. One of the effects of prolonged intensive training is to enhance self-awareness and it has long been debatable whether athletes become neurotic or simply represent a group of natural neurotics who are physically talented.

One further aspect of self-awareness is crucial in the management of competitors – 'perceived exertion'. 'Perceived exertion' is the athlete's subjective impression of the workload. This can be expressed on a verbal scale ('nil to flat out') or numerically, as on the scale devised by Borg. 'Perceived exertion' correlates well with pulse rate, cardiac output, oxygen uptake, workrate and catecholamine production. It therefore forms a reliable, cheap and convenient way to self-monitor fitness and exertion.

Distortion of 'perceived exertion' can, however, be due to mood and personality variations, fatigue or exhaustion, drugs or hypnosis. As the demonstrable 'fitness' and the workload offered are unchanged, perceptual distortion gives interesting insights into the interrelated physical and psychological aspects of

sports performance. In practical terms, the athlete who reports undue effort is probably fatigued or stale and needs a rest or change in training.

Other individual differences in perception may be linked to game skills. Some people are naturally better at more narrowly defined skills in a closed environment, e.g. shooting in a gallery, others in more open situations where wider environmental factors must be taken into account. There are possible personality differences, correlating with arousability and anxiety, which lead to different processing of given stimuli. People may augment, reduce or selectively distort sensory input and it is thought that differences in perceptual sampling underlie skill variations in ball games.

Motivation, arousability and control of anxiety are central factors in sports performance. The traditional diagrammatic representation of the inverted 'U' applies, as shown in *Figure 10.2.*

It is essential that the player is aroused to just the right level for competition. Some have difficulty in getting 'up' for the big match, others need to be relaxed from overarousal.

Underarousal may be due to personality, typically extroversion, or a result of disinterest, e.g. minor competition, or the end product of staleness, fatigue or depression, when the athlete has lost all interest.

Overarousal is common in introverts. It may follow overstimulation with drugs (e.g. caffeine), pep-pills or even pep-talks, or it may be an early sign of staleness due to excessive training or competition before the athlete breaks down to apathy and depression.

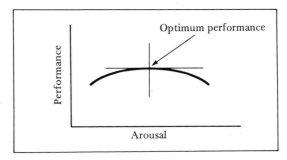

Figure 10.2
Interrelation of arousal, performance and optimum performance

Anxiety is reduced by exercise, as is most dramatically experienced in the sudden abolition of nervousness by the starting gun or whistle.

As tested anxiety levels have not been shown to differ greatly between winners and losers, it may be true that successful performers have superior control over their anxiety levels and more consistently arouse themselves to optimal levels of competition.

The coach's traditional pep-talk may be helpful, harmful or possibly largely irrelevant. It will follow from the previous pages that each subject has a particular personality and motivation and that failure to realize this causes antagonism between player and coach. Not all football managers realize that a simple cash or disciplinary stimulus can be unhelpful! If there is to be a pep-talk, it should take account of the individual player's needs, e.g. sub-group talks by different coaches, or be concerned with tactics in an emotionally neutral way. Most experienced players probably ignore invective – and proffered advice! It should be remembered that the coach giving his pep-talk is sometimes the most aroused person present and may, unconsciously, be resolving his own, rather than his team's, emotional problems. It should be remembered that 'for better or worse, the athlete should probably establish his own performance objectives'. No coach will motivate a gold medal into a sportsman who simply doesn't want one.

Motivation probably falls with age, maturity and achievement. An Olympic Champion can hardly be expected to get anxious about his club championship. While age is not a guarantee of emotional maturity, there is some truth in the dictum that 'the end point of competitive sport is to wean the player off the need for competition'. Some individuals will be helped by sport to acquire a personal maturity and viewpoint which is no longer aggressively self-assertive. Others will divert the lessons learned in sport into other competitions, such as work; a further group will continue to be competitive indefinitely and indiscriminately.

While this range may represent normal individual differences in interest and motivation, it is common, in some sportsmen, to find a degree of almost pathological motivation. In the young this may show as an insatiable pursuit of victory at any cost, in the old as a sad reluctance to accept realistically the gradual changes of ageing.

The social determinants of motivation underlie an individual's attitudes. A society tends to indicate its own answers to the questions 'Why compete?' or 'Why participate at all?'. Cultural factors exert an influence on the range of sports and recreations available and individual selection of any one may be more influenced by opportunity than biological aptitude alone. Some societies go to great lengths for all sports to select by aptitude as part of national policy while others adopt a *laissez faire* attitude.

Even the Olympic movement reflects society's sporting dilemma. While stressing as a central tenet the essential value of participation – taking part rather than winning – it has the simple motto '*Citius, Altius, Fortius*' (Further, Higher, Stronger), the quintessence of elitism and winning!

The sportsman finds himself living and playing in a society which has given sport its place in cultural life and largely pre-set the value systems. Values change, however, and the major shift in the twentieth century has been the mass democratization of sport, followed closely by its increasing politicization and professionalization. This in turn leads to a tendency to opt out of overzealous sport and into a new movement based on the alternative values of mere participation and the use of exercise, not as a vehicle for aggressive competitive emotion, but as a method of general and spiritual health improvement. Even in competitive sport, many players will not mind losing if they have performed well – they derive as much joy from a personal best as from their placing.

Motivation to win may be strong because of various personal or group pressures but it is not always recognized that many are driven to win by a fear of losing which has its origins deep in the individual's background and upbringing. Personal differences in motivation may underlie the interesting phenomenon of the record-breaker who cannot win a major, slower competition. Perhaps inappropriate motivation, rather than success-phobia, is the central problem.

The clinical psychologist studies the athlete by observation and interview. This may be backed up by questionnaires of the inventory type as mentioned earlier. The individual's personality is assessed and his problems identified. This analysis may be simple or extremely complex, involving long-term consultation and discussion with others close to the sportsman. Group questionnaires can also be devised to indicate the different psychological needs and attitudes within a team or community.

Common problems for the psychologist relate to failure of performance. Typically, a sportsman who is demonstrably fit and physically capable of a certain level of achievement habitually fails to compete successfully. This may be due to medical, physiological or psychological causes, or very commonly combinations of all three.

The psychologist must assure himself that his patient is free from illness or inappropriate training faults such as overtraining or wrong scheduling of sessions, regardless of whether there is a significant psychological problem. Only in this way, which clearly involves teamwork with coaches, team managers and doctors, can the athlete gain maximum benefit. The simple assumption by coaches that failure to thrive on a given training programme is due to psychological faults is wrong. Each player is different and needs slightly different training and management once the basic group essentials have been achieved.

Conflict is common in younger players between the demands of home and school, school and play, exams and competition. Psychosomatic symptoms and performance failure are common, and should be readily explicable if all aspects of the athlete's life are considered. In the older player there may be conflict of motivation – self against family or self against other interests.

Some athletes fear success. They train hard, they perform well but never quite win the greatest prizes.

While it is rather harsh in the intensity of today's extremely competitive arenas to brand losers as success-phobic – and the commonest reason for losing will always be that the winner is better – athletes who habitually fail to do themselves justice may benefit from the help of a psychiatrist or clinical psychologist.

In this context, it is far more useful to adopt the concept of over- or underachievement than to deal in absolute times, distances or ranking lists. Some players or teams habitually underachieve, others rise above themselves; the same teams can change completely from day to day, or from manager to manager. A close victory by a given team may be a major triumph, a bitter disappointment or a serious warning of team failure of performance. Many judgements in this field are highly subjective, but the complexities of human performance reflected in sport need considerable understanding and skilled management by qualified experts working together to help the individual or team.

Injury-prone sportsmen are well known to every coach and doctor. Proneness relates to personality type and risk-taking and detailed analysis of personal motivation is needed to change the individual's habitual behaviour. In females, injury-proneness may correlate with the changes of the menstrual cycle.

Some sportsmen resist coaching either individually or as team members. The main effect is that individuals, often skilled and senior, may disrupt team morale by adverse influence on younger colleagues. Others seem attracted to cheating, by drugs or devices wherever available, and construct elaborate webs of excuses and pseudo-moral justification around themselves. It is unlikely that there would be any drug or doping problems in sport if athletes were not psychologically pushed into feeling the need to boost performance unfairly. Again, the psychologist will identify the personal conflicts leading to stress and social difficulty.

Therapeutic approaches

Behavioural methods are widely employed to help athletes modify harmful or inappropriate behaviour. The essence of this approach is to modify behaviour consciously in discussion with the athlete, by actions put into practice rather than with words alone or even drugs. Some useful approaches are outlined below.

Control of anxiety and arousal, the key to competitive success, can be helped in several ways. Biofeedback techniques measure individual physiological aspects of stress, e.g. pulse, muscle tension, tremor or sweating. By giving the patient a visual or sound display, these techniques allow him to practice muscular or mental relaxation, thus gradually lowering his anxiety level.

There are various systems of relaxation including certain massage techniques, progressive muscular relaxation exercises, meditation, yoga and autogenic training, all of which are used to help control anxiety. Techniques vary with individual preference, availability and capability.

Autogenic training is widely used in Eastern Europe. It combines rehearsed relaxation techniques with suggestion and self-motivation which can bring the athlete to peak performance well equipped within his own mental resources.

Some athletes need help in gaining self-confidence or in working out aggressive tensions not necessarily related to their sport. Verbal and physical techniques are available in each case, allowing the athlete to leave his problems at the stadium gate if he cannot fully resolve them.

Mental rehearsal involves the psychologist's talking the sportsman through his previous or future crises. It may be used to unravel the origins of performance failure when suppressed fears or doubts can be demonstrated and expressed. The technique is useful in preparing the athlete for a vital event by helping him to 'rehearse' the expected stress and all its variations in advance so as to be better placed for the event itself.

Hypnosis is dependent upon the subject's being receptive. Skilled help may improve relaxation, aid arousal or help to resolve inner conflicts of personality or motivation. While some physiological functions can be influenced, e.g. pain response, the power of hypnosis significantly to enhance personal or team performance is uncertain.

Sportsmen often need psychological help when injured. Some revel in the 'macho' martyrdom of the injured state but many see the collapse around them of their dreams and perhaps several years of dedicated preparation. Coach and psychologist should think of psychological first aid to the failing sportsman as keenly as they do of ministering to physical injury.

'The game beyond'

Much interest has developed in the use of sport as a method of attaining psychological benefit, spiritual growth and philosophical development. Concepts of awareness, self-discovery and self-expression, have led to further concepts such as 'the inner game' and 'peak experience'. The concept of relaxed concentration seeks to disinhibit the subject from restraining tensions so that he is then totally relaxed and concentrated 'into' rather than 'on' personal performance. The worldwide 'Runners Movement' has developed partly through this concept.

'Peak experience' is a trance-like state which may, paradoxically, occur at both ends of the running spectrum, as well as in any other exercise or game. The jogger pursuing his daily rhythmic exercise may learn to relax so completely that he gains a trance-like 'high' from his movement. On the other side, the champion athlete experiences a day when 'it all comes right' for him. Somewhere beyond his known capability he finds an automated trance-like state which takes him to his personal victory beyond pain and ordinary feeling, yet with enhanced awareness.

Many pundits have sought to explain these states in relation to drug-induced experience, others to religious, spiritual or meditational states. Some authorities have defined 'the runner's high' in terms of an addiction in some susceptible individuals to the relaxant hormones produced by the brain – the endorphins – with appropriate withdrawal symptoms affecting runners as they do drug addicts.

While such concepts may not be immediately relevant to a particular competition, they are beginning to form a major part of individual motivation and interest and may play an important role in the popularization of mass-participation exercise programmes in the future.

Psychiatric aspects

Psychological disturbance may alter sports performance, and sport and exercise may have significant mental effects on individuals.

Psychological good health is not necessarily a prerequisite for good sports performance and a sportsman may come to his game suffering from mental disturbance or frank illness. This may create difficulties for colleagues playing with him or for his team manager. Unduly aggressive or sensitive attitudes may disrupt team morale. In individual events, unpredictable results and manipulative and demanding behaviour may invoke hostility and it is not rare for a talented player to be dropped from a team because of his ability to undermine everyone else's confidence.

More commonly, personality traits rather than illness present problems in sport. Reference has been made to motivational problems and excessive competitiveness. The differences in psychological demands of sports events give scope for a wide range of personalities and attitudes and some normally unacceptable traits like aggression or risk-taking can in some competitive situations be an advantage.

Anxiety states are common. If a sportsman's basic mood is too anxious, then his arousal mechanisms are distorted. He also tends to become fatigued because the constant nervous activity throughout his body pre-empts too much of his energy and leaves him depleted at competition. Anxiety may be treated both by behavioural methods (*see* above) and careful use of sedatives and tranquillizing drugs.

Depression is extremely common and may fluctuate with moods of elation or be combined with anxiety. It is a common cause of loss of form and is effectively the same as 'staleness'. Tell-tale symptoms may include insomnia, early wakening, loss of appetite, moods of despair and marked diurnal mood swing, together with somatic symptoms and fatigue with apathy.

Depression may follow overexertion, typically a long and stressful season or run of matches without enough relaxation and with spells of prolonged overarousal. Nervous exhaustion may be caused and it becomes difficult to overcome apathy and start training.

This same state is extremely common after organic illness, notably viral illnesses such as influenza, hepatitis or jaundice and glandular fever. This should be widely accepted as a natural aftermath of such illnesses and adequate time permitted for a gradual resumption of training and return to competition. Attempts to 'run off' such symptoms are almost always unsuccessful and often cause prolonged depression. The body's immune system may show evidence of such disorders.

Time naturally heals most minor depressions; however, any prolonged, severe or chronic depressive states need urgent expert medical treatment, usually starting with antidepressant medication. The importance for the athlete of rest and relaxation must always be acknowledged. Experiments have shown that a planned moderate exercise programme can dissipate anxiety and also improve depression, in some instances at least as well as the usual drug therapy. This may be because many endogenous depressives have abnormally low adrenal hormone (cortisol) levels during their illness. Treatment restores normal levels. Exercise, by boosting cortisol levels naturally, may achieve similar results in this group.

Drug therapy may affect performance. For instance, sedatives may impair mood and movement accuracy and stimulants may cause overarousal. Drugs themselves may interact with each other or with food or alcohol. There may be times when active drug treatment may make it unwise to pursue certain sports where key criteria of performance are likely to be affected, such as for instance, visual acuity, sweating responses, muscular tone, tremor, wakefulness and concentration or reaction times. It is important that the sportsman asks his physician or psychiatrist for specific guidance on these matters when drugs are prescribed and also that due attention is paid by the prescriber to the prevailing doping regulations in sports.

11 General medicine

Infective illnesses

In certain illnesses physical exercise is dangerous because pathological processes may be worsened causing complications or even death.

In infectious diseases, particularly if there is fever, exercise should be prohibited, or at least very severely reduced because viral infections cause inflammation of the internal organs including the lymphatic system and heart; myocarditis is one of the causes of sudden death during exercise.

Bacterial infections, such as tonsillitis or otitis, may permit limited exercise provided that the infections are well controlled with antibiotics and any fever which may have occurred has subsided. While limited performance may be possible in events requiring more skill than cardiorespiratory effort, however, toxic impairment lasts until full recovery. An early return to sport seldom produces a satisfying result, either for the individual or the team. Many have learnt the hard way that premature return to strenuous exercise simply prolongs full recovery.

In many viral illnesses, particularly glandular fever or influenza, exercise prolongs convalescence and possibly increases the risk of depression. Also, strenuous exertion during the incubation phase of certain illnesses increases the severity and complications. This is particularly so with infective hepatitis (jaundice), poliomyelitis, where activity may actually induce and exacerbate the degree of paralysis, and possibly during glandular fever,

though this is often hard to define owing to the insidious onset of that condition.

With glandular fever, exercise during the active phase may, apart from the hazards of myocarditis, lead to sudden death from rupture of the spleen. The low-grade hepatitis present in glandular fever interferes for a considerable period with general health, athletic performance and alcohol tolerance. Alcohol should be avoided for at least 6 months.

The duration of convalescence varies with each illness and individual, but the highly trained athlete tends to show a remarkably quick return to form once he has achieved full recovery. It is a disservice to let him short-cut convalescence from illness. Medical advice should be sought in case of doubt and a safe rule is to allow a gradual, rather than abrupt, return to training.

Inoculations – at home

In early life, most Western children are given full protection against diphtheria, pertussis (whooping cough), tetanus ('lock jaw') and poliomyelitis, with booster doses through childhood and schooldays. Naturally occurring smallpox has been declared eradicated by the World Health Organisation and vaccination should now be unnecessary, except for certain laboratory personnel.

Many schoolchildren are given BCG inoculation against tuberculosis after Mantoux testing and it is routine practice in most hospitals to give tetanus toxoid to all open wounds as a further preventive measure, even after primary inoculation. Athletes, in particular, are exposed to tetanus spores in the ground and inoculation is essential. The full duration of protection is uncertain but booster doses are recommended at 5-yearly intervals.

Because of the risks of assembling and travelling in large numbers, athletes should ensure that all their inoculations are complete, that regular boosters are arranged according to the prescribed schedules and that the all-important tetanus protection is fully maintained as this is not only an extremely severe and distressing illness but a preventable form of death.

Inoculation abroad

Foreign travel may require protection against more exotic conditions. For travellers to Southern Europe, Asia, Africa and Southern and Central America, typhoid and cholera inoculations give some protection. They may cause unpleasant general aching with mild fever but this may be minimized without loss of protection if smaller doses are given into the skin instead of into deeper tissue.

Yellow fever inoculation is required for a limited zone of tropical African and American countries only. This must be given in advance of travel and will not therefore interfere with competition.

Malaria

Because malaria is such a resilient disease, great emphasis must be placed on preventive measures. There were signs that malaria had been brought under control by concerted worldwide action, but in recent years it has started to spread again and many strains have become resistant to one or more antimalarial drugs. Without leaving the plane malaria can be caught through one infected mosquito bite while the traveller sits in a tropical airport in transit. Anyone travelling in a malarial zone is advised to check on current requirements for the particular country he is to visit because prevalent mosquito strains and associated drug resistance vary

from area to area. Antimalarials must be taken before arrival, throughout the stay and for a prescribed time after leaving endemic areas. The parasite lodges in the body and drugs only work during some stages in its life cycle, possibly after the victim has left the original country of infection.

Infective hepatitis

Gamma-globulin by injection may be advisable for travellers to countries where there is a particular risk of infective hepatitis. Enquiry should be made of travel agencies, embassies or airline medical services for up-to-date recommendations.

Alimentary system
Aphthous ulcers (mouth ulcers)

Aphthous ulcers occur sporadically in the mouths and throats of vulnerable subjects. The cause is probably viral and there is as yet no cure for these spots which break down to form painful, white-topped ulcers which usually last for 7–10 days before clearing spontaneously. They are sometimes associated with general ill health, gastrointestinal upsets or stress.

Indigestion

Indigestion is commonly related to exercise. Sharp upper abdominal pains may be due to dyspepsia, with irritation of the lower oesophagus by gastric acid due to hard straining, e.g. vigorous exercise too soon after a meal. Peptic ulcers occasionally occur in athletes. Some notable champions have suffered them and there may be a relationship between the extreme stresses of top-class competition and peptic ulceration through oversecretion of the stress-related corticosteroids which themselves cause ulcers. Occasionally heartburn, or acid regurgitation, may be due to a hiatus hernia where the diaphragm does not fully separate the lower oesophagus and thorax from the abdominal cavity. Raising intra-abdominal pressure, e.g. by straining, or lying flat or head downwards, makes some of the stomach slide up into the thorax. This causes reflux of gastric acid with the characteristic burning pain.

In all these conditions, milk or antacid preparations relieve symptoms and, in hiatus hernia, positional adjustment is important – the subject should sleep with the head of the bed slightly raised and should take care to avoid bending forwards or straining, e.g. as in weight-lifting which raises pressure in the abdominal cavity.

Flatulence is usually due to anxiety or inappropriate diet. In precompetition nervousness, overaction of the sympathetic nervous system causes temporary functional disorder of the gut with an assortment of symptoms including flatulence, nausea, indigestion or diarrhoea. Most athletes need at least 1 hour between meals and exercise; the greater stress of competition requires much longer, between 2 and 4 or more hours because of prolonged digestion time. The timing of meals is important and individuals should experiment to find what suits them best. Fizzy drinks, fatty or rich protein foods should be avoided as their slower digestion keeps the stomach full of undigested residues during exercise.

Peptic ulcer

Peptic ulceration may be related to stress or may be coincidental in people who happen to be athletically active. Ulcers in the stomach or duodenum cause indigestion and occasionally bleeding. This causes vomiting of blood (haematemesis) or the passage of black altered blood in the stools (melaena). These symptoms call for full medical investigation of the disease and the anaemia which often results. The stress of intensive training and competition should be avoided in peptic ulceration but modest exercise as a relaxing activity can be encouraged.

Occasionally necessary are the operations of partial gastrectomy (removal of about one third of the stomach) or vagotomy, which cuts the vagus nerve supply to the stomach and thus reduces the production of acid. These operations are usually successful but the post-gastrectomy syndrome is a complication and may cause anaemia, diarrhoea, bloatedness, or premature fullness after small meals. Another possible effect is dumping, in which food is rushed through the stomach remnant generating a rebound secretion of insulin 1 or 2 hours later which causes hypoglycaemia, or sudden lowering of the blood sugar. This condition may severely limit athletic exercise. Many patients whose dyspepsia leads them to gastrectomy and its complications tend to be tense, introspective and competitive – all traits which militate against a relaxed approach to athletic competition. It may be difficult for such people to acquire a more philosophical approach and the solution might be a change of sport, perhaps even to outdoor recreation alone.

Appendicitis

Appendicitis is usually an acute and obvious condition with low right-sided abdominal pain leading to fever, vomiting and dehydration. Occasionally, less dramatic pain in the right lower quarter of the abdomen may, often without much good evidence, be labelled as subacute or chronic appendicitis. The differential diagnosis may lie between inflammation of the appendix or of the ovary, or other less common abdominal conditions. Such pain can also be confused with adductor muscle strain, particularly at the pubic origin, which is referred upwards from the groin (*see* page 185).

Diverticulitis

Diverticulitis is a common age-related condition in which naturally occurring diverticula, or pouches, develop in the muscular wall of the lower colon. Stagnation of bowel contents and constipation lead to infection, or diverticulitis. Prevention and treatment includes adequate dietary intake of roughage, or fibre-containing foods, such as bran and vegetable matter. The mere presence of diverticula does not limit exercise although it should be remembered that the sweat losses of heavy exercise often lead to dehydration which, in turn, exacerbates any tendency towards constipation. Dehydration can be avoided by adequate fluid replacement.

Constipation

Constipation is the frequent accompaniment of dehydration due to profuse sweating during exercise in warm conditions. It may occur in sportsmen such as long-distance runners whose habitual activity may easily lead to a degree of chronic underhydration. General undereating, for instance in weight-conscious young women, may also cause constipation. It is doubtful whether constipation in itself causes much in the ways of symptoms but consciousness of constipation may be distressing. Sportsmen travelling abroad to competition in unaccustomed heat often become constipated due to simple dehydration. They should be advised to drink more, and be thankful that they have not been smitten with traveller's diarrhoea! Under such circumstances, saline purgatives, such as magnesium sulphate or Epsom salts, should not be taken because of their further potential dehydrating effect.

Diarrhoea

Diarrhoea may be caused by infective or chemical factors or by anxiety. The latter rouses the sympathetic nervous responses and prematch diarrhoea is well known. As a rough guide, nervous diarrhoea is clearly related to the stress of impending competition or, at a time of stress, may cause loose stools first thing in the morning. Diarrhoea occurring repeatedly through the day, or at night, is usually due to infective or other organic causes.

Infective diarrhoea is one of the commonest illnesses throughout the world. Severe diarrhoea, particularly with blood or mucus in the stools or with fever, can be rapidly disabling with toxaemia, dehydration and loss of electrolytes into the gut which

lead to weakness. Therefore, training and competition should be avoided even though the symptom of diarrhoea may be controllable.

Traveller's diarrhoea Traveller's diarrhoea commonly affects groups of athletes travelling abroad for competition. It is, by definition, a short, sharp, self-limiting condition due to infection by types of the common bacterium *Escherichia coli* which differ from those that occur naturally in the athlete's home environment and to which he is unaccustomed. Attacks usually consist of acute diarrhoea, without much abdominal pain and without fever; they last from literally one loose stool to a couple of days. Provided that no other symptoms are present, the diarrhoea is easily controlled by avoidance of solid food for 24 hours; bowel sedatives, such as codeine phosphate, kaolin, loperamide or Lomotil, and adequate fluid replacement must be maintained.

As traveller's diarrhoea may seriously impair athletic performance, simply by the coincidence of timing, the greatest possible care should be taken to avoid the illness. The crucial factor is avoidance of unsterilized water, milk or drinks, salads and fruits which may be infected from water, or food such as ice cream, cream or cold meat which may not have been cleanly prepared. In most major competitions, e.g. Olympic or Regional Games, such great attention is paid to catering arrangements that traveller's diarrhoea should not occur as a result of eating and drinking within the official venue. On lesser travels, however, athletes may be tempted by food or drink freely available outside a closely disciplined environment and slices of melon, ice creams or meat and salads are frequent causes of infection.

The role of prophylactic medication is controversial and iodochlorhydroxyquinoline (Enterovioform) has been abandoned because of neurological side effects. The sulphonamide drugs have been widely used and advertised as preventive measures either alone or in combination with streptomycin (e.g. Streptotriad) but there is no convincing evidence of their superiority over dietary discipline. Moreover, both streptomycin and the sulphonamides are potent causes of allergy. Because any conscientious athlete will observe dietary precautions for the avoidance of more severe gut infections, the use of prophylactic drugs is best avoided.

Acute diarrhoea should be treated with rest, simple drugs and fluids. At present, codeine phosphate is permitted under some doping regulations but there have been problems with this compound in the past because its metabolites appear in the urine as those of the forbidden opiates. As the regulations are under frequent review, the rules covering a particular competition should always be checked by the team managers well before departure so that there is absolutely no doubt about what is, and is not, allowed.

Specific diarrhoeas The traveller may acquire a more severe form of infective diarrhoea such as dysentery, amoebiasis or cholera. Symptoms are prolonged and may include fever, toxaemia, vomiting, dehydration and bloody diarrhoea. Specific diagnosis and treatment are urgently needed.

A frequent infection in both tropical and temperate climates is giardiasis; the parasite *Giardia lamblia* is found in food and water. Episodic diarrhoea and dyspepsia with abdominal ache may persist indefinitely, although diagnosis may be difficult because the parasite may be excreted only intermittently in the victim's stools. Specific treatment with metronidazole (Flagyl) is required.

Dietary diarrhoea Dietary fads may cause diarrhoea. All sugars can cause diarrhoea if taken in large quantities. For long-distance runners, fructose was popular as a form of sugar-based energy which was thought not to lead to the rapid insulin secretion and hypoglycaemia associated with glucose. A high concentration does cause osmotic secretion of water into the bowel, however, leading to diarrhoea.

Ulcerative colitis

Ulcerative colitis is a disease which affects the colon and rectum. Abdominal pain, fever and diarrhoea with blood and mucus cause varying degrees of anaemia and toxaemia. In the more toxic phases of the disease, exercise is impossible because of general disability but in milder stages, limited exercise is safe. Between exacerbations, no restrictions are necessary and international performances of outstanding merit have been recorded. In some patients stress may precipitate attacks and, for them, the strain of competition may have to be avoided.

Respiratory system

Funnel chest (pectus excavatum), with its depressed sternum, may force the heart further over into the left chest. Some restriction of expansion and vital capacity will limit potential performance but exercise can be encouraged.

Pigeon chest (pectus carinatum) is associated with longstanding early life obstructive airways disease, particularly chronic bronchitis or asthma. Functional limitation and exercise tolerance depend on the disease and not necessarily on chest shape.

Kyphoscoliosis, a variable degree of hunchback deformity involving a lateral curvature of the thoracic spine, for example, may be of slight degree and cause no limitation of function, but in more severe degree it can cause impairment of lung function, including underventilation and ventilation–perfusion imbalance.

Ankylosing spondylitis is a rheumatic disease, usually affecting younger men, in which there may be rigid fixation of the ribcage with gross impairment of the chest expansion and hence of pulmonary function. Exercise is definitely not contraindicated (*see* page 106) but the degree of achievement possible will be limited.

Inflammatory chest disease, e.g. acute or chronic bronchitis, bronchiectasis or airways disease, e.g.

asthma or pulmonary fibrosis, or silicosis cause functional impairment of the lungs and the exercise permitted will depend on medical assessment of the degree of illness and lung impairment.

Exercise-induced asthma is common and is discussed on pages 30–31.

Exercise improves lung function and patients with many chest diseases will benefit from some exercise. Attention is drawn to doping regulations which affect many drugs commonly used in chest conditions (*see* Chapters 12 and 13).

The nervous system

The central nervous system is divided into motor, sensory and autonomic systems. The motor system initiates and controls voluntary movement and is also the final stimulating pathway for reflex, or uncontrolled, movements. Voluntary movement is initiated in the motor cortex of the brain and impulses pass via the spinal cord and segmental nerve roots from the cord to the peripheral nerves which reach the muscles and other tissues.

The sensory system returns sensation via closely parallel pathways to the sensory cortex of the brain. In addition to heat and touch, a sense of position and movement is conveyed from the peripheral parts of the locomotor system to the brain through the proprioceptive nerve endings in the moving parts. These impulses are the basis of the body's automatic three-dimensional spatial awareness of itself and are crucial to the games player.

Reflex movements short-circuit the full route of information to and from the brain. Drastic stimuli such as pain and heat pass from the limb to the spinal cord and stimulate the spinal reflex arc which causes protective withdrawal from harmful stimuli. A similar reflex acts in the tendon jerks which are elicited as part of the clinical examination. Here the tendon, such as the patellar or Achilles, is tapped and abruptly stretched. The spinal reflex makes the appropriate muscle contract quickly in response to

this overstretch and hence the movements of kick or foot pronation, respectively, are elicited.

The central nervous system is incompletely developed at birth and early-life movements are crude, uncontrolled and reflex. During early life, the movements are gradually controlled by the development of inhibiting reflexes from higher centres in the brain, particularly the cerebellum. Fine control is gradually achieved of both static posture and movement.

As with all other biological functions, there are considerable differences in individual ability to achieve and control fine movement or posture. This will lead to differences in ability between individuals in many sports. For instance, the pistol-shooter clearly needs to maintain an extremely accurate, as well as steady, posture and co-ordinate this with his visual sense. The tennis-player will need all the attributes of locomotor and cardiovascular fitness relevant to his sport but, in addition, he must have a high degree of spatial awareness and co-ordination in order to reach the 'unreachable' shots. Some of this ability is trainable but it is clear that inherited giftedness must be one of the final limiting factors in sports achievement.

Handedness (left or right) is an inherited characteristic, although it may be influenced by early-life conditioning. Higher skills are achieved with the dominant hand which is controlled by the opposite side of the brain. While damage to the appropriate side of the brain, or limb, usually leads to gross impairment of function, some individuals have a considerable capacity for complete rehabilitation. This is shown, for instance, by the example of Takac who won gold medals in Olympic pistol-shooting, one in 1936 with his right hand, the others in 1948 and 1952 with his left hand, following right-hand amputation in 1938.

The autonomic nervous system is the pathway for the brain's control of automatic visceral function and, in contrast to the motor system, is mostly involuntary. It is controlled by the hypothalamus in the brain and works through two mutually antagonistic subsystems, the sympathetic and the parasympathetic nervous systems. The sympathetic nerves emerge from the thoracolumbar segments of the spinal cord and follow either blood vessels or peripheral nerves to reach the viscera as well as blood vesels, muscle and skin. Sympathetic stimulation is through the release of adrenaline at the nerve endings and the general reaction is to prepare the body for exercise by accelerating the heart rate, dilating the respiratory airways and diverting blood from the viscera to the muscles.

The parasympathetic nervous system, in contrast, emerges by the nerves of the cranial and sacral levels. The tenth cranial nerve, the vagus, supplies the viscera. The parasympathetic stimulus is transmitted at the nerve endings by the release of acetylcholine. Blood is diverted from the muscles to the viscera, so that bodily activities appropriate to rest are able to proceed, including digestion and bladder, bowel and sexual functions, all of which are inhibited by sympathetic activity.

Sympathetic stimulation and emotional stress inhibit one of the bladder's normal reflexes and, instead of accommodating itself to its contents, it becomes unduly sensitive and triggers the urge to keep passing urine, felt as 'prematch' nerves. Once competition begins, full sympathetic inhibition of the bladder takes over and may continue for a considerable time after competition – witness the extreme difficulty often obtained in getting from athletes the necessary urine specimen for dope control.

Headache

Headache is common after severe or unaccustomed effort, particularly in untrained subjects. Occasionally, severe throbbing headache may follow hypoglycaemia in both diabetics and non-diabetics, even after its correction with sugar. The mechanisms of headache include vasodilation and the sharp increase in blood pressure associated with exercise. Headache at rest is commonly due to referred pain from neck structures such as cervical spondylosis and muscle spasm or injury in the trapezius muscle. This condition is often eased by exercise including simple jogging which does not require great trapezial activity. It should also be noted that headache is often due to tension or depression, or local infection such as sinusitis.

Migraine

Strictly speaking, migraine consists of a preliminary aura of visual symptoms such as distortion, blurring or partial blindness, or speech slurring and sensory disturbances, including tingling in part of the hand or side of the face, followed by the gradual development of severe unilateral headache. The migraine syndrome includes many variations and partial manifestations of these symptoms including 'sick headaches' and abdominal pain in young children.

A full understanding of migraine has yet to be found but certain precipitants are well established. These include anxiety, tension and depression, certain foods including those rich in amines such as cheese and chocolate, certain wines (particularly red) and external stimuli and such as flashing lights. Fatigue is an important factor in some sufferers and family history plays an important part. Some 10 per cent of the population suffer from migraine or its variants.

The tension associated with sporting events may precipitate some attacks but other sufferers thrive on tension and get their attacks in the relaxed aftermath of stress, classically during the quiet weekend after a hectic week.

During an attack, some subjects are capable of continuing to participate, although this may be impossible in certain sports if there is visual impairment; other subjects are forced to withdraw because of general distress. Once the headache is established, some subjects may continue with impunity, while others find that the combination of vasodilation, causing vascular headache, together with the rise in blood pressure and further vasodilation due to exercise produce an intolerable effect.

Treatment along classic lines is difficult to apply in the sporting context without withdrawal. Tablets, suppositories or injections are not usually readily to hand on the field of action! Prophylactic therapy with regular medication reduces the frequency of attacks. General sedation helps some people considerably but in respect of doping regulations care should be taken with the choice of sedative or tranquillizer. Drugs like clonidine (Dixarit) act on the walls of the arteries, damping down their degree of response to the chemical stimuli which finally trigger the migraine attack. There are no appreciable side effects in the small dosage used for this purpose and there is no conflict with performance or doping regulations. Other drugs, e.g. pizotifen (Sanomigran), antagonize the bioamines which trigger the attack and are also free from dope control problems.

In susceptible subjects, migraine can be precipitated by exercise and this tendency is exacerbated by the lower oxygen content of air at high altitude. Severe exercise may be followed by some of the premonitory signs of migraine, e.g. fortification spectra, without necessarily the full attack. Blows on the head, including heading the ball at soccer, can cause attacks and a player may have to give up such sport if attacks continue.

Migraine is a highly variable condition but there is no general contraindication to exercise and some international sportsmen suffer regularly from this complaint.

Poliomyelitis

In Western countries it is usual to protect the population with oral polio vaccine but in the developing countries polio is still common. It is well established that exercise during the incubation period exacerbates or causes the paralysis and localizes it particularly to the exercised muscles. As this may include the diaphragm and cause irreversible respiratory paralysis, polio should be seen as a preventable disease and nobody should be without full immunity.

Encephalitis

Many viruses can cause encephalitis of varying degree, from minimal to fatal: the Coxsackie, herpes simplex and mumps viruses are well-established examples. The depression commonly following viral illnesses, often trivial, may be partly explained by mild encephalitis and it is possible for well-trained athletes to suffer 'staleness' associated with the post-encephalitis syndrome for at least 1 or 2 years. Diligent investigation of athletes who present with prolonged loss of form will often pinpoint its origins in a viral illness.

Epilepsy

Epilepsy consists of transient electrical disturbances of brain function leading to major or minor disturbances in consciousness and body function, typically with the occurrence of convulsions followed by unconsciousness (grand mal). Lesser forms of epilepsy include petit mal; this may amount to no more than a transient lapse in conscious awareness which may not be apparent to observers, though it is clearly important to the subject should it occur at a time when sustained concentration is needed at work or play.

Temporal lobe epilepsy may involve sensory hallucinations such as visions, smells, tastes or sounds, in addition to convulsions. The causes of epilepsy are not all clear but some cases follow childhood fevers or infection at any age of the nervous system. A notable sporting cause is closed head injury and this is a real possiblity in contact sports.

Most epileptics are well controlled by medication but there are some drawbacks due to side effects of the drugs used. The widespread use of phenobarbitone as an anticonvulsant should always be declared at competitions which involve doping control. So much have attitudes to epilepsy changed over the years that it is usually possible for the controlled epileptic to be allowed a driving licence after a symptom-free period, usually 3 years. Epileptics are capable of very high level athletic achievement, including international athletic selection. In some patients, fits are triggered by illness, hypoglycaemia, excessive fatigue, stress or alcohol. Some epilepsies are precipitated by visual stimuli such as the flickering of television screens, disco lights or driving through the alternating light and shade of a sunlit avenue of trees. Patients will usually learn to cope with all these possibilities and there is no reason, subject to certain provisos, to exclude them from sport.

The main danger of epilepsy is that the victim may suffer not from the mere fact of his fit, but from the consequences of collapsing in a dangerous environment. Epileptics should not risk falling from ladders, high diving boards or mountains. They are not allowed to be exposed to motorsport or flying.

Swimming and epilepsy The risk of drowning need not prevent the epileptic's swimming. The British Epilepsy Association, together with the Co-ordinating Committee on Swimming for the Disabled, recommend that the epileptic seeks his doctor's permission to swim and a reasonable degree of control should be expected. Because uncontrolled fits in water may lead to drowning, it is essential that the epileptic should only be allowed to swim if accompanied by a responsible companion who must be a strong swimmer and capable of life-saving. The environment should be safely manageable for both parties. It is usually safe for the controlled epileptic to swim in an indoor swimming pool. The companion must be totally committed to the continuous observation of the swimmer. It may be more practical to observe continuously from the side of the pool and this may permit the observer to reach the victim more rapidly than if he is actually in the pool but too far from the victim to gain a clear view of circumstances.

Petit mal may cause a swimmer suddenly to sink. Grand mal makes the swimmer become unco-ordinated and jerky head movements may occur. The urgent aim is then to reach the swimmer and keep his head above water. Because of the violent uncontrolled movements of the convulsion, control from behind is easiest and once the convulsion is over, the swimmer should be removed from the pool to complete his recovery. Resuscitation is necessary if breathing has stopped. Other points of importance are that a third person be generally present in case an emergency arises, and it is safest for the epileptic to wear a brightly coloured swimming cap to facilitate observation.

Practical problems make it difficult to achieve one-to-one observation of swimmers in groups and normal school swimming sessions cannot provide enough safe observation unless additional staff or volunteers such as parents take over part of this function. It must be stressed that different criteria apply in outdoor swimming. Epilepsy is more likely in cold-water swimming and the practical difficulties of safe observation, life-saving and possible resuscitation in rivers and the sea are so obvious that these environments should normally be prohibited to the epileptic swimmer.

Boxing and brain damage

Repeated blows to the head cause small haemorrhages, leading to chronic brain damage (traumatic encephalopathy). The 'punch-drunk' syndrome consists of gradual personality deterioration with misplaced euphoria, aggression and forgetfulness, with signs including unsteadiness, slurred speech and tremor, progressing to dementia. Stricter regulation of boxing, with shorter bouts, such as the recent reduction of championship bouts from 15 to 12 rounds, should reduce the incidence of punch-drunkenness but the fact remains that the cumulative damage to brain cells from blows to the head is an integral part of boxing and long-term brain damage is inevitable. Brain scan and EEG (electroencephalogram) tests are helpful in assessing the degree of brain damage.

In addition, acute brain injury and death may

occur due to concussion, skull fracture or haemorrhage. Padded floors and corner posts are essential protective measures. Any boxer who is knocked out should be medically observed for 24 hours in case of delayed cerebral haemorrhages and most authorities advocate at least one month's rest from boxing following unconsciousness.

Urogenital system

Kidneys

The kidneys lie on each side of the middle of the body and, at rest, filter about a quarter of the cardiac output. Most of the plasma is filtered by glomeruli but nearly all of it is then reabsorbed in the renal tubules.

The body's water content is finely regulated by a balance of hormones. Pituitary-secreted vasopressin is responsible for reabsorption of most of the filtered water, leaving the excess – or the bare minimum required for the dilution of waste products – to descend the ureters for excretion via the bladder. The blood minerals are similarly filtered but reabsorbed under the influence of the mineralocorticoid hormones.

Glucose is normally completely reabsorbed, none appearing in the urine. In diabetes, glucose is not properly reabsorbed and its excretion takes an appropriate volume of water for its osmotic dilution and leads to excessive production of urine (polyuria) which causes thirst and dehydration.

Kidney function is sensitive, through neurohumoral mechanisms, to blood volume, blood pressure, the pulse pressure of the blood flow and the concentration of the blood. It also regulates the acid–base balance (pH) of the blood and is responsible for the elimination of the waste products of metabolism, including urea, uric acid, creatinine and the mineral phosphates and sulphates.

Renal function may be investigated by plain X-rays or following the injection of dyes which are selectively concentrated in the kidney. Blood tests reflect renal function in the concentration of waste products, notably urea. Urine tests for protein and glucose are part of the routine examination.

Response to exercise Exercise causes a drastic reduction in renal blood flow leading to a temporary reduction in urinary volume. Occasionally, prolonged severe exercise may precipitate acute renal failure, particularly in a hot climate and in dehydrated subjects. Renal shutdown is an extreme medical emergency and needs specialist control of fluid and dietary input until renal function recovers. This possibility is ever-present in extreme heat as with long-distance running in hot climates.

In view of the increasing popularity of distance events, race organizers should not only make fully adequate provision for drinking stations and medical attention, but should also draw the attention of participants to the dangers of dehydration and possible renal failure. At present, the spacing of water stations is restricted in some long-distance races but it is strongly advocated on medical grounds that all such restrictions be removed so as to encourage fully adequate fluid intake throughout the events.

Dehydration Dehydration is a further hazard of hard training for some sportsmen. An athlete training for 4–8 hours/day, or running up to 200 km (120 miles) in a week, may from time to time find it difficult to keep up his fluid intake. Initially, urinary concentration conserves as much fluid as possible, urinary volume dropping to a minimum with possibly a slight rise in the concentration of blood urea. Later, the athlete may present with a renal tract complication, such as stone formation, or simply fatigue and loss of form. Diagnosis may be difficult without a full history and estimation of diet and fluid intake.

It is difficult to give acceptable figures for the blood urea measurement. Levels as high as 60 mg/100 ml are known under these circumstances and the highest reading in the medical literature is 90 mg/100 ml, though this was during a transcontinental run.

Dehydration, certain metabolic diseases and excessive milk and alkali consumption all predispose to renal stones. The athlete should keep well hydrated and urine volume and colour are good guides to a correct balance. Sufficient fluid should be drunk to achieve an output of $1-1.5\,\ell$/day of urine, much of which should be pale.

Proteinuria Some people filter protein when upright, possibly due to renal vascular changes. Provided that this condition, orthostatic proteinuria, is proved, no further action is required. The first morning urine specimen after rising is clear of protein but subsequent specimens through the day, with the subject vertical, show the presence of protein, often with some accompanying cells. In contrast, proteinuria may be a sign of renal disease and its discovery on routine examination must always be fully investigated.

Haematuria Blood in the urine is always pathological. Red discoloration of the urine is not necessarily due to blood, however, and may follow consumption of certain dyes such as the drug phenolphthalein or vegetable dyes such as beetroot. Some rare conditions may cause a normal-coloured urine to become discoloured on standing.

Blood may appear in the urine directly as fresh blood cells, or indirectly through its pigment haemoglobin (haemoglobinuria).

Haematuria, or the presence of fresh blood in the urine, may be due to bleeding in the urinary tract or from inappropriate filtration of blood cells which are normally neither filtered nor reabsorbed during the blood's passage through the renal blood vessels. Bleeding into the renal tract may be due to direct damage to the kidney by a blow from a fist, ball, boot or implement. Such a blow directly bruises the renal tissue and, for a few days, fresh bleeding causes haematuria. Rest and plenty of fluid are usually all that is required and exercise should not be permitted until the complete cessation of haematuria. Contact sports should probably be avoided for at least a week or two after this if there is a serious chance of a further blow.

Bleeding into the renal tract may also be due to tumours or infections of the kidneys, ureters, bladder, prostate or urethra and must always be taken seriously, even if it seems obvious that exercise haematuria is the cause. Urinary tract infections usually cause pain and an urgent desire to pass urine. Prostatic infection in the older male may be associated with some difficulty in initiating or maintaining a good stream of urine. Medical investigation is important, particularly in the older runner, because of the cumulative risk of renal damage from infection or prostatism plus exercise-induced dehydration.

Inappropriate filtration of red cells is common in severe exercise. Almost any significant degree of effort leads to the appearance of some protein in the urine and, shortly after exercise, casts and red cells are usually found on microscopy of the urine. This condition is usually transient; a specimen passed immediately after exercise shows a few cells and protein casts but the next specimen will be clear.

Beyond this, under increasingly severe and prolonged exercise, there is a whole spectrum of urinary contents. Most subjects never show more than a few cells and casts. Others progress to considerable degrees of haematuria with microscopy showing all the elements of the blood, red cells and white cells, as well as casts and protein in the urine.

The clear relation of such haematuria to the immediately preceding bout of exercise usually invites a diagnosis of exercise haematuria. This is relatively common in the small world of very-high-mileage runners. It is puzzling that a small group of otherwise entirely fit distance runners may suddenly develop haematuria which, for an indefinite period may, or may not, be repeated under similar circumstances. Often, a few episodes lead to medical investigation, including internal examinations of the urinary tract, all of which are usually found to be completely normal.

In the absence of demonstrable disease there is no reason to stop sport but some athletes become unnerved by haematuria. It should be possible to drop the intensity of exercise temporarily and find a threshold level below which there is no haematuria. In other cases, the haematuria clears up as quickly as it started and its circumstances remain mysterious, with no serious consequences.

In practical terms, the 'totally fit' athlete who develops haematuria after severe exercise should be medically examined , including particularly blood pressure, blood urea and full urinalysis. Although his urine may be completely clear between bouts of exercise, which usually also means no symptoms during training, haematuria may nevertheless occur after exceptional sessions or races and he should be continuously observed. Any new symptoms or change in pattern of events call for specialist investigation of the urinary tract.

It is particularly important that this syndrome should not be mistaken for acute glomerulonephritis in which there may be an identical urinary appearance.

A preceding sore throat or febrile illness calls for totally different management with immediate prohibition of exercise pending full investigation for acute nephritis with throat swab, blood and urinary investigations. There is some confusion in the medical literature, occasioned by the expression 'athletic pseudonephritis' which describes cases of apparent glomerulonephritis, some with preceding sore throat, but with totally normal results on full medical investigation and rapid clinical recovery. It seems much simpler, as well as safer, to regard athletes as potential victims of serious renal disease no less than the general population and who should be investigated fully along the same lines with the additional feature, confined to the physically active, of a mechanical filtration defect associated with heavy workloads. This, under certain functional circumstances, may be seen as a physiological fault consisting of a whole spectrum of urinary findings from a few cells to massive haematuria and not clearly linked with any other disease process.

Return to training after renal tract illnesses should always be slow enough to confirm full recovery. Precipitate exertion may cause a recurrence of symptoms; this is particularly true after acute glomerulonephritis.

Haemoglobinuria Rarely, the blood pigment haemoglobin causes reddish discoloration of urine without the presence of any cells or protein. Red cells are broken down in the bloodstream by intravascular haemolysis in capillaries subjected to severe jarring. This may occur in the feet of hard-surface runners, or the hands of the karate player constantly delivering blows. The condition is more common in men than in women. Alleviation of impact by suitable padding or running on softer surfaces is easy to effect and the condition has no long-term significance.

Myoglobinuria is discoloration of the urine by myoglobin, the oxygen-carrying pigment of muscle cells which is released into the circulation only after severe muscle injury of the type unlikely to be found outside the vehicular sports such as motor racing or hang-gliding.

Analgesic nephropathy The habitual use of some analgesics causes renal damage which, initially, produces protein and cells in the urine. It can eventually lead to renal failure however. Phenacetin is the drug most specifically incriminated, but there have been several reports of a possible association with aspirin. Casual use of these drugs is unlikely to be dangerous in this respect since prolonged continuous dosage is required to cause nephropathy.

Venereal diseases

Urethritis with discharge and pain on passing urine occurs in some of the venereal diseases, particularly gonorrhoea, non-specific urethritis and Reiter's syndrome. There is a considerable risk that the infection will spread to joints and immediate accurate diagnosis and antibiotic treatment is required. Athletic activity is unwise during the active stages of infection because of the risk of general spread.

Sexual activity

The physical aspects of sexuality are unimportant in terms of energy consumption or fatigue but this does not apply to the infective or emotional consequences which are the important factors for the athlete. Associated problems such as social disruption and lack of sleep may be counterproductive.

The young athlete should be reassured that sex is normal, its expression depending on individual and cultural factors. Older, and theoretically wiser, team managers and coaches should be careful not to impose their own guilts and inhibitions upon their charges. Disturbance of an athlete's normal routine, in sex no less than other aspects of life, may upset his track performance. Such managerial actions as the barring of wives from team quarters seem at times to place the joy of athletic recreation on a par with the rigours of imprisonment and probably say more about the manager's attitude than his team's normal physical and emotional development.

Emotional aspects of sexuality may cause considerable difficulties for some athletes. For instance, the sportsman struggling with examinations, competition and courting, or the newly-wed couple trying to adjust to each other's life pattern against a background of competitive stress, may each suffer considerable tensions.

Too many medical writers have dismissed discussion of sex in sport with the trite observation that the act of intercourse only uses as much energy as a short sprint. In contrast, many coaches and managers have traditionally felt it necessary to ban sex for a full 6 weeks before competition! The most relevant factor should be the attitudes and commitments of the individual athlete. It is well known that superlative athletic performance can follow uninhibited sexual conduct or, on the other hand, can be derived from prolonged periods of

monastic withdrawal. Individual variation is the key in preparation for competition and a sympathetic understanding of a wide range of differences is vital for any conscientious coach or medical adviser.

The most important aspect of team care in this respect is that the adviser should try to remain emotionally neutral and offer guidance on entirely individual lines based on the need of the individual athlete in matters of sexual conduct, including advice about masturbation, VD, birth control and emotional relationships.

Some aspects of sex and sport worry athletes. In the male, depression of sperm production to the point of temporary (though unreliable) impotence, may be caused by tight underclothing, including jock-straps. This is promptly reversed on changing to looser clothing which lowers testicular temperature. A similar sperm reduction is caused by anabolic steroid or male hormones, both of which are forbidden by doping regulations in any case. The sheer fatigue associated with heavy training may lead to impotence or unsatisfactory sexual performance, notwithstanding any endurance benefits derived from the training itself. The answer to this problem will lie in appropriate adjustments of personal relationships such as modifying or avoiding sexual activity at a time of maximum fatigue.

The problems of female athletes are discussed in Chapter 6. There has been much speculation about the sex ratio of children born to active athletes but there is no clear statistical evidence that shows a predominance of children of one gender.

Skin conditions

Blisters

Blisters are probably the commonest of all sports injuries, affecting either the feet from footwear or the hands from gripping implements. Blisters are often due to wearing new or unaccustomed footwear, such as is often handed out free to teams before competition. Hot and humid conditions, indoors or outdoors, increase the chance of blistering and may be avoided by the use of prophylactic talc, resin or zinc oxide plaster. Once a blister his occurred, the most effective method of continuing competition is to de-roof it with a sterilized needle or blade after thorough skin cleansing with antiseptic. Spirit, Friar's Balsam (tincture of benzoin) or a similar preparation is applied to the raw surface which is then directly covered by a zinc oxide plaster raw to the skin. An intervening layer of lint simply provides a mobile surface which can continue rubbing and cause further blisters.

Blisters may be prevented to some extent by applying surgical spirit regularly to the hand or foot surfaces to cause hardening. Some sportsmen use Vaseline to prevent foot or groin skin chafing but others find this unpleasantly messy.

Heat rashes of a non-specific type are common and need no specific treatment. Skin hygiene, including thorough cleansing and drying after training, together with adequate ventilation from loose clothing, is the best method of prevention. Prickly heat (miliaria) is an intensely itchy skin response to hot and humid conditions which cause temporary blockage of the sweat ducts. Management depends on graduated rather than sudden exposure, cool loose clothing and skin hygiene and cooling.

Warts

Warts are benign viral conditions and are only important to the sportsman if they occur at a particularly strategic site, e.g. the spinning finger of a cricket bowler. Normally, warts respond to treatment with a silver nitrate caustic stick, or podophyllin paint, but in more troublesome sites can be effectively removed by surgery, or electrical or cryo-cautery.

Verruca

Verruca or plantar wart is a similar viral condition which occurs on the undersurface of the foot. Treatment is similar but verrucae are notorious for

their chronicity and tendency to recur. As they are infective and spread in baths or changing rooms, it is only fair to the community to limit spread by not sharing common facilities or at least by applying a thoroughly waterproof protective plaster to the area around the wart.

Acne

Acne is common in athletes during adolescence. It is usually due to infection of the hair follicles by the body's own naturally occurring staphylococcal bacteria. It is worsened by the combination of sweating and dirty clothing. Thorough washing and drying of the skin after training is important. Sufficient changes of sports clothes and towelling should be available to avoid the usual changing room joke of age-old clothing almost rigid with the sweat of a hundred training sessions! Antiseptic skin creams or oral antibiotic treatments are occasionally needed but the possible side effect of diarrhoea which may impair performance should be considered in the active athlete.

Fungal infections

Fungal infections are extremely common in sport. These cause athlete's foot (tinea pedis) or 'dhobie itch' in the crutch (tinea cruris) which spreads easily in changing rooms and on wet floors. The degree of severity varies from a local itchy discoloration to a very irritating pustular eruption with secondary infection. In extreme cases, the feet are too painful to allow training. Treatments include potassium permanganate foot baths, Whitfield's ointment (salicylic acid and benzoic acid in a base of carbo wax), Monphytol (boric acid, chlorbutol, salicylic acid, methyl undecenoate and propyl undecenoate in a liquid preparation applied by brush) or many of the dusting powders such as Mycil (chlorphenesin). These dusting powders can be used prophylactically and, because the fungus may persist in shoes and socks, they too may be powdered. Prevention includes the cleansing of changing room floors and careful washing and drying of feet after sport.

Pruritus

Pruritus is an itchy rash which occurs in the sweaty skin-fold areas of the groin and natal cleft. In vulnerable subjects it is worsened by tight clothing or non-sweat-absorbent material such as nylon. Secondary infection following skin tears due to scratching is common. *Candida* infection (thrush or moniliasis) may be a cause or complication in females and, occasionally, in diabetics.

Treatment is by antibiotics or fungicides where indicated and symptomatic, with steroid skin creams or ointments applied after thorough washing and careful drying of the affected parts. Suitable modification of clothing should be considered with special attention to effective sweat absorption and evaporation.

Haemorrhoids

Haemorrhoids, or piles, are varicose veins at the anus and are common in both sexes and may be accompanied by symptoms similar to pruritus. Symptomatic treatment is along similar lines to that for pruritus and specific treatment of the piles may be indicated. Initially this may be by simple ointments or suppositories, and then more definitively, in selected cases, by injection, ligation or surgical treatment.

Certain illnesses and the athlete
Gout

Gout is an inherited condition in which the body fails to complete the metabolic breakdown of its protein waste to the usual end product of urea which is excreted in the urine. Because of a deficiency of the enzyme responsible for the conversion of uric acid to urea, the process stops short at uric acid. Sporadic accumulation of uric acid in the blood and tissues leads to its deposition as crystals in and around the joints, causing an extremely painful form of arthritis. This is more likely to happen if the athlete is dehydrated. Blood tests may be completely normal between attacks but show elevation of the serum uric acid level during the attack. Medical treatment consists of dietary regulation, to avoid provocation of the metabolism with rich protein foods or alcohol, and drugs which encourage the excretion of uric acid or its precursors.

Gout is controllable and a co-operative patient need not stop sport. If the disease is not properly controlled, however, the slight increase in uric acid production caused by exercise may precipitate symptoms of joint or muscle pain or even further acute attacks.

There is sometimes confusion over the diagnosis of gout because in the population there is a wide spread of serum uric acid (s.u.a.) level. A raised s.u.a. level in a 'totally fit' subject does not mean that he has gout nor necessarily that he will develop it, although there is a correlation between the highest s.u.a. levels and the eventual development of clinical gout.

The relation between s.u.a. and soft-tissue injuries is also unclear. Some studies have correlated the incidence of overuse injury, particularly tendinitis, with a raised s.u.a. level and furthermore have claimed clinical response to treatment with antigout drugs. On the other hand, a knowledge of the normal variation in population levels of s.u.a., together with due allowance for a harmless natural slight elevation of perhaps 1 or 2 mg/100 ml in the very actively exercising population will make the clinician very wary of the diagnosis of gout in these circumstances.

Most experienced clinicians feel that there is no indication either for routine s.u.a. testing of athletes or antigout medication for injuries which have, after all, a mechanical explanation and which nearly always respond effectively and without recurrence to routine treatment. An indication for investigation of the uric acid level would be an athlete who habitually suffered soft-tissue soreness, stiffness or minor injuries, or whose injuries habitually and inexplicably failed to respond to standard therapy.

Ankylosing spondylitis

This is an inflammatory arthritis in which there is a strong inherited predisposition. Youngish males are affected, females rarely. Typically, a young man presents with non-traumatic backache and general malaise. Early examination may show no specific feature. Occasionally, there may be considerable limitation of spinal movement as well as poor chest expansion. Blood tests show a raised ESR and a characteristic antibody structure. The X-ray shows characteristic changes leading finally to 'bamboo spine' with calcification of the ligaments supporting the spine, together with complete bony fusion obliterating the sacroiliac joints.

Clinically, there is a very wide spectrum of ankylosing spondylitis from the virtually symptomless chance finding of typical changes on X-ray, through mild occasional attacks of backache and stiffness, to the advanced forms in a small minority with considerable spinal deformity. Functionally, limited rib movement causes reduced chest expansion but this rarely embarrasses respiration because of the diaphragm's continuing freedom to move. The most serious complication is the development of aortic valve incompetence in a few patients leading to heart failure (*see* Chapter 4).

Treatment of ankylosing spondylitis relies heavily on anti-inflammatory drugs, particularly the non-steroidals, and an active exercise programme throughout the disease except when severe exacerbations make this impossible. Many men with ankylosing spondylitis find themselves encouraged to pursue active recreation, but the choice of sport should avoid those with a sustained flexed spinal posture, such as cycling, or a high risk of back pain and injury, for example, weight-lifting. The aim is to keep the spine in an anatomically correct position so that if increasing fixation of the spine cannot be prevented, then at least a good cosmetic and functional position is finally achieved. Wherever possible, swimming should be encouraged because of its general cardiorespiratory merits as well as its specific benefit for the back, shoulders and hips.

Exacerbations of the disease cause increased backache and stiffness and call for a temporary rest from effort. Disproportionate breathlessness may be due to anaemia but the possibility of developing aortic valve disease should be borne in mind. The peripheral joints, particularly the knees, may rarely develop a temporary arthritis but this almost invariably settles without specific treatment or adverse sequels.

Osteoarthritis (osteoarthrosis)

Osteoarthritis (OA) exists in two forms and is a universal response to ageing. Over two-thirds of the population are found to have typical X-ray changes by the age of 60. OA is not a disease in a commonly understood infective sense but is a mechanical deterioration of the joints. The mere presence of OA in joints is not an indication of clinical symptoms and many people with extremely severe OA changes on X-ray live a long life, free of any joint symptoms. Frequently OA is discovered in middle or old age in association with, for instance, backache, and the X-rays quite obviously antedate the clinical symptoms by perhaps 10 years or more; the patient may become symptom-free for an indefinite period after treatment.

The cause of OA is thought to be a failure of joint lubrication leading to increased friction and mechanical wear of the cartilage. Reactive bony spikes, or osteophytes, are formed at the edge of the joint which itself becomes distorted. Symptoms may supervene at any stage in the process and probably relate more often to coincidental sprains or mechanical stresses than simply to the degree of OA present.

The second type of OA, which may be a variant of the same condition described above, is the accelerated degenerative change seen in a joint damaged by previous disease or injury.

Arthritis and sport It is well established that OA can follow previous damage to joints. However, it is not established that athletic activity, without injury, leads to premature degeneration in any joint. In fact, there is strong suggestive evidence that the opposite holds true, namely that regular rhythmic mechanical stimulation of the joints is one of the crucial factors in the maintenance of their correct nutrition and lubrication. Exercise like running, swimming or cycling serves to keep the active joints fit rather than to wear them out. Hence, it is essential to treat immediately and thoroughly any suspected joint injury at any stage in life in order to prevent subsequent reactive OA. It is also important to encourage regular exercise as a way of deferring degenerative change.

In the clinical treatment of symptomatic OA, anti-inflammatory drugs, physiotherapy and regular exercise programmes each have an important place.

Rheumatoid arthritis

Rheumatoid arthritis (RA) is a generalized inflammatory disease affecting many joints as well as the body's connective tissue. The patient suffers characteristically inflamed, painful and stiff joints, as well as general malaise. There is probably an inherited predisposition to RA, which may start at any age.

Detailed management is outside the scope of this book but, during the acute phase, exercise is impossible or grossly limited by pain. During the convalescent phases, physiotherapy and regulated exercise programmes play an important part and much attention is paid to the restoration and maintenance of full muscle function so as to give maximal support to the inflamed joints. During quiescent phases, exercise should be encouraged as a means to maintain maximum fitness because much RA suffering is due to remediable muscular weakness.

Diabetes

Diabetes mellitus affects about 1 per cent of the British population. Most patients suffer mild forms which come on in middle or old age; also there is a strong hereditary factor. Diabetes is sometimes precipitated by illness or emotional stress, such as bereavement, or the therapeutic use of steroids and certain other drugs. The latter fact should serve as a further warning against the indiscriminate use of anabolic or cortico-steroids for sporting purposes.

In diabetics the pancreas does not produce enough insulin to cope with the metabolism of glucose which, therefore, tends to accumulate in the body with severe metabolic side effects. Also in some cases, the body may become resistant to its own insulin. Paradoxically, in the presence of more sugar than it can handle, the body behaves as if it lacks glucose and the metabolism both produces further glucose by gluconeogenesis in the liver and switches to using fat as a fuel. In consequence the blood sugar level rises and glucose is freely excreted in the urine, taking with it, by osmosis, a large volume of water and creating excessive urinary output, thirst, fatigue and general debility.

Raised body glucose levels predispose to infection from bacteria, viruses and fungi, particularly through candidiasis (moniliasis, thrush) causing sore throats and pruritus (*see above*). The characteristic acetone-like smell of the breath is associated with metabolic fat burning (lipolysis) and is similar to that found in normal subjects during periods of starvation when they, too, switch from a sugar to a fat-burning metabolism.

In milder maturity-onset diabetes, there is often obesity and mild symptoms of malaise or infection which respond to diet alone or to treatment with tablets. In classic diabetes, onset occurs at any age and the progression to coma is relentless. Control is subsequently by insulin and regulation of diet. Insulin may be given in one or two daily injections and it lowers the blood glucose level. The speed and duration of action of the various insulins varies, however, as does the response of individual patients.

Efficient control is monitored through simple dipstick tests of the urine which indicate the presence and concentration of sugar; more precise monitoring is by blood tests of glucose concentration. If diabetes is untreated, ketotic coma develops and the blood glucose level rises. Insulin is needed, always with saline transfusion, as coma only occurs with considerable dehydration. In contrast, excess insulin causes extreme lowering of the blood glucose level to cause hypoglycaemia. Hypoglycaemic coma develops suddenly when a diabetic runs out of sugar in the presence of much insulin. Unconsciousness is accompanied by heavy breathing and possibly twitching and the ketotic odour is usually absent. The urgent need is for sugar.

If a known diabetic is found in coma, an attempt should always be made to administer sugar, e.g. sugar in water by mouth in emergency. If the coma is due to insulin, then response to sugar is usually rapid and the danger of brain damage due to hypoglycaemia is averted. On the other hand, should the coma be due to excessive sugar, then a little more will not harm the patient.

The diabetic sportsman has practical problems. Exercise burns glucose and lowers the blood sugar levels. The anticipated amount of exercise has therefore to be provided for in his daily calculation of diet and insulin requirements. Practical considerations and experience suggest that intermittent sports are more suitable for the diabetic because they permit him to interrupt his game briefly for a quick refill of carbohydrate as and when necessary. Clearly, this is easier than setting out on a marathon-type endurance event with the risk of running into the sudden confusional state and possible collapse of hypoglycaemia. The diabetic should take particular care to start his competition adequately fed and watered. Sugar or chocolate should be to hand in case hypoglycaemia develops. Patients may become dizzy, faint, suddenly tired, confused, blurred of vision, irritable or, in a co-ordinated game, their play simply 'falls apart'.

The diabetic should notify his fellow players of his condition so that, in case of emergency, they will be able to help out if he becomes impaired.

A long-term commitment to exercise is a useful addition to diabetic control and may help to prevent complications; however, the key to good health lies in meticulous control of diet and medication and immediate treatment of any infections or skin wounds.

Death and sport
Drowning

The commonest cause of death in British sport and recreation is drowning, usually caused by negligence. For instance, non-swimmers go boating without life-jackets, or float out to sea on inflatable mattresses or find themselves suddenly out of their depth from one stride or stroke to the next. Seaside notices are ignored in areas where strong currents are dangerous. Ignorance of even the simplest life-saving procedures may prevent effective resuscitation, even when the victim has been rescued from the water. Universal encouragement of swimming competence, instruction in life-saving and strict enforcement of safety measures such as life-jackets and seaworthy boats would all prevent many deaths.

Exposure

Exposure deaths are also unnecessarily frequent. The combined effects of wind and rain cause lethal chilling of the inadequately clothed body of the casual walker or rambler. In many places weather conditions are liable to rapid change and the unprepared walker or climber who sets out on a fine morning can perish within a few hours during a cold, wet afternoon. Young people are at risk because of their relatively greater surface area. Spare layers of clothing, with water- and windproof outer garments, should always be carried where sudden weather changes may occur or where help may not rapidly be forthcoming, for example, when climbing or rambling in mountain areas. A small supply of emergency food such as chocolate and nuts should be carried. Schoolteachers in charge of groups of children should be particularly aware of dangers, precautions and rescue procedures.

Trauma

Sport-related death may follow brain injury, as in boxing falls or kicks on the head, and implemental injury, as with cricket bats or balls. A sudden blow on the chest may be fatal, for instance in contact sport or vehicular accidents. A cricket ball blow may also lead to sudden cardiac arrest or fatal ventricular arrhythmia. Immediate resuscitation is vital, starting, paradoxically, with a smart blow on the chest if no pulse can be detected.

Vascular problems

Most other sports deaths are due to cardiovascular diseases or abnormalities. Sudden rupture of a cerebral artery may cause death at any age, with or without exercise. The relation of rupture to effort is probably coincidental, although the final trigger mechanism in a weakened artery may well be the sudden rise in blood pressure due to vigorous exercise.

Coronary thrombosis may also occur during sport at any age. Many premature victims of heart attacks have, in fact, reported cardiac symptoms such as chest pain or undue breathlessness on exertion in the period preceding death and prevention was therefore a real possibility. As the chance of a heart attack increases with age, these symptoms are even more important in middle-aged and older sportsmen. For instance, rugby referees may have a greatly increased risk of coronary thrombosis leading to death during games but they usually experience fair symptomatic warning which, unfortunately, is often ignored. Similarly the dangers of squash in the middle-aged and overweight are well established.

Sudden cardiac death in the young is more usually due to a structural abnormality of the heart's own blood vessels. This is usually unheralded and undetectable without symptoms and is an inevitable but very rare hazard affecting a few unfortunate subjects.

Infection

Exercise can be fatal during the active phase of many infective illnesses due to myocarditis (cardiac inflammation). Two crucial warnings are that if there is either a raised temperature or a muscular aching, then exercise is absolutely forbidden because there is a strong correlation between these symptoms and myocarditis.

12 Medication

The practice of taking medicine is so widespread that it is desirable for the effects of drugs to be more widely understood, particularly as dope control regulations ask for a declaration by athletes of any medication being taken, apart from the defined doping substances.

While most drugs have positive actions, a few remedies have minimal demonstrable pharmacological action and are probably active by placebo, or suggestion, effect. The trend in modern medicine has been away from the traditional pharmacopoeia full of herbal tonics towards refined chemicals with clear-cut actions.

The placebo action must be taken seriously with medication, as well as diet. In many trials, about 30 per cent of patients respond either in a manner unrelated to the chemistry of the administered drug or in a positive way to an inert pill and this effect of suggestion constitutes the placebo response.

Drugs have positive actions which are used for therapy and negative side effects which may be trivial or severe enough to outweigh the benefits. Side effects are often dose-related and may cause subtle inconvenience by interaction with other drugs or foods to produce symptoms which are not recognized as being due to the drug.

Some of the commoner drugs and usages not described elsewhere are as follows.

Antacids and indigestion

Self-medication with antacids for indigestion is common. Milk drinks are popular and alkalis such as sodium bicarbonate or neutral mineral salts of calcium, aluminium or magnesium may also be added. Excess of bicarbonate and milk may lead to alkalosis, in which the body's pH becomes excessively alkaline. Moderate doses may not cause much disturbance but alkalis are best avoided because of the compensatory renal and respiratory changes which alkalosis causes. Unfortunately, the antacids have other effects on the bowel; some cause constipation, others, particularly magnesium salts, are effective mineral laxatives, an effect not particularly welcome to the sportsman. The increasing use of carbenoxolone (bio-gastrone, duo-gastrone) for peptic ulcers may lead to weight gain due to salt and fluid retention and the corresponding potassium loss may cause muscle weakness. Powerful gastric acid suppressors (e.g. cimetidine, ranitidine) are used for short courses of treatment for proven ulcers, but side effects may include diarrhoea or dizziness.

Other popular drugs for indigestion are the antispasmodics (e.g. propantheline, belladonna) which sedate the gut and relax some of the painful spasms associated with indigestion and ulceration. They mimic parasympathetic nervous system cholinergic action but the characteristic side effects may cause difficulty. Blurring of vision may seriously impede target visualization, dry mouth is always unpopular, palpitations may be confused with organic heart disease, particularly in anxious sufferers from dyspepsia, and there are dangers of prostatic obstruction and glaucoma in older people.

Diarrhoea

Diarrhoea is usually self-limiting and self-treated with simple chalk, or kaolin, mixtures. Medically prescribed codeine phosphate, Lomotil and loperamide (Imodium) present few problems apart from slight sedation, dry mouth and dizziness in some individuals. It should be remembered that Lomotil is a mixture of a synthetic narcotic, diphenoxylate, with a small dose of atropine which in overdosage will present its own side effects of blurred vision, palpitations, dizziness and dry mouth.

Laxatives

Laxatives are widely abused. One of the commonest causes of constipation in athletes is simple dehydration due to sweating without adequate fluid intake. Simple vegetable purgatives such as cascara, rhubarb or senna, work by stimulating the bowel muscle and are harmless in reasonable dosage. Dietary fibre has a useful laxative effect, partly through bulk formation and partly through maintaining hydration of the stools. Methyl cellulose acts similarly. Saline purgatives such as the magnesium salts work osmotically by drawing extra fluid into the bowel to dilute their own concentration. While heavy usage is unlikely to lead to harm, it is pointless since adequate body hydration through sufficient intake of drinks will provide an effective remedy. The general effect of diarrhoea is to lead to some loss of potassium as well as fluid and, for this reason, successful sport may be compromised biochemically as well as socially.

Heart disease

Many patients with controlled heart disease are able to enjoy limited recreation once their cardiac rhythm or failure has been controlled. No general rules can be given but the individual management of each patient must be a matter for discussion with the physician (*see also* Chapter 4).

Diuretics

Diuretics are widely used in the control of heart failure and hypertension. In cardiac conditions, the individual physician must decide the patient's safe limits of exercise. However, many patients are now taking diuretics for long-term control of moderate hypertension, which is unrelated to symptoms, in order to reduce the chance of strokes and heart attacks. In the absence of any other contraindications, exercise is positively desirable for this group of people because it should promote further relaxation and is itself a blood-pressure-lowering activity.

Diuretics cause increased urinary excretion of sodium, potassium and water. This may lead to significant potassium loss and it is common practice to add supplementary potassium if diuretics are taken daily or on alternate days over the long term. There are many diuretics, varying between individuals in their effectiveness and consequent mineral losses. Potassium supplements, if necessary, can be given separately or as combined preparations.

Typical diuretics include chlorothiazide and hydrochlorothiazide, bendrofluazide, chlorthalidone, frusemide and ethacrynic acid. A further problem is that all diuretics may precipitate an attack of gout due to retention of uric acid and patients with gout should increase their medication when starting diuretic therapy.

Diuretics have been abused to achieve acute weight loss, e.g. by wrestlers or boxers trying to 'make weight' for contests. In the short term the fluid excreted will simply be replaced but, and this is a major consideration, the competitor may be dehydrated and thus inefficient in the contest. Apart from chronic mineral loss and dehydration, this is obviously a false approach to weight limits. A player will do best at his best weight, not at an artificially contrived one.

Another important use of diuretics is in the control of cyclical weight gain due to salt and fluid retention in some women. Occasionally, a few days of mid-cycle or premenstrual weight gain are associated with breathlessness, a feeling of fullness or clumsiness, oedema and, rarely, joint swelling. These effects may be alleviated by hormonal adjustment or, quite simply, by taking diuretic pills for a few days as necessary at mid-cycle or premenstrual phases. For such diuretic usage, no potassium supplementation is required.

Hypertension

Mild hypertension, or raised blood pressure, with a diastolic level no higher than about 105 mm Hg, often responds to weight reduction, cessation of smoking, mild sedation and a diuretic. Moderate hypertension with a diastolic reading of up to about 115 mm Hg, is treated by specific antihypertensive drugs such as methyldopa (Aldomet). This treatment is usually satisfactory but the side effects of drowsiness and lethargy may cause a change to alternatives including the beta-blockers or agents such as clonidine (Catapres) which itself may cause sedation, dry mouth and some fluid retention.

More severe blood pressure is treated by the strongest hypotensive agents with both potent action and more troublesome side effects. These are usually related to postural hypotension, i.e. a drop in blood pressure with giddiness on sudden change of position, particularly getting up from lying or sitting. Diarrhoea and sexual difficulties occur with some of these drugs. Individual medical advice should be sought on permitted severity of exercise. It should be

remembered that isometric exercise, e.g. straining, weight-lifting and so on, causes quite drastic rises in blood pressure and is therefore undesirable in the hypertensive person who is trying particularly to lower his higher levels of blood pressure. Isotonic repetitive exercise, e.g. walking, jogging, running, cycling, swimming, would all be more suitable exercise for such patients.

Beta-blocking drugs

The beta-blockers have recently been introduced over a wide range of therapy. The sympathetic nervous system exerts its effect through the nerve endings which use noradrenaline as the final transmitter chemical (*see* Chapter 11). The body has three types of sympathetic receptors each with different responses.

The alpha-adrenergic receptors cause constriction of the bronchi, skin and gut blood vessels and sphincters, causing a rise in blood pressure, relaxation of the gut and dilatation of the pupil. This response is produced by noradrenaline, given by infusion, and other drugs such as phenylephrine. The response is blocked by the alpha-specific blockers such as phenoxybenzamine (Dibenyline) which is of no practical use in sport. A non-specific stimulation of all the alpha- and beta-receptors is achieved by sympathetic stimulating drugs like adrenaline itself or ephedrine.

The beta-adrenergic receptors may be generally stimulated by isoprenaline and blocked by propanolol (Inderal) or sotalol (Beta-cardone, Sotacor). Subdivision is made into beta$_1$- and beta$_2$- receptors. Stimulation of the beta$_1$-receptors increases heart rate and the force of cardiac contraction and this cardiac stimulant effect is blocked by beta$_1$-specific blockers such as oxyprenolol (Trasicor) but, in addition many of these drugs have extra non-specific stimulant effects on the sympathetic system.

Beta$_2$-adrenergic stimulation causes bronchial relaxation and dilatation of small arteries. These effects, obviously useful for exercise in asthmatics, are stimulated by the specific beta$_2$ sympathomimetic drugs salbutamol (Ventolin) and turbutaline (Bricanyl or Brethine).

Beta-blockers are widely used in the treatment of angina, cardiac arrhythmias, high blood pressure and to block the nervous reactions of anxiety. The side effects include the precipitation of heart failure in cases where the cardiac muscle is in a poor state and, more importantly from the athlete's point of view, constriction of the bronchi in the asthmatic.

Another little-known side effect is the liability to cause hypoglycaemia by beta-blocking the adrenaline-induced mobilization of glycogen in glycogenolysis. Lowering of blood sugar may be prolonged and a cause of distress after exercise; the lowering is not rapidly and satisfactorily corrected by giving sugar in the usual way.

Tranquillizers and sedatives

Tranquillizers are discussed in relation to doping regulations in Chapter 13. Sedatives and tranquillizers counter the effects of anxiety, including sleeplessness, lack of concentration and tremor. Their effect on individuals is variable, however, and oversedation is counterproductive to athletes. Sleeping pills, or hypnotics, may create similar problems due to side effects – prolonged drowsiness, headaches and hangovers.

Apart from doping regulations, care should be taken with all forms of sedation and the competitive sportsman should not, for the first time, be given any sedative near enough to competition for adverse side effects to upset his performance. In the long term, it is better to try to help the sportsman to come to terms with anxiety through psychological training techniques. Short-term anxiety may be helped in some individuals by selective use of the beta-blockers which may simply counteract the somatic symptoms such as anxiety, sweating and tremor caused by sympathetic overstimulation, without also exerting a general sedative effect.

Travel sickness and antihistamines

Travel sickness may distress some athletes on short trips but most of the remedies used for this purpose have unwanted side effects. Anti-emetics such as metoclopramide (Maxolon, Primperan), or antihistamines with anti-emetic effect such as dimenhydrinate (Dramamine), promethazine (Avomine, Phenergan) all have such effects which include drowsiness and blurring of vision. Apart from causing danger while driving, these side effects may interfere with fine control of sporting performance. Also, these drugs interact dangerously with alcohol and other sedatives. The 1984 British National Formulary (BNF) advocates small doses (300–600 μg) of hyoscine for travel sickness which, despite the same side effects, is a shorter-lasting drug and therefore less liable to interfere with skilled activity after the journey.

Periactin (cyproheptadine) is an antihistamine with appetite stimulant effects useful in some medical patients. This preparation earlier enjoyed a vogue among athletes in association with body building and strength training but is now generally discredited in this respect. In a group notorious for its gluttony, it is difficult to imagine the power athlete who needs appetite stimulation!

Antidepressants

In recent years, antidepressant consumption has assumed extraordinary proportions in Western countries and here there are practical points to remember. First, all effective antidepressants have side effects, which may include drowsiness, dizziness or fainting associated with hypotension, blurring of vision, dryness of mouth, constipation and sweating, all of which may settle with time and adjustment of dosage.

Secondly, the antidepressants may react severely with other medication or foods, including drugs used in hypertension, antihistamines, travel sickness pills and tranquillizers. Particularly dangerous is the interaction of one group of antidepressants, the MAOIs or monoamineoxidase inhibitors, with a wide range of drugs and foods, including alcohol, cheese, chocolate and the sympathomimetic amine constituents of many common cough and cold mixtures.

The biochemical effects of exercise should be considered in patients on antidepressants as it may lower the need for medication. There are both tranquillizing and antidepressant effects associated with exercise, particularly regular exercise programmes. Some studies have shown exercise to be as effective as either of these groups of drugs. Of course, in the wide spectrum of human variation, it is not surprising that exercise may effectively overstimulate some subjects and this is further discussed in Chapter 10.

Any patient on antidepressants is doubly warned against taking chances with the prohibited doping substances, particularly so because of the added danger of drug interaction.

Antibiotics

Antibiotics impair sporting performance and attention is drawn to the dangers of exercise during infective and febrile conditions (*see* Chapter 11). Most illnesses which require antibiotics obviously preclude vigorous exercise. In some instances, for example long-term prophylaxis of rheumatic carditis with penicillin or sulphonamide, some activity consistent with the cardiac limitations is permitted.

The practical problem for the sportsman and his doctor is the safe limits of practice or competition allowed during the treatment of a septic condition, e.g. otitis or tonsillitis, particularly during an important competition or a team trip abroad. Antibiotics are started as soon as the diagnosis is clearly established. Exercise is not permitted during the first part of the illness during which symptoms and fever abate. The athlete often looks and feels well within 36–48 hours of starting therapy, although there are still physical signs of sepsis. The team physician's skills are required in the assessment of each individual case.

In highly skilled events, for instance shooting, competition may be feasible and even highly successful. The more stamina and strength required, however, the more likely that premature resumption of hard activity will lead to poor performance and, occasionally, to exacerbation of symptoms. Too often, the symptom-free but incompletely recovered sportsman competes without harm, far below his best. Clearly, no general rule can be laid down but avoidance of strenuous effort during any illness usually turns out to be the quickest path to full recovery.

The side effects of antibiotics include skin rashes and diarrhoea. Enthusiastic treatment of minor diarrhoea with antibiotics is strongly contraindicated. Drug prophylaxis of this condition is probably unnecessary. Prophylactic antibiotics have not been validated and the condition is self-limiting and shortlasting. Two of the drugs most commonly used, the sulphonamides and streptomycin, e.g. as contained in Streptotriad, are liable to cause drug sensitivity reactions.

Cancer

The presence of cancer, whether diagnosed and treated or not, is not necessarily inconsistent with sport and recreation. Many patients with limited or controlled disease have no reason to lose the pleasure of sport. Two practical limitations on exercise relate to the disease process itself and its therapy. Cancer may invade key organs and impair function sufficiently to limit exercise capacity. Surgical treatment may create new problems which may or may not allow return to particular sports. Radiotherapy may cause a spell of distressing general symptoms during which, in any case, sport will not be desired but successful radiotherapy may leave the patient cured and fit. Cancer chemotherapy of whatever sort is liable to give distressing side effects which may themselves be the main reason for any limitation of exercise.

Skin

Skin problems are common and some are discussed in Chapter 11. Griseofulvin is an oral antibiotic occasionally necessary for fungal infections resistant to local preparations. Capsules have to be taken, in some cases, for about 6 weeks; however, for grossly infected toenails the period may be up to 1 year. With this drug there is undesirable interaction with alcohol and a small chance of general side effects including headache. If side effects are troublesome, surgical treatment of the nail-beds is preferable to prolonged medication.

It is common practice to harden the skin against the effect of rubbing and blistering and simple surgical spirit or methylated spirits are effective. The treatment of warts and verrucae is described in Chapter 11. Conditions such as eczema and psoriasis may need long-term corticosteroid skin applications and a small proportion of steroid is absorbed in such instances. This is not usually of any significance from the athletic point of view and certainly not from the doping aspect.

The prophylaxis of fungal infections such as athlete's foot is best achieved by the combination of thorough washing and drying of feet and footwear with the use of antifungal dusting powders such as chlorphenesin (Mycil), zinc undecenoate (Mycota, Tineafax) or tolnaftate (Tinaderm). The active infection may be treated by these or alternative formulations of creams or ointments, including benzoic acid compound ointment, Whitfield's ointment (salicylic and benzoic acids in wax) or a suitable paint such as Monphytol (boric acid, chlorbutol, salicylic acid, methyl undecenoate and propyl undecenoate).

Sunburn

Sunburn is an important problem for many touring teams unaccustomed to hot sunshine. First, overexposure should be avoided by graduating the daily exposure, starting with no more than 15 or 20 minutes per session. Secondly, one of the ultra-violet-light-filtering creams should be used, such as mexenone (Uvistat) or the many commercial alternatives widely availabe. Swimming and sweating both cause these barriers to be washed off and they should be freely reapplied.

Anti-inflammatory drugs

Anti-inflammatory drugs are widely used for a whole range of aches and pains, injuries and arthritis. Many drug trials have shown that anti-inflammatories promptly started at the time of sports injuries can accelerate recovery, particularly by relieving early symptoms and allowing quicker progress in remedial exercise programmes.

Aspirin remains a highly effective, remarkably safe and cheap drug. The disadvantage of consequent indigestion is modified by the use only of soluble aspirin taken in drinks. A rather stronger action can be gained by combinations of soluble aspirin with small doses of codeine in aspirin and codeine tablets BP (Codis, and others). Those athletes upset by aspirin may gain relief from paracetamol tablets or proprietary equivalents (e.g. Panadol) which are freely available over the counter. The cheapest forms of these preparations in the UK are soluble aspirin tablets BP, aspirin and codeine tablets BP and paracetamol tablets BP – all are available cheaply from pharmacists in reasonable quantities.

Other anti-inflammatories are available only on prescription though ibuprofen has been deregulated and is available in several brand names.

It is an unfortunate fact that all effective anti-inflammatories have side effects, usually including gastrointestinal disturbance which can include serious ulceration or perforation of the bowel. Diarrhoea is a common side effect of some of the more powerful drugs in this group and some – particularly phenylbutazone (Butazolidin) and oxyphenbutazone (Tanderil) – may cause fatal anaemia as well as peptic ulceration and so should not be used casually. Phenylbutazone may cause fluid retention and is particularly unsuitable for patients with cardiac failure or women athletes with a marked tendency to cyclical weight gain due to fluid retention.

Indomethacin (Indocid) may cause flatulent indigestion and abdominal discomfort and often causes odd mental symptoms including heavy-headedness, disorientation, choking or dizziness. Such effects call for immediate cessation of this drug.

Stiffness

Stiffness may affect some athletes unduly at times of heavy or unaccustomed training. It also becomes more of a problem with the older sportsman or jogger where stiffness a day or two after effort is more distressing than any symptoms associated with the event itself. Anti-inflammatory medication is highly effective, whether in the form of soluble aspirin or the more complex drugs. Phenylbutazone is widely used in race horses to give permanent anti-inflammatory cover to the tissue micro-traumas. Indiscriminate high dosage or long-term use of anti-inflammatories for this purpose cannot be advised because of the very real danger of side effects. The commonest of these, gut disturbance, is aggravated by alcohol, so that the sportsman easing into his post-game consolation of anti-inflammatories and alcohol may find himself even worse off!

While anti-inflammatories are useful for some individuals much troubled with post-exercise stiffness, every effort should be made at a long-term approach. Such approaches include adjustment of training to less provocative extremes together with a determined commitment to regular, rather than occasional, exercise. As fitness improves, small, frequent training loads nearly always relieve stiffness. Occasional excesses remain distressing. Some individuals are undoubtedly far more prone to stiffness than others, however, although there is no evidence to link this to any form of rheumatism or arthritis.

Other useful measures include muscle relaxants, e.g. diazepam (Valium), and hot soaks, cold showers and massage, all of which have their advocates. Unfortunately, alcohol does not seem effective, perhaps because its vasodilatory effects exacerbate existing tissue congestion, particularly if the legs are still and dependent throughout medication. Regular slow stretching techniques as part of a thorough warm-up help to prevent stiffness. Each stretch should be held for at least 10–15 seconds and repeated equally thoroughly immediately after exercise to minimize subsequent stiffness. Short-duration rapid or jerky stretching movements are ineffective and may increase stiffness by stimulating efficient contraction rather than relaxation of muscles.

Alcohol

Alcohol is a source of energy, providing from about 0.3 to 4.0 Cal/ml (1.26–16.74 kJ/ml) of drink but this is not available as effective energy for the athlete. These are 'empty calories', not usually associated with other nutritious substances and may cause weight gain if not accounted for in the diet.

Metabolically, alcohol has been shown to have no effect on maximum oxygen uptake or the intracellular energy pathways during exercise. Alcoholic drinks tend to dehydrate the subject and unbalanced alcohol intake is therefore undesirable, particularly in hot weather where it may seriously delay efficient heat acclimatization in travellers. Alcohol should therefore be particularly avoided before endurance events, e.g. marathons, where dehydration is already a major problem.

Reaction times are known to be slowed with minimal blood alcohol levels; while this varies between individuals, complex tasks are more impaired initially although all skills deteriorate as alcohol levels rise. As skill, including hand/eye co-ordination, deteriorates, strength, bravado and aggression increase as alcohol's depressant action progressively disinhibits cerebral control. While minimal levels of alcohol may impair skills, it is true that some subjects may find a welcome control of nervous tremor, only to run foul of dope control regulations in some sports. Alcoholic hangovers are shown to impair visual acuity, as well as concentration and stamina.

A further disadvantage of alcohol is that its action as a peripheral vasodilator enhances skin flow and interferes with the normal autonomic control of sweating which may be particularly unwelcome during hard effort in hot surroundings.

Moderate amounts of alcohol are an effective and enjoyable relaxant. The potency of cross-reaction between alcohol and other drugs may be considerably more serious than the effect of alcohol alone and there are particular dangers in mixing alcohol with many of the sedatives, tranquillizers and antidepressants.

Finally, alcohol must never be drunk out of doors to protect against cold exposure. The resultant skin flush increases heat loss, possibly fatally. It can, however, safely be drunk to warm up again indoors after cold exposure.

Corticosteroids

Corticosteroids are widely used in the treatment of soft tissue injuries and some forms of arthritis. The corticosteroids, e.g. cortisone and hydrocortisone, are not anabolic and act by suppressing the inflammatory response of the tissues to injury. These steroids have catabolic, or tissue breakdown, effects in contrast to testosterone and the anabolic steroids.

It is not known why steroid injections are so effective, one possible explanation being that they stop the inflammatory process while the injury heals. Particularly favoured is the chronic injury where anti-inflammatory cover from an injection may allow some chronic fibrous adhesions to be torn and a new healing process started, converting a chronic injury into a new acute one which may heal satisfactorily.

Local use of steroid injections, properly indicated, is a highly effective treatment option which is further discussed in Chapter 19. Side effects include non-response and, rarely, infection. About a fifth of injected patients suffer worsening of pain for up to a couple of days after injection, often followed then by swift improvement. The majority of patients suffer no such flare-up. The small quantities of steroid injections are slowly absorbed and do not give rise to general side effects. The misconceived use of systemic corticosteroid therapy for stiffness or sports injuries, however, risks all the dangers of steroid therapy including adrenal suppression and weakness. Thus, patients on corticosteroid therapy for disease may find themselves weakened in sporting terms although paradoxically their steroid-induced euphoria may make them feel particularly well.

Enzymes

It is not possible to become allergic to corticosteroids but allergy can arise to substances injected with steroids such as hyaluronidase or local anaesthetic. Hyaluronidase (Hyalase) is a natural enzyme with a useful local effect in helping to disperse exudate and to spread injected drugs further. Because of its production from sheep tissues, danger of allergy exists, particularly after repeated use. There is, therefore, no indication for its routine use with all steroid injections, only in specific cases where exudate dispersal or fibrous breakdown is required.

Oral enzymes are claimed to disperse inflammatory

tissues, although claims have always been hard to prove in clinical trials. Such compounds as Ananase, Chymoral Forte and Varidase are available. It has been shown that the use of such compounds prophylactically in boxing has helped to minimize the accumulation of bruising and swelling which, in competitions where successive rounds must be fought, may otherwise cause premature withdrawal of a victorious competitor. These drugs are available on prescription only.

Skin preparations

Various anti-inflammatory skin creams are available. These usually work by counter-irritating the skin over injuries to produce analgesia. Other preparations, singly or in combination, introduce various drugs through the skin to give a therapeutic effect in the tissues themselves.

Simple counter-irritants include Wintergreen, e.g. methylsalicylate ointment or liniment BPC; turpentine liniment, BP, containing turpentine oil with camphor in solution; or white liniment BPC,

containing turpentine oil only. Commercial preparations include Algesal, Algipan, Bayolin, Bengue's Balsam, Cremalgin, Movelat and Transvasin.

Creams containing dispersant enzymes include Bayolin (containing heparinoid) and Movelat (including corticosteroid extracts as well as heparinoid).

There is evidence that sympathomimetic agents can be absorbed by the skin from such creams and may give positive dope tests.

DMSO (dimethylsulphoxide) is an extremely potently absorbed chemical which may transport other compounds through the skin. These dangers have led to its removal from routine clinical use.

Skin sprays

Skin sprays delivered from aerosol cans, e.g. PR spray, Skefron and Medi-Cool, deliver volatile substances locally to the skin surface, the rapid cooling of which produces temporary analgesia, but no further anti-inflammatory effect.

13 Doping

Doping in sport is defined as: 'the use by, or distribution to, a sportsman of certain substances which could have the effect of improving artificially the athlete's physical and/or mental condition and so augmenting his athletic performance'.

There is nothing new about doping in sport but what has changed during the twentieth century has been the systematic attempt to search the pharmacopoeia for helpful chemicals. In addition, this has often been without full consideration of side effects or disadvantages. Drugs like strychnine and morphine, with their considerable dangers, have been widely used.

In horse racing, over the years, there have been similar trends but the racing authorities have been considerably quicker in setting up detection mechanisms than have their counterparts in human sport. Most international federations, spearheaded by the International Olympic Committee, have their own comprehensive doping regulations. The standard classification of doping substances is into stimulants, narcotic analgesics and anabolic steroids.

Stimulants

Stimulants include a wide range of different drugs and many naturally occurring compounds like cocaine and caffeine have a stimulant effect. Manufactured drugs such as amphetamine also have similar properties in that they have a direct stimulant action on the central nervous system and often on the cardiorespiratory system as well. Both such stimuli may enhance performance.

The side effects may overstimulate the sportsman and remove warning signs of fatigue or temperature control so that mental excitement forces him to continue his performance despite naturally occurring warnings of overheating and excessive fatigue. Death from exhaustion and heat stroke is well documented in overstimulated sportsmen. Caffeine is so widely present in normal diet, including tea, coffee, colas and other soft drinks, that its prohibition was introduced only in 1982 and made quantitative. The forbidden level of 15 micrograms/ml (μg/ml) is set at some 10 times the average level in the normal population. Such a high level is most unlikely to be reached by taking the drinks mentioned above and would thus infer that caffeine supplements had been taken in the form of tablets or injections.

Sympathomimetic amines form a sub-group of the stimulants and comprise drugs which have actions that mimic closely the naturally occurring adrenaline type of hormones which mediate the sympathetic autonomic nervous system responses of the body. They have a direct stimulant effect on the cardiorespiratory and nervous systems and, because of side effects, sympathetic overstimulation is unwelcome to the sportsman.

Unfortunately, sympathomimetic amines are commonly present in many medicines, including antiasthmatic and antiallergic medications, cough mixtures and nasal sprays: ephedrine is, for example, widely used in this way. Strictly speaking, detection of any of these substances in a competing athlete leads to disqualification and it is most important that the sportsman and his doctor are fully aware of the drug regulations governing their particular sport. Positive steps should be taken to avoid forbidden substances not only as artificially used dopes but as part of normal medication. The commonest conditions causing difficulty are asthma, hay fever and allergy (*see* Chapter 11) and it is important to adjust medication in line with permitted drug usage well before arrival at competition so that full confidence can be established.

A further group of stimulants includes a miscellany of drugs ranging from strychnine to nikethamide. Strychnine heightens awareness of one's surroundings and improves peripheral colour vision but in high dosage is a dangerous nervous system toxin. It was formerly a constituent of many tonic mixtures but has now fallen out of use.

Many stimulants, such as nikethamide and bemigride, do have a place in modern medicine as respiratory stimulants and are often used during resuscitation.

Narcotic analgesics

These include all the narcotics from morphine down to its derivatives, even including codeine which is metabolized along similar pathways. The analgesic properties of this group are useful but their habit-forming propensity makes them potentially dangerous. It may seem odd to use such drugs at high performance levels but there is a long history of morphine injections being used for their temporary but powerful stimulant effect, e.g. towards the end of a long cycling race, this being followed by the profound sedative or narcotic response. The cyclist could, therefore, inject himself towards the end of a long day's racing to achieve his final kick and follow this promptly with speedy and effective relaxation.

Apart from side effects and doping control problems, many of the narcotic analgesics are governed by strict legislation under the Dangerous Drugs Act (and similar foreign legislation) so that mere possession under non-clinical circumstances is a criminal offence.

Codeine has caused dilemmas for administrators. It is a widely used component of simple analgesics, e.g. aspirin and codeine tablets, Codis, and so on, and, as tablets of codeine phosphate, is extremely useful in the management of traveller's diarrhoea, so common among athletes. However, the technical problem has been that drug testing shows it to be metabolized along similar pathways to morphine and confusion in identification may be possible. Although the position has changed in recent years because of the demands of team doctors wanting to use codeine safely and freely, further changes are possible.

In 1982 there was still conflict between the regulations of the International Olympic Committee which prohibits codeine and the International Amateur Athletic Federation which specifically permits therapeutic use of codeine. Team officials and athletes should be familiar with current regulations in their own particular sports.

Anabolic steroids

These are the scourge of modern sport. Anabolic means 'building-up' of the body's tissue. The body contains natural hormones which have an anabolic effect and promote growth, healing and tissue build-up in training and use. These hormones include the pituitary growth hormone and the male hormone testosterone which is also present in small amounts in women through secretion from the adrenal cortex.

Testosterone has potent anabolic effects but is also the main promoter of virilization and excessive use leads to side effects. This is not necessarily flattering to male competitors but may be disastrous for females with development of male-pattern hair growth, deepening of the voice and massive muscle development, together with suppression of female hormones.

The body's complex control mechanisms ensure that the circulation of a hormone provides a feedback to its own controlling organs which regulates further secretion. If an excess occurs, the controlling organ reduces output. If, for instance, testosterone is given, suppression of natural levels occurs. If this continues long enough, there may be prolonged or irreversible suppression of the male organs when administration is stopped, although all will apparently be well (or even better!) as long as the full doses of testosterone are administered to the subject.

Anabolic steroids are chemical derivations of natural male hormone which have a purer anabolic and lesser virilizing effect. Variation between drugs and individuals is unpredictable and side effects may occur, particularly if large doses of anabolic steroids are given to either sex. For instance, the normal therapeutic dose of Dianabol in medical practice is between 5 and 25 mg/day but athletes are well known to use doses of 250 mg/day or more. The documented side effects include suppression of sperm production and development of liver cancer. The virilizing effects on women are all too distressingly obvious to those who have seen them. Adolescent growth stunting can occur through premature fusion of the bones' growing epiphyses.

How do anabolics work? While the reluctance of all concerned to be open in this matter is understandable, two clear facts emerge. First, anabolic steroids do work, remarkably effectively in many cases. Secondly, it is not known how they work.

For many years research has tried to elucidate the reasons for improved performance claimed by anabolized athletes. Muscle bulk can be increased considerably by taking anabolic steroids; however, it has been shown that the extra bulk consists of mineral and water, not bigger, better muscle fibres. No gains in strength have been demonstrated from anabolic steroids alone and there is universal agreement that, whatever anabolics may do, extremely hard physical work is the key component which is the final mediator of athletic performance. Diet, heavy training and anabolics may be the effective combination.

Some studies have denied a training effect due to anabolics while others have claimed significant improvements. These differing results are almost certainly due to wide discrepancies in the populations studied; there are probably different effects at different levels of fitness as well as at different intensities of training. Sheer increase in body bulk may help certain performances, particularly where momentum is required, e.g. during rotational techniques of throwing the hammer or discus where bigger bodies can generate greater prerelease momentum and hence expect to throw further. Skill plus bulk still needs strength for full performance, however, hence the need to accompany any programme with extremely heavy physical training.

How then do the anabolic steroids work? Early debates tended to crystallize into two camps. On the one side, the coaches and athletes who experienced benefits showed a paranoid encapsulation within their world because of the prohibitions and attitudes of administrators. On the other side, many officials took the view that because, for instance, an experiment showed no clear improvement in performance due to steroids alone, all other factors being eliminated or equalized, there was no actual effect to be had apart from rendering the muscles swollen with salt and water.

The years have led to some changes in attitudes, although it is true to say that the sporting side of the fence remains ambivalent – torn between a professed desire to be chemically clean and an urge to make the most of any available aids going, pausing only to cock a snook at the 'backward' doctors and scientists whom it is deliberately trying to outwit. It has emerged that the major effects of anabolic steroids are undoubtedly those related to the ability to perform and recover from heavier training and competitive loads than in the unaided state. Such is the language used that one is drawn to the conclusion that there is probably a tonic effect being exerted and that this is probably at the mental or general hormonal level, rather than merely in the locomotor system. It is possible that the anabolic steroids, especially in higher doses, interact with the body's endogenous steroids to produce the euphoriant effect analogous to that seen in clinical medicine where steroid euphoria, even mania, is well documented.

Thus, looking at the overall effect of anabolics as related to appetite for, and recovery from, work, one should consider perhaps the most relevant side effect for most anabolic users. This is that disproportionate increases in strength between the locomotor tissues, e.g. muscles and tendons, may lead to an increased incidence of soft-tissue injury, and this may be the commonest side effect of anabolic usage. The bizarre and admittedly rare glandular side effects whose scare value has been so contemptuously brushed aside by so many athletes for so long may be of less significance.

There is proceeding throughout the world of organized sport, massive financial investment in dope detection and prohibition. Such measures call for major long-term education and indoctrination of populations so that people may possibly revert to the simpler, purer, concepts of yesteryear. For those less optimistic, the prospect of almost unlimited long-term expenditure on prohibition and further research seems all too sadly inevitable.

Testosterone

While detection methods have allowed extremely accurate and reliable detection virtually to outlaw the use of anabolic steroids within about a month of competition, athletes have responded by a switch to testosterone itself which is not detected by tests specific for synthetic anabolic steroids. However, they overlook the fact that as anabolic steroids are specifically outlawed at present and testosterone is one of the most potent anabolics, they are already highly liable to disqualification under present regulations.

Because it is difficult to state exactly the precise limits of normality occurring in athletic populations, it is not easy to specify a level of testosterone in the body above which an athlete can be disqualified.

Hence indirect methods have been developed which measure whether the discovered level of testosterone is natural or unnatural.

As messenger hormones (LH or ICSH) bring about the secretion of testosterone, there is a naturally occurring normal ratio of LH to testosterone. If excessive testosterone is given, the feedback mechanism causes the LH to fall and a new ratio is found in which LH is too low in relation to a high level of testosterone. Were the athlete to be naturally endowed with a large testosterone output, the LH: testosterone ratio would remain 'normal'. Hence a theoretically simple test exists to detect the artificial testosterone user. The only problem with widespread implementation of this and, no doubt, further subsequent developments in response to more enlightened cheating, is cost and manpower.

More recently pituitary growth and other hormones have entered the doping arena, with the possibility of serious medical side-effects as well as detection difficulties.

The IAAF Doping Control Regulations are reproduced in full as Appendix 1. It will be seen that extremely careful regulations and protocols are prescribed for the collection and registration of urine samples and their subsequent analysis, together with the neutrally observed cross-checking of any positive samples which make the technical analysis virtually foolproof. Indeed, it is true to say that all the protests which have arisen following positive dope tests have confined themselves to criticisms of collection of the specimen, not the scientific procedures.

Marginal doping problems

Small amounts of alcohol may have a sedative effect but the pharmacological action of alcohol is one of inhibition. It inhibits the central nervous system inhibitors, so that the normal constraints to uncontrolled action are removed and wilder, uncontrolled actions are unleashed: hence, the use of alcohol to promote aggression prior to or during competition. Alcohol in sustained competitions such as archery or shooting is unreliable because the need to maintain a constant performance, perhaps for 2 or 3 hours twice a day during 3 or 4 days, makes it difficult to control the alcohol level. Intermittent consumption leads to fluctuating blood alcohol levels with a variable level of sedation, and common experience is of a tendency to deterioration and unreliability of performance.

Tranquillizers are now so widely used by the population that they are naturally of interest to sports people. A sedative effect may clearly help some nervous subjects in archery or shooting but it has been shown that performance can be improved if these competitors are weaned off the tranquillizers and at the same time carefully taught good relaxation techniques. In other words, the best form of control and sedation in an accurate technique sport is self-control, including self-induced conditioning and relaxation. Tranquillizers may flatten the mood too much or give an unreliable or permanently slightly below par level of performance and are therefore, in any case, not ideal.

Beta-blockers selectively inhibit some of the sympathetic system nerve endings. They control 'exam nerves' or 'stage fright' and should therefore help fine sporting technique performance. Experience has shown, however, that response is uncertain and variable between subjects so that, while beta-blockers are not prohibited, they may not actually help competitors and it is important that there is close co-operation between physician and competitor in assessing individually the use of beta-blockers.

Female oral contraceptives are not prohibited. The performance of female competitors varies considerably between subjects at different times of the menstrual cycle, possibly to a major degree. Thus, the same woman can be a world-record beater one day and a failure a few days later. A great benefit of 'the pill' is the levelling-out of wide fluctuations in mood, body weight and fluid retention (*see also* Chapter 6). Unfortunately, many women find the resultant flattening of mood tends to average out performance

to something both reliable and below the best possible for that performer. Theoretically, it would be ideal to manipulate the menstrual cycle in a way which would always deliver a women to her major competitions in the perfect phase of her cycle. This is not feasible, so the choice may be between accepting the peaks and troughs of the natural cyclical fluctuation without medication, or experimenting with different types of pill to try to find the best combination of hormones for the individual sportswoman concerned.

Dope detection

As illustrated in Appendix 1, there are clear protocols for the collection and analysis of specimens. These, incidentally, take account of differences in the pH, or relative acidity/alkalinity of the urine, manipulation of which has been a time-honoured evasion trick by some sportsmen who have used a combination of forced urinary output through diuretic pills and artificial adjustment of the urinary pH to produce apparently clear urine at testing. Experienced testers now know how to overcome this problem!

There are two main testing techniques. Testing for anabolic steroids is through screening by radioimmunoassay techniques and detailed identification of any anabolics found, together with screening for all other drugs by gas liquid chromatography–mass spectrometry (GLC–MS).

Radioimmunoassay techniques depend on the production of animal antibodies to anabolic substances. The addition of any body fluid containing anabolics to the prepared testing material leads to an antibody–antigen reaction which can be identified as positive. Because doping regulations require the explicit identification of the particular substance, not merely the generic detection of an anabolic, such a positive test would lead to GLC–MS techniques for detailed identification.

Gas liquid chromatography and mass spectrometry are analytical methods which depend upon detailed spectroscopic analysis of samples subjected to flame photometry. Each chemical substance emits its own characteristic wavelength which can be measured and identified by reference to known standards.

Positive tests are obtainable from microgram quantities of chemicals. For instance, a whiff of nasal spray tonight may still give a positive test after tomorrow's football match. So effective is this method of detection that the use of stimulants and narcotics is virtually unknown in top sporting competitions where testing is expected, however prevalent doping may be at lower levels.

Summary

The rather negative problem of doping control has become an unfortunate and expensive necessity but is clearly a reflection on the personal values and judgements occurring in today's sport which, sadly, is only a reflection of today's society. Unless radically new attitudes towards doping can infiltrate society, there seems little chance that dope control technology and expenditure will decline in the foreseeable future.

14 Failure of performance

Failure by athletes to produce their expected level of performance in training or competition should be carefully analysed. The commonest causes of failure are overambitious expectation, undertraining and inappropriate training. 'Staleness' is a complex combination of mental and physical factors.

The role of the coach, teacher or parent is important in keeping the athlete to reasonable perspectives. The commonest reason for defeat is losing to a superior opponent and this may be difficult to accept if unrealistic targets and attitudes are adopted. 'Bad luck', 'we were robbed' and 'the referee was biased' are all possibly true reasons for defeat, but are more often indications of failure to analyse defeat realistically. The coach or parent's pressure may represent more the projection of ambitions upon the young athlete than a critical appraisal of the latter's ability or personal motivation.

Medical factors

Illness is the most important factor to be considered because of its possible threat to health or even life. Virus infections are common and may lead to inflammation of lymph glands, lungs, muscles and the heart itself with the possibility of sudden death (*see* Chapters 4 and 11). A frequent sequel is post-viral depression, possibly due to mild encephalitis, which may be confused with 'staleness' but may last indefinitely, although normally it is self-limiting to a week or two.

Bacterial infections include sore throat, earache, nail infections, boils, acne and carbuncles. Before the antibiotic era, dental abscesses and chronic tonsillitis were prominent causes of athletic failure. In all such infections medical cure restores full fitness. Chronic fungal infections, especially of the feet or nails, may undermine health and lead to secondary bacterial infection. In many parts of the world chronic tuberculosis is an insidious low-grade illness; many tropical diseases cause chronic long-term anaemia and lassitude rather than acute illness.

Anaemia may reflect illnesses or dietary deficiency and may impair performance by lowering the blood's oxygen-carrying capacity. Rarely, it may be caused by the sport itself – chronic pounding of the feet or hands leading to destructive haemolysis of the red cells.

There is no universal standard for normal haemoglobin (Hb) levels in the blood. 'Normal' Hb represents the local laboratory's average finding for the particular sex and age group. The physiological changes in training (as also in pregnancy) may cause low Hb findings in groups of athletes compared with local norms (*see* Chapter 4). In the absence of symptoms of lassitude, undue fatigue, lack of stamina or pallor, scepticism should be the rule. No amount of iron supplements – nor of vitamin B_{12} or any other supplements – will raise the Hb level in an athlete whose body stores are full. Iron supplements often have gastrointestinal side effects which may themselves upset the athlete.

Normal dietary considerations apply, and female

menstrual loss of iron should be fully provided for, as discussed in Chapters 9 and 6. The particular fluid and mineral requirements must be met for prolonged performance in hot conditions, as dehydration and salt deficiency impair performance.

Diabetic athletes need careful management during sport since hypoglycaemia (low sugar, excess insulin) impairs concentration, judgement and performance (*see* Chapter 11).

The nervous system's need for sugar as its main nutrient explains the use of sugar supplements at half-time in team games and during prolonged intermittent events such as pole vaulting or competitions which involve several contests in one session. Falling blood glucose levels cause a fall-off in performance as the event proceeds.

Psychological factors

The psychological key to competition is the athlete's effective balance of his arousal in relation to the required performance. This is discussed in Chapter 10 and illustrated by *Figure 14.1a*, in which it is clear that optimum performance occurs when the degree of arousal is most appropriate.

Arousal is trainable, and autogenic training, relaxation or meditational techniques are widely used. The coach's pep-talk must be appropriate to each individual and overaggressive arousal may be counterproductive to an individual or a team.

'Staleness' may reflect depression, recent illness, anxiety and overarousal, or the general state of overtraining (*see* Chapter 5). Sleep deprivation may be an important factor, especially when combined with travel-fatigue and excessive competition – a common pattern at top levels of sport.

Physiological factors

Mental and physical appropriateness to the chosen sport are fundamentally important – the Sumo

wrestler is not going to do a 2 m high-jump! Many distressed athletes brought to the clinic have nothing whatever 'wrong' with them but are clearly in the wrong event or sport. Better education of coaches is the main answer to this problem which occurs even at the highest levels. Examples include the international 800-metre runner whose somatotype is ideal for 5000 metres, or longer racing, and the international gymnast who has rapidly outgrown her sport at puberty but is still expected by her coach to maintain her previous position.

For every biological characteristic considered – including muscle fibre type, enzyme efficiency, oxygen uptake, somatotype, limb length, proportion of shin to thigh length, percentage of body fat or even time taken for 800-metres run – the frequency distribution curve applies, as shown in *Figure 14.1b*.

Successful performance can be seen, therefore, as a result of many variables coming together. For instance, the frequency distribution curves for any two functions may be portrayed as by *Figure 14.1c* (or

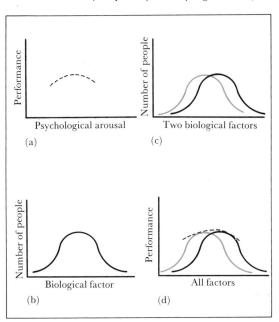

Figure 14.1
Factors which affect performance

by plotting two different points on one single curve).

Ideal performance implies that all the appropriate variables interrelate perfectly in the individual, so that *Figure 14.1d* indicates approximation of all the important biological functions, including optimum arousal on the crucial day. Expressed differently by using only one curve, all the points on the curve come together so that the athlete's body build is matched by his biochemistry.

Failure of performance at the peak of career fitness should be seen in such biological terms. The athlete with 'perfect' lungs and chemistry may not be able physically to beat one with 'near perfect' lungs and chemistry, but who has superior limb leverage. Motivation is only one of the biological variables and 'failure' to win a given event may nevertheless represent total biological success in the loser's performance – no cause for the widespread dejection so often seen in losing finalists.

15 Sports injury

In sport and recreation there is always conflict between the heights of intensive competitive performance and the general concept of 'Sport for All'. Overemphasis on success has turned many sportsmen away from the higher levels of competition and created a greater interest in recreation, outdoor pursuits and leisure activities.

Sport has long been used as a political weapon and some nations – the German Democratic Republic, for instance – have incorporated sporting aims into their state constitutions. Others, like the UK, have taken a much more casual attitude to official provision but have, nonetheless, made government commitments which have been improved, in financial terms, over the years. Realization that laziness is associated with ill health has led a number of governments to adopt some level of 'Sport for All' recreational provision as a public health measure.

Automation has brought more leisure time and all sporting activities have grown since the Second World War. Increasing demands are made on all sports facilities and many forecast a possible move by society towards compulsory provision of recreational facilities at, and even during, work. While there is still notable underparticipation in sport by identifiable groups, including school leavers, females, immigrants and underprivileged groups, there is a corresponding recruitment of others by media campaigns reflecting an increased concern with personal health and well-being. It is difficult to get accurate figures for sports participation but many estimates suggest that between 15 and 20 million people (up to about one third of the population) in Great Britain take some form of regular recreational exercise.

Safety in sport

Sport often supplies excitement in a drab daily life and it is inevitable that 'Sport for All' leads to sports injuries for all. A British Sports Council survey published in 1955 gave the injury rates of particular sports; the figures ranged from 36.5 injuries per 10 000 man hours of play in soccer down to only 0.3 in swimming. The latter rate ignored drowning, however, which, in most published surveys, exceeds the sum of all other recreational deaths put together. The important thing about risk factors is that they should not be ignored but that society should regard them with the utmost respect and take what precautions are possible to mitigate unnecessary suffering. For instance, the risk of some rugby injuries is related to foul play and there may be a need for changes in the rules and certainly stricter refereeing to eliminate this group of serious and unnecessary injuries. Seeking to suffer and parade injuries in the name of sport is a rather immature concept and society would surely not enjoy its sports less with reasonable protective equipment.

Rules are framed with the intention of ensuring fair play and avoiding unnecessary injury risks or dangers. It is imperative that they be strictly respected and enforced. Unfortunately, violence among spectators and on the fields of play has led to considerable public provision being made towards ground security and discipline. Only by constant education of players and inculcation of fair values by coaches and teachers can society hope to ensure a happier long-term state of play in sports.

The increasing intensity of sport has led to wider recognition of overuse injuries. In general, sports injuries may be classified into those caused by external trauma and those due to overuse. External trauma is caused by impacts such as being kicked or struck, or by falling. Overuse relates to the repetitive, usually stereotyped, performance of limited movement patterns. These are usually highly specific for the sport concerned, e.g. tennis serving, running, kicking or jumping, and they lead to localized breakdowns in the body's locomotor system. Overuse accounts for between 20 and 30 per cent of all sports injuries, varying from under 5 per cent in contact sports to almost 100 per cent in long-distance swimming or running. Today's youngsters are doing as much training as yesterday's adult champions. Whereas a middle-distance runner 20 or 30 years ago would have trained perhaps between 20 and 50 miles/week, many ordinary club athletes are today running well in excess of 80 miles/week (120 km/week). This brings not only extra injury risk but a phenomenal increase in the mental and physical commitment given to sporting activity. This has considerable implications for competitiveness as well as the consequences of success or failure.

Over 5 per cent of all British hospital casualty attendances are due to sports injuries and each sport has its characteristic injury profile. Certain sports are notorious for causing more serious injuries. For instance, ski-ing produces serious fractures because of the speeds involved, and riding causes a worrying number of serious head and spinal injuries.

Death in sport, although rare, is usually due to direct severe head and neck injury caused by falling or being struck. Also, drowning and exposure in water sports or coincidental sudden death due to cardiovascular disease are prime causes.

Safety and prevention of injury in sport is essential and often a matter of common sense. Many water deaths are due to such stupid incidents as: five persons in a two-man dinghy on a rough sea; failure to wear life-jackets; sailing in frail boats; or excessive alcohol intake. All these are totally avoidable and call for constant vigilance and relentless education, particularly among instructors of the young. Simple measures of public policy such as requiring all schoolchildren to learn to swim seem obvious but have yet to be adopted. Indeed, many Education Authorities have even cancelled provision for swimming to save money.

Other safety measures in sport include the provision of padded boxing ring floors and posts which have achieved much in preventing further gratuitous insult to the smitten brain of the falling boxer. Likewise, flexible flag-posts and padded goal-posts have softened some collisions in field sports. Hard gymnasium landings or jumping pits also call for adequate padding.

Sports equipment may itself cause injury. It is ironic that protective items like American football helmets can become used as offensive weapons, although rule changes have outlawed the practice of 'spearing' opponents. Recently in Britain a runner's leg was hit by a falling athletic hammer not restrained by the proper cage and a number of schoolboy deaths have been caused by javelins landing in children's bodies instead of the turf provided. Only by constant publicity and education is it possible to make any impact on the cavalier manner in which young players fool around with what are potentially highly dangerous weapons. Too often the teacher in charge of school games seems unaware of the dangers of the situation and a great deal more has still to be done for the education of such staff. For instance, high-jumping is dangerous without a well-padded and protected landing area and children should not be exposed to this event, particularly the 'Fosbury flop' style, without both supervision and suitable landing areas. The same applies even more forcefully to the pole vault where the greater distance to be fallen enhances the risk of injury. The injury rate is probably small only because so few take up this event. The trampoline is always popular with youngsters but two paraplegias have occurred in world-class pole vaulters in recent years during trampolining at which they were expert and experienced. Tragedies occur each year because people fall on to the edge of the trampoline instead of into the padded middle. Alert catchers must be present whenever trampolining is undertaken. It is inevitable that racquets will cause a certain number of injuries within enclosed court spaces but careful consideration should be given to eye protection in the case of squash where the ball is notoriously liable to cause severe eye injury. While the risk may be acceptable to the normally sighted, the minimum protection called for in the spectacle wearer is a shatter-proof spectacle or goggle.

Cricket has become a strangely different game in recent years with the changes in protective gear, particularly helmets. The philosophy of this increasing protection is interesting as exponents describe considerable gains in confidence at playing more aggressive shots, for instance the hook off the eyebrows, without fear of serious injury. On the other hand, the availability of protective equipment may change the nature of the game by inviting more aggressive play.

Synthetic surfaces have added much to modern sport performance. Running tracks are consistently faster than the old cinder tracks, though there is some apprehension about increased injury risks because of the mechanical properties of these surfaces. For instance, the introduction of brush spikes, consisting of multiple short spikes brought new problems: unfortunately, their traction turned out to be so great that the tendency to leave the leg behind on the bends caused more leg injuries and that shoe style had to be abandoned!

Other synthetic surfaces have enabled players to continue high-level training in all weathers and have added to the intensity of training loads. Because they are usually harder than the softer turf they replace, they give rise to more foot injuries. The synthetic turfs have, in hot climates, caused characteristic injuries, particularly abrasions, because of the tough fibres which replace the natural grass. New footwear has had to be designed and an incidental side effects is that synthetic turf stadia in warm climates may be so much warmer than the naturally evaporating turf which they replace that they cause heatstroke in the players, particularly where they are already heavily dressed with protective gear as in American football. On the credit side, the synthetic surfaces have lower maintenance costs and are always usable.

Protective clothing has developed in parallel with modern materials and technology. It is not now sufficient to wear just a simple skull-cap but it is essential that the mechanical design of such a device is the result of thorough research. For instance, the insides of protective helmets may be supported in different ways by springing or direct padding, but in each case the impact resistance must be maximal. Design features have to be carefully planned. For instance, earlier models of American football helmets were found to be associated with severe neck injury if the face-piece was grabbed by an opponent and the neck thrust into extension. This called for softer and lower-cut padding at the back of the head and incidentally, a drawing-in of the face-cage and an outlawing of face grabbing.

Apart from helmets for all risk sports, including cricket, boxing, cycling and riding, scrum caps, ear bands, goggles, shatter-proof spectacles and soft contact lenses have all brought safety and high achievement. Attention has still to be paid to clothing and many of the synthetic fibres are unsuitable for hot and humid environments. Unfortunately, ease of laundering may not make up for the loss of the sweat absorbency and coolness of traditional cotton, although attempts continue to overcome some of these disadvantages with design features such as more open-meshed weave.

Much attention has been paid commercially to shoe and boot design but this is still, in many instances, far from satisfactory. The average sportsman still tends to be held to ransom for unnecessarily expensive sports shoes. Many of these are not entirely satisfactory for their purpose and some are positively dangerous. Constant attention and modification is necessary to features such as stud length and sharpness, and also to wear on the sharp front of a boot sole plate.

16 Muscle injury

Muscles provide power for the body's movements. They are firmly attached to bone and transmit the pull of their contraction over one or more intermediate joints through noncontractile tendons inserted into bones. They may work intermittently and violently as in athletic activity, extremely finely as in the control of delicate movements such as shooting, or almost permanently in the regulation of body posture during waking hours. Muscles contract in response to spinal reflexes or in response to detailed control from the brain via the spinal cord and peripheral nerves. There is a constant feedback to the brain and reflex centres through the sensory nerves and all body movements are in patterns involving complex and co-ordinated contraction of some muscles together with automatic reciprocal relaxation of their antagonists. Fine movement patterns are learnt throughout life and one of the functions of all skill training in sport is to perfect the neuromuscular patterns of sports movement so as to render them increasingly reflex and reliable in the face of athletic stress. Muscles need a rich blood supply and both strength and capillary vascularity are improved by training.

Muscles may be damaged by direct blows, which may cause bruising and some disruption of fibres, or by self-induced tears.

Muscle tears

Muscle tears may be complete or incomplete (*see Figure 16.1*).

Complete muscle tear

Complete muscle tears may be seen dramatically in the upper-arm biceps muscle when the long head of the biceps is torn and bending the elbow up causes the unattached end of the muscle to appear as a lump halfway down the forearm (*see Figure 21.8*). A similar appearance is seen at the front of the thigh where the rectus femoris muscle may be damaged in a direct blow or torn in a kick, or at the back of the thigh in the hamstring muscles which are often torn in sprinters.

Partial muscle tear

Partial muscle tears (*see Figure 16.1*) involve only part of the muscle's substance. The tear may occur deep in the substance of the muscle (central) or towards the edge of a muscle bundle (peripheral). It is not immediately possible to differentiate between a peripheral and a central tear; the sportsman simply hobbles off the field with a 'pulled muscle'. After a day or two however, the two types may be distinguished.

Central muscle tear

At this time a central tear is usually more painful, loss of function is more evident and bruising is unlikely unless there is associated superficial contact injury.

Peripheral muscle tear

In contrast, a peripheral tear allows drainage by gravity of the haematoma, or bruise, along tissue planes and often spectacular bruising appears a few centimetres away, while the original site of the injury is much less tender. Confident movement returns rapidly.

Treatment

The practical importance of differentiation between these lesions is that central tears may take about three times as long to return to full training as peripheral tears which can drain and heal more quickly. Good management should permit recovery in about 3 weeks for the average central tear or 1–2 weeks for the peripheral tear.

The first principle is 'R–I–C–E', starting with *Rest*.

The aim of first aid is to stop bleeding and minimize tissue damage, so that there is minimum delay to recovery. As the tissues are torn, bleeding and unstable, any further movement, massage or manipulation may increase the initial bleeding. Therefore, rest is logical for the first day.

Ice cools the tissues and diminishes the bleeding. It should not be applied directly to the skin, however, but always with a towel or cloth intervening so as to avoid the danger of ice burns. If ice is not available, then a cold soaked towel or running water from a tap is highly effective.

Compression is produced by firmly bandaging the affected part so as to constrict the tissues sufficiently to stop further bleeding but not enough to stop circulation altogether.

Elevation is raising the affected part so as to allow free drainage by gravity of the tissue congestion.

Rehabilitation

After the first 24 hours the principle of muscle rehabilitation is clear. The aim is to stretch the

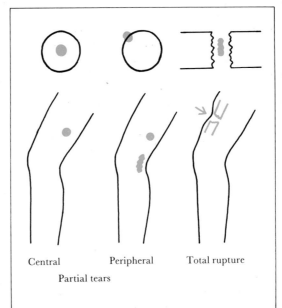

Figure 16.1
Muscle tears

Central   Peripheral   Total rupture

Partial tears

muscle back to its full range of movement, passively then actively, guided by pain tolerance. After that, progressive resisted movement is the key to full recovery. Passive treatment like heat or massage cannot of itself mend tissues – only exercise restores muscles!

The use of anti-inflammatory drugs soon after injury and ice or ultrasound treatments during rehabilitation may sometimes accelerate healing.

After the first day, the more treatment that is applied, the better. The truth of this is evident in the experience of any professional team where it is found that two to six or more treatments daily produce better and quicker results than a casual session once or twice a week. 'Treatment' will in most cases mean the patient's *own* conscientious performance of stretching exercises throughout the day – not just a few minutes once daily!

The fitness test

It is most important to return the sportsman gradually to his training and a test of his muscle function must be carried out before full training is resumed. This fitness test consists of putting him through his paces in the gym, or on the field, under realistic circumstances similar to the movements required in his game, whatever that may be. It should also be a golden rule that no one be allowed to play a game until he has survived full training.

Complications

There are occasional complications of muscle tears. It is very rarely necessary for a surgeon to have to aspirate a major haematoma, and even rarer for a cyst or abscess to form in a neglected muscle tear.

Myositis ossificans is an ill-understood condition which may follow a direct blow to the periosteum, or bone lining, under the muscle. This, by releasing bone cells into the deep muscle bruise, may lead to the formation of plaques of dense bone, usually in the thigh, rarely around the elbow or other sites. The warning sign of myositis is early and excessive pain and loss of movement, together with a swelling or dense or woody feeling of the deep tissues. For instance, in thigh muscle injury, inability to bend the knee past a right angle after 48 hours may indicate a longer disability time and a significant risk of myositis. Suspicion of this condition calls for urgent medical help and diagnostic X-rays. Myositis needs absolute rest for some weeks; active interference makes it much worse. Subsequently, once the new bone has become stable, active physiotherapy is resumed, or occasionally the deposit must be surgically removed.

Myositis ossificans sometimes leads to disastrous functional limitation but the usual result is remarkably good. Most cases are minor and recover fully over the course of some months, especially if rested early on.

Cramp

The commonest causes of cramp are vascular changes, due to tight garters, fatigue or unaccustomed muscle strain, for instance in swimming, where temperature changes may also play a part. Salt deficiencies and dehydration in certain circumstances cause cramp but it is a mistake routinely to load any victim with salt and water. Relief of tight clothing, rest, change of temperature, massage or stretching of the affected muscle may all help. Thorough warm-up and stretching exercises before competition are effective preventive measures. Resistant cases of habitual cramp should be checked for adequacy of diet but, again, it should be emphasized that the cause is usually unknown in scientific terms. Vigorous sweating in hot temperatures, indoors as in fencing or outdoors as in football in hot climates, obviously calls for salt and fluid supplementation. Other cases may require symptomatic relief by medication. Muscle relaxants, such as diazepam (Valium) may be effective and the time-honoured remedy of quinine sulphate is occasionally effective. Leg cramp may be a symptom of certain spinal disorders and treatment should be directed accordingly.

Highly trained muscle tends to be tense and bulky. It may be tender on palpation and there is often crepitus, or crackling, at its musculotendinous areas.

Muscular relaxation may be a considerable problem for some very highly trained or overtrained athletes and coaches should pay as much attention to relaxation as to heavy training exercises.

Fibrositis

This is a painful condition, due to local muscle spasm, which occurs in the neck, shoulder-girdle and back. It is induced by unaccustomed effort, poor posture, cold, exposure to draught and muscle tension due to anxiety. No tissue changes have been shown microscopically or chemically.

Symptomatic relief is gained from: warmth; exercise, especially isometric (static) contractions; massage, including frictions; injections of local anaesthetic and analgesic or anti-inflammatory tablets. Soluble aspirin is cheap, safe and effective.

Prevention is best achieved by careful attention to warm-up and prevention of chilling during or after exercise, together with regular training to improve muscular efficiency. There is no doubt that some people are particularly sensitive to fibrositis and it may occasionally be associated with gout or the rheumatic diseases. Referred pain from adjacent joints or the spinal nerves should not be overlooked as a cause of local painful muscle spasm.

Stiffness

Stiffness in the muscles, as well as the other soft tissues in the locomotor system – tendons, ligaments and joint capsules – may be due to unaccustomed exercise. In the untrained, any strenuous effort may cause stiffness in the stressed muscles; in trained athletes, overload is the key factor especially relative to the athlete's prevailing state of preparation. Changes of training type or running surface may induce stiffness although the actual exercise load is not increased. The same predisposing factors as for cramp and fibrositis may play a part: rarely, gout or rheumatic disease is a causative factor. Some individuals are more prone to stiffness and the severity as well as the tendency to suffer increase with age, it being common to suffer more severe stiffness for a longer period after exertion with increasing age.

The causes of stiffness are not clear. The main competing theories concern micro-trauma and metabolic factors. The micro-trauma theory suggests that minute tissue ruptures occur and cause the release of tissue chemicals, including prostaglandins, which give rise to pain and inflammation. Metabolic causes which have been postulated include local accumulation of waste products, but none has been demonstrated and the main substance, lactate, is rapidly removed. There is possible evidence of excess muscle enzyme accumulation, with some studies suggesting a link between LDH (lactic acid dehydrogenase) levels and symptoms of stiffness over several days following severe exercise. A further possibility is that in some subjects there may be an exaggerated response of the immune system to the cellular changes of exercise and increased levels of circulating immune complexes have been reported in groups of athletes.

The most effective remedy for stiffness is to train regularly and specifically for the event. Warm-up and stretching routines are important, gradual acceleration and deceleration are less liable to cause symptoms than drastic changes in pace, and avoidance of post-exercise chilling is wise. The athlete should shower and change as soon as possible after exercise – not hang around in sweaty clothing prone to drastic cooling by evaporation, especially in cool windy conditions.

Warmth relieves stiffness. Light exercise may speed recovery but many subjects cannot train when stiff and find that further exercise merely increases symptoms. In this case rest for one or more days is necessary.

Drugs should be avoided in the long term because stiffness is a reflection of incorrect training which is easily amenable to correction without chemical interference. Acute distress can be relieved by soluble aspirin or any other anti-inflammatory medication. Muscle relaxants and tranquillizers may be helpful and, paradoxically, either hot soaks or cold showers help many victims. Locally applied counter-irritant preparations, such as oil of wintergreen or rubefacient ointment, have a time-honoured place in sports therapy. Alcohol has conflicting actions; it may cause beneficial relaxation, or it may increase leg symptoms by causing tissue congestion.

17 Tendon injury

Tendons connect the contracting muscles to the bone which is being moved. They have a sparse blood supply and metabolism but, due to compactly aligned collagen fibres, have a high tensile strength. Tendons have limited elasticity and loss of this with age predisposes to injury. Most tendons have a fibrous sheath containing synovial fluid as a lubricant which allows free sliding movement. The body's two largest tendons, the Achilles and the patellar, do not have such a sheath and present slightly different medical problems. Tendon injuries cause pain on movement, in the line of the tendon. Serious injury may rupture a tendon, more commonly inflammation occurs.

Tendinitis

Tendinitis is the simplest injury, consisting only of slight pain on movement and tenderness on being touched. This is a common response to unaccustomed or excessive exertion and usually settles within a day or two with no special treatment *apart from rest.*

Tenosynovitis

Tenosynovitis occurs in injury or some rheumatic diseases, for instance as 'trigger finger' with localized inflammation on the flexor tendons, or spontaneously arising in the wrist extensor tendons (De Quervain's disease). Tenosynovitis is usually a response to overuse, industrial, domestic or athletic, and the cause is obvious. The affected tendon is swollen, tender, crepitant and extremely painful on movement. Examples include the forearm tendons in canoeists or racquet players, the tibialis posterior or the toe extensors in runners, and the peroneal tendons rubbing against the boots of fell-walkers.

Rest is the correct immediate treatment and rapidly relieves symptoms. Simple padding, strapping or splinting may be highly effective. Relief of pressure points, such as keeping shoe-backs away from the ankle, may bring dramatic relief. Ice treatment is simple and effective. More resistant cases may be treated by ultrasound, steroid injection or, very rarely, by surgical decompression of a badly scarred tendon sheath.

Peritendinitis

Peritendinitis is the equivalent condition of the major tendons which have no clear-cut lubricated sheath. The soft tissues around the Achilles and the patellar tendons may become chafed by constant pressure or use so that there is inflammation and obstruction to the free movement of the tendon.

For example, unaccustomed running may cause inflammation of the soft tissues round the Achilles tendon at the heel. This is often worsened by the pressure of a high shoe-back pressing into the tendon during the take-off phase of running when the foot thrusts down into the full plantarflexion (*Figure 17.1*).

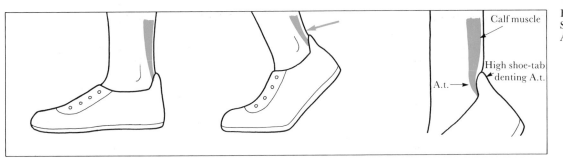

Figure 17.1
Shoe-tab pressure on
Achilles tendon

Total rupture

Total rupture of tendons is unusual. It may happen to the finger extensors in some rheumatic conditions. Traumatic avulsion of a tendon may occur, for instance at the base of the terminal phalanx in 'mallet finger', caused by a ball's striking the outstretched fingertip, where the extensor mechanism is distrupted and the terminal phalanx held flexed (*see Figure 21.16*). More dramatic ruptures occasionally occur at the major tendons. For instance, the patellar tendon may be forcefully disrupted during a football tackle, a violent thrust at squash, or a jump or landing. The Achilles tendon may rupture spontaneously at any age or during athletic activities, particularly during a sudden or violent change of pace. It is particularly liable to occur when footing is lost, as in treading awkwardly onto a kerb. The diagnosis of total rupture is usually self-evident. Major disability is obvious and the affected tendon simply does not work. While prompt strapping and splinting is usually satisfactory for the 'mallet finger' type of injury, surgical repair is usually necessary for major tears. There is no doubt that a functionally satisfactory result may be gained by simple plaster immobilization of Achilles tendon rupture but the time scale required for this and the final functional strength of recovery are unacceptable for athletes and the sooner surgical repair is carried out, the better the result.

Partial rupture

Partial rupture of a major tendon is quite common. Total rupture of the Achilles tendon is accompanied by a sensation of 'snapping' and pain, together with total loss of Achilles function such as tip-toeing and thrusting. Partial rupture, however, often produces a similar pain and snap but with the Achilles tendon intact on examination. Lesser cases are associated with pain and a weakness in thrusting the foot during running. Careful palpation may show a localized tender lump on the Achilles tendon which tends to move between the examining fingers as the ankle is gently flexed up and down through its full range of movement. Soft-tissue X-ray may confirm the classic appearance and in the young and active patient surgery is indicated without further delay. Older and less impetuous patients may, however, be willing to accept a prolonged spell of restricted activity rather than surgery. Many veteran athletes have returned successfully to long-distance running after a partial Achilles tendon rupture followed by between 6 and 12 months of avoidance of running, followed by careful return to progressive training loads. There is no evidence that any type of physiotherapy or drug treatment is useful in this condition but surgery gives good, quick results. Only occasionally is the rupture so complicated that an elaborate plastic repair operation is required and although this may jeopardize full recovery the needs of daily living activities are able to be met.

Focal degeneration

Focal degeneration lies between tendinitis and the tendon ruptures. Repeated overloading of the tendon leads to disruption of collagen fibre alignment with development of small focal areas of rupture and degeneration. These may be associated with local ischaemia (impairment of blood supply) and surrounding fibrosis and lead to more major ruptures. Focal lesions of this sort commonly occur in both the major tendons – the Achilles and the patellar ('jumper's knee'). Steroid injections into the tendon are avoided because this weakens the collagen and predisposes to ruptures. Focal lesions respond to rest if mild or superficial but fail to settle in many intensive sportsmen. In such cases, limited surgical decompression may bring dramatic relief with quick recovery. The small necrotic focus of tissue is excised through a minimal incision, stitches are rarely required into the tendon and active rehabilitation starts at once.

Tendon insertion strains

Tendon insertion strains, where the tendon joins the bone, may cause much difficulty. For example, the wrist extensors in racquet players or the tibialis anterior or Achilles tendon insertions at the foot may be particularly difficult to treat. This is because of difficulty in localizing and diagnosing the lesion or because of the patient's failure to rest adequately during recovery. Splinting or strapping, ultrasound, ice therapy and steroid injections may all help.

Treatment

Rest is nearly always the treatment of choice for tendon injuries. Further movement increases tissue damage. Physiotherapy is unpredictable, although ultrasound and ice often help. Anti-inflammatory drugs are usually unnecessary and local steroid injections are best used in chronic well-localized lesions which have not responded to rest. Surgery is usually indicated for tendon ruptures or decompression of locally stenosed tendon sheaths.

18 Bone, joint and ligament injury

Bones

The skeleton is laid down initially as cartilage. During growth, centres of ossification appear from which the hard bony skeleton is progressively developed. During adolescence, the crucial growth phase occurs when these centres fuse with each other and the ends, or epiphyses, of the bones join up firmly to the main shafts (metaphyses) to give the final adult form. Bones consist of a dense outer calcified cortex and a soft inner medulla which contains the bone marrow. X-rays of long bones look like white tubes because of the thicker surface of cortex on each side of the bone as it is struck by the X-rays tangentially. It is often difficult to interpret X-rays in adolescence because of confusion between possible fracture lines and the incompletely fused bone ends.

Fractures (*Figure 18.1*)

Simple fractures may occur across or obliquely along the bone. They are due to direct blows or rotational forces. Greenstick fractures in children combine a fracture with some bending of the young bones. Comminuted fractures cause fragments rather than one clear break. Compound fractures involve a break in the overlying skin, for instance when the footballer's tibia comes through his shin. These injuries are liable to infection, especially from the soil of sports fields.

Fractures are X-rayed to establish the extent of the break and then treated by manipulative reduction to the correct alignment and immobilization, usually for several weeks, in a plaster cast. Some minor fractures, e.g. fingers, are held by strapping, while some major ones are kept in traction frames to hold the new bone at full length. Many unstable fractures can be internally fixed surgically by pins, nails, screws or plates. On rare occasions, to accelerate healing a simple fracture is held firmly together by compression plating and screws. Recently, electrical stimulation of slow healing or ununited fractures has been introduced using implanted or surface electrodes.

Fractures take from 4–6 weeks up to several months to heal. Callus is laid down at the fracture site and then gradually remodelled towards the original shape. A period of functional rehabilitation after healing is essential because the affected limb becomes considerably weakened by immobilization. A fracture site may ache for years after recovery due to remodelling but this does not preclude full athletic activity once the initial healing is complete.

Opinion varies about the wisdom of the resumption of contact sports by sportsmen with metallic plates and screws still in place. In practice, the sportsman should make it clear to his surgeon that he is intending to pursue contact sports, so that a full appraisal of each case can be made.

It is sometimes difficult to diagnose fractures early, particularly in busy casualty departments where acute injuries are readily dismissed if there is an apparently normal X-ray. The scaphoid fracture at the wrist is the best known diagnostic catch, where

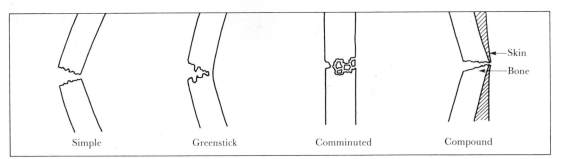

Figure 18.1
Fractures

Simple   Greenstick   Comminuted   Compound

Skin
Bone

initial X-ray of the sprained wrist is normal, only to be followed some weeks later by the appearance of an obviously necrotic area in this bone.

Stress fractures

Stress fractures are the characteristic occupational hazards of the sporting bone. These are analogous to the metal fatigue which occurs in aircraft wings. Stereotyped movements put very localized stresses on a bone which finally cracks. At the same time, this tiny crack starts trying to heal itself. The characteristic 'crescendo' pain, related to the sporting movement, comes on sooner and more severely in each session as time goes on, lasting longer after each session eventually to become continuous. Initially, X-ray is often normal (*Figure 18.2*). Later, it shows callus formation at the edge of the cortex where healing starts to occur. If the early history and X-rays are ignored, a stress fracture may progress to comminution without warning. For this reason, a typical history and tenderness over the affected bone should lead to at least 3 weeks of rest from sporting activity, regardless of the X-ray findings. In this way, an initial brief rest, followed by a gradual reintroduction to training loads, may achieve full recovery without risk.

The commonest sites of stress fracture are in the metatarsal bones of the mid-foot, the fibula just above the outer side of the ankle, and the tibial shaft where there may be confusion with shin soreness. Less

frequently, stress fractures may occur elsewhere in the foot, in the femur, ischium, spine or elbow. The usual treatment required is simply 3–6 weeks' avoidance of the provocative stereotyped sports movement. Other sports training or activities are usually possible and immobilization may be indicated only for the untrustworthy patient!

The patient should be warned that symptoms usually subside within about 10 days when there is an obvious temptation to resume sport. This usually brings the symptoms right back.

Tomography is another useful X-ray technique in which a number of views of the affected bone are taken at slightly different angles to give a more three-dimensional picture which may show irregularities.

If plain X-rays are repeatedly normal in the face of a strong clinical history and bony tenderness on examination, radioisotope scanning techniques may be used. A small amount of radioactive substance is taken by the patient and then concentrated in the bone. Areas of excessive bone cell activity such as fractures or incipient fractures show up readily on the radioactive bone scan picture produced and these may confirm the diagnosis. This technique is not dangerous because only minute doses of short-lasting isotope are used.

While most stress fractures heal uneventfully, allowing resumption of full training within 3–6 weeks, some athletes do not heal quickly and it may sometimes take up to a year for full healing – the reason for this delay is not known. Occasionally the

Figure 18.2
Progression of stress
fracture as shown on X-ray

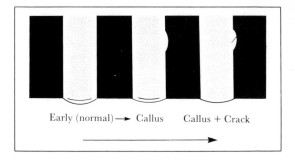

Early (normal) → Callus   Callus + Crack

fracture gap becomes filled with dense scar tissue which does not calcify properly to heal as bone. The surgeon can drill this fracture to revitalize the area which can then proceed on its original healing path.

Joints

Bones join each other at joints which can be of very different shape, depending on the function at each site. For instance, the ball and socket type of joint is almost completely round at the hip but at the shoulder, where a greater range of movement is required, the socket is incomplete. There are hinge joints such as the elbow or ankle which can also allow very complex further combinations of movements such as glidings and rotations of adjacent bones. Such versatility, for instance, allows the forearm to rotate about its hinge movement, or the foot to shock-absorb and rotate on uneven ground about is simple ankle hinge movement.

Joints such as those at the ribs or collar bone connect and stabilize adjacent parts of the body and have a simpler structure with a small cartilage plate between the bone ends.

The sacroiliac joints are elaborately interdigitated like jig-saw puzzles and, while allowing some 'give', are virtually impossible to disrupt.

Synovial membrane lines the joints and secretes the lubricating and nutrient synovial fluid. The bone ends in the joint are lined with cartilage which is also nourished from within the bone and slides against the cartilage of the adjacent bone in the joint. Some joints contain additional internal cartilages which add to the stability and padding of the joint and these cartilages often give rise to disabling symptoms by forced displacement, for instance in the knee.

Joints have a firm fibrous capsule which contains the fluid and synovium and is reinforced and stabilized by closely applied ligaments, which are tough bands of condensed collagen. In the knee, there are internally placed ligaments and the general stability of many joints is further enhanced by the muscles and tendons which run past the joint.

Joint injury

Direct blows may cause simple bruising in or around joints.

Sprains are stretching injuries caused to the joint structures. The capsule, lining and adjacent ligaments can all be damaged. A synovial effusion causes pain and swelling due to tension caused in the joint by excess synovial fluid secreted by the lining. A haemarthrosis, or bleeding into the joint due to tearing of blood vessels in the joint structures, is always painful and serious.

It may be difficult to know if effusions are clear or bloody, or if haemarthrosis is due to a fracture in the joint. Needle aspiration and X-ray of the joint are helpful in making an accurate diagnosis.

Arthrography is the technique of joint X-ray using injected dyes or air to produce clearer definitions on the picture (the arthrogram). Arthroscopy is the internal inspection of a joint using a small fibre-optic torch. Its advantages include the avoidance of unnecessary surgery and greater precision in diagnosis. Limited operations such as the removal of loose bodies or pieces of damaged cartilage may be performed through specially adapted arthroscopes but open operations remain essential for most serious injuries.

Joint instability

Injuries may damage the mechanical supporting structures of a joint such as ligaments or bone, or the nerve supply to the capsule. In this case the sprain heals but the nerve endings may remain damaged and give the brain false information about the joint's position and stability. The athlete feels unsure of his joint and it may 'give way' with, or without, obvious cause.

Examination may show the instability to be mechanical, e.g. due to an undiagnosed ruptured ligament which must then be repaired: or the joint may be mechanically intact, in which case remedial exercises are given to re-educate the athlete's nerve endings as with the wobble board in the rehabilitation of the sprained ankle (*see Figure 26.6*).

Arthritis

Normal use and sporting activity preserve joint structure and function in the long term. Exercise by itself does not increase the chance of arthritis in later life. Active joint movement encourages joint nutrition and lubrication and thus preserves good function. Severe or neglected joint injuries do, however, predispose to later life arthritis and the immediate diagnosis and efficient management of all joint injuries is vital.

Treatment

Serious joint injury has to be rested, usually with strapping and supporting splints. Sometimes a short spell of plaster-cast immobilization is necessary to allow inflammation to settle. Aspiration of tense effusions eases pain. Analgesic and anti-inflammatory drugs relieve symptoms. Physiotherapy aims to restore uninhibited movement patterns by progressive resisted exercise and uses ice, heat, or ultrasound to relieve pain.

Manipulation is sometimes used after joint injury or surgery. The aim is to tear small fibrous adhesions which bind the synovium and thereby inhibit movement. If a joint is manipulated, this must be followed with active exercise to capitalize on the improved range of movement.

19 Principles of treatment

In severe injury, the player must be removed from the game. Some damage may have been overlooked, for instance more serious brain injury in the concussed player, and further harm may occur. In soft-tissue injuries, further haemorrhage and tissue damage may prolong disability. The injured player is not likely to be of much use to his team while hobbling about and rules allowing substitutes should prevent further injury to the player without penalizing his team.

Minor soft-tissue injuries

Immediate assessment of the player may show that a minor knock has been sustained from which there will be rapid functional recovery within minutes, safely allowing further play. Many minor injuries cause momentary pain due to direct contusion of tissue but the pain wears off rapidly. With other injuries, the pain eases off with continued exercise but then returns after the game. The cause of muscle 'stiffness' is uncertain but probably includes minor muscle tears which result in aching and stiffness after play. Bleeding must be stopped and wounds cleaned and dressed as soon as possible to reduce haemorrhage or infection. Medical opinion is divided on the correct time and place for stitching skin wounds, particularly in respect of return to play. It is recognized that the provision of some wound repair may fall to paramedical personnel, for instance during touring where qualified medical help may not be readily available. This is the exception rather than the rule.

Nevertheless, therapists should remember their legal obligations and liabilities and unduly strident critics should remember that much stitching is done in British hospitals by non-medically qualified staff.

The first principle in the management of minor sports injuries is to minimize the tissue damage in the first 24 hours. The principles of rest, ice, compression and elevation (R–I–C–E, *see* page 136) are all aimed at reducing further haemorrhage and tissue exudation. This allows a firm sealing of blood clots to form which thus provides the basis for sound tissue healing over the next couple of weeks. Cold applications are safest and most effective. Cold running water, cold-water-soaked towelling, ice cubes or chemical ice packs are all effective.

Ice should not be applied directly to the skin because of the possibility of ice burns. A layer of damp towelling is a simple precaution, a further layer of towelling can contain the ice around the limb and the application of ice may usually last about 10–20 min per session.

Commercially available cooling sachets are effective but relatively expensive; they consist of two separated chemical components which are shaken vigorously together to release a cooling reaction which is then applied within the supplied package to the affected part.

Massage and tissue manipulations are strictly forbidden at this stage as the intention is to spare the tissues from further mechanical forces liable to cause further tissue disruption. Analgesic and anti-inflammatory pills may be helpful. There is evidence that anti-inflammatory drugs taken within the first 3 days after injury may increase comfort and accelerate return to full activity. The more powerful drugs are available only on prescription but soluble aspirin remains both highly effective and cheap and is available 'over the counter'. The chief disadvantage of aspirin is its tendency to cause indigestion but this effect is minimized if taken dissolved in water. Aspirin should not be taken together with alcohol. A daily dose of up to six or eight soluble tablets (up to 4 g) for 2 or 3 days is usually both effective and safe.

Some enzyme preparations which aim to dissipate the inflammatory products released by injury and promote healing are available on prescription. Trials have remained inconclusive but there are strong claims that the prophylactic use of enzymes may reduce the amount of bruising in boxing where multiple contests are necessary in many competitions and otherwise successful boxers have often to drop out because of bruises sustained in an earlier victory.

A number of creams and ointments are claimed to accelerate the healing of soft-tissue injuries but these are, again, extremely difficult to assess in trials.

After the first 24 hours the principle of rehabilitation is one of progressive resisted exercise. While the initial damage and pain may restrict movement, it is important to re-establish a full range of movement at each affected joint as soon as possible and this is done by gentle movement of the affected limb by patient, coach or therapist. These movements are repeated several times daily and at the same time static contractions of the muscles are started. Such movements restore tone to the affected muscles and start bracing the limb and joints in preparation for active movement.

Active movements are encouraged within as wide a range as the pain allows. Thereafter the range and power of active movement is increased until the point comes when there is no difference between the remedial exercise and the active movement of training.

Physiotherapy

Both physiotherapy and training are based on progressive resisted muscular exercise. All other modalities of physiotherapy treatment are concerned with facilitating these active movements. In all controlled trials, advantages have been shown where early exercise has followed injury or surgery. Muscle bulk and function declines rapidly with rest or immobilization.

Heat

Whilst cold packs create analgesic and relaxant effects, heat, from all sources, is used to encourage relaxation prior to active movements. Radiant or infra-red heat from lamps warms the superficial tissues directly. However, a similar effect is obtained effectively and cheaply by application of hot packs or a hot water bottle. The traditional but messy kaolin poultice, cotton wool, Thermagene or extra clothing and blankets are alternative ways of applying heat.

Shortwave diathermy (SWD) uses the tissue-healing effects of a high-frequency AC current, applied by either condenser plates beside, or coils wound around, the affected area. Tissues may be heated to a depth of some 5–6 cm. SWD is especially effective in chronic soft-tissue inflammation.

Microwave exploits the heating effects of short-wavelength electromagnetic waves but does not penetrate as deeply as SWD.

Ultrasound

Ultrasound therapy (ultrasonics, u.s.) applies mechanical energy from high-frequency sound waves, above the audible range, to the tissues. The reaction between energy waves and the different tissue planes creates a localized effect which both heats the tissues and agitates them mechanically. Ultrasound stimulates the formation of fibrous tissue and must be correctly applied through a properly tuned machine.

Pulsed electromagnetic energy (e.g. Curapulse,

Diapulse) produces tissue heating and mechanical effects, the pulsed application allowing a higher dosage to be used than with continuous treatments. These machines are expensive and their benefits still uncertain compared to those of other modalities of treatment.

Electrical stimulation

Faradism and galvanism involve direct electrical stimulation of the muscles during their re-education. However, electrical stimulus is no substitute for natural exercise of the muscle itself under voluntary control. There are many occasions where injury leads to considerable lack of confidence and co-ordination of muscular movements, and a short course of faradism may be invaluable in re-educating confidence and neuromuscular control. Particular applications for faradism include the retraining of the patient to use an injured thigh muscle efficiently and the teaching of intrinsic foot muscle exercises after injury or in cases of poor foot posture.

Electrical devices are commercially available in the form of vibrators and stimulators. Low-voltage electrical stimulation of the tissues creates a tonic feeling accompanied by relaxation. Whether this does full justice to the case for vibrators is uncertain. A number of simple faradic machines are sold as pulsators or transcutaneous nerve stimulators (TNS machines). These have simple electrode attachments and can be strapped or placed over the various muscles to provide a modest electrically induced contraction as required. Although these have a limited but useful place in muscle and nerve home re-education programmes, they are not substitutes for professional rehabilitation programmes. The use of transcutaneous nerve stimulation is well established in analgesia. A stimulating current passed over a painful area leaves an after-effect of pain relief which may last for a considerable time.

A vital point constantly to bear in mind is that no equipment is a substitute for determined self-motivated exercise programmes which alone retrain the injured tissues effectively.

Massage

Manual therapy has long held pride of place among therapists and their grateful patients. Massage may help to drain inflammatory exudate from injuries in the early stages and friction massage may help to keep the soft tissues well mobilized during later stages of healing or in chronic scarring. Much as athletes enjoy the relaxing effects of massage, however, it must be emphasized that it is a passive technique and is no substitute for either muscular training or a thorough precompetitive warm-up and active stretching of the muscles before competition. Reliance on passive warm-up or stretching is unwise because it cannot give the same degree of mechanical, vascular or biochemical preparation to the tissues for competition.

Manipulation

Other manipulative techniques are designed to free mechanical blocks in the musculoskeletal system, usually at the sites of joint injuries. There are different schools of manipulative techniques, including osteopathy, and these range from vigorous manoeuvres used by some practitioners to the gentler mobilizing techniques widely used by most physiotherapists. The advantage of gentler mobilizing manipulation is that the patient's full muscular control and co-operation is sought so that any new positional correction achieved by manipulation is well maintained each time by the patient's own muscles. More violent manipulations, particularly under anaesthetic, have the serious disadvantage of pushing the body into a new position but not necessarily creating soft-tissue control of the newly gained position, with the result that many patients initially relieved by manipulation then relapse. Again, manipulations are not a substitute for conscientious exercise programmes. Joint mobility in the athlete can only be gained by long-term mobility exercises, never by the short-term expedient of overstretch. The temptation to compete soon after a manipulation should always be resisted because of the potential temporary short-fall in muscular control of the joint range.

Traction

Traction is widely used by physiotherapists through a collar on the neck or corset on the lower back for cases of disc prolapse. Traction has been shown to stretch the spine and pull back extruded intervertebral discs towards their proper resting place, thus relieving pressure on the adjacent spinal nerve roots.

Traction is also widely used as an effective non-specific treatment in chronic backache without signs of nerve pressure. This is because many people suffer backache due to damage to the intervertebral discs which does not show up on normal X-rays or go so far as to cause pressure on adjacent nerves. Also, traction often has a non-specific pain-relieving effect when applied to any tissues. Traction should always be followed by a supervised programme of remedial exercise. No attempt should be made at active sport, particularly weight-training, until full recovery has been reached.

Surgery

More complex treatment may be required in some soft-tissue injuries. Scarring after an injury may be so great that the surgeon has to remove some tissue obstruction to allow recovery of full movement. For instance, massive scars in the thigh or hamstring may so tether the muscle that it cannot move freely to full range. Excision of the scar tissue or associated cysts is necessary to untether the muscle which can then recover satisfactorily. Occasionally, adolescent avulsion injuries may not progress satisfactorily without operative repair. In chronic tenosynovitis, localized decompression of scar tissue in a tendon

sheath is often effective. When all else has failed, the technique can, for instance, be used in the forearm extensor muscles in for example canoeists or racquet players.

Steroid injection

Steroid injections have a prominent place in sport therapy. Most soft-tissue injuries recover completely given sufficient time and full functional recovery is almost invariably the rule in the general population. In sport, however, the time scale and intensity of movement required in training and competition may be such as to justify attempts to accelerate the natural time scale and seek therapeutic short-cuts. Some doctors are notoriously quick on the draw with steroid injections but there are certain well-established indications for this therapy. Steroid injections consist of one of the synthetic cortisone derivatives such as hydrocortisone, methylprednisolone, or triamcinolone, usually mixed with a local anaesthetic. This has the twin effect of easing the patient's distress at once and confirming to the doctor that the correct area has been effectively infiltrated. Occasionally a spreading agent, hyaluronic acid (Hyalase), is mixed into the syringe. This is best reserved for cases of chronic scarring because Hyalase helps to break down adhesions, but allergic reactions are possible since Hyalase is derived from animal proteins.

The aim of the steroid injection is to deliver the anti-inflammatory steroid precisely to the point of a clearly defined injury. The more accurately the injection is made, the better are the results. Good results are often obtained by injecting localized inflammations in ligaments or on tendons. Disappointment often follows widespread indiscriminate infiltration of whole areas.

The best results from steroid injections often occur in chronic soft-tissue injuries where physiotherapy has failed. Injections are particularly effective at the musculoperiosteal origin of muscles, for instance at the elbow in 'tennis elbow' or the upper shin in some cases of shin soreness, or at the distal insertion of the tendons, for instance at the wrist or foot. They are also highly effective in chronic ligament strains. Chronic tenosynovitis, e.g. in the forearm extensors, often responds well and bursitis, such as sub-acromial bursitis at the shoulder, or calcaneal bursitis at the heel, often responds dramatically.

Contraindications to injection

Injections should not be given if there is diagnostic doubt or if there is infection present.

Injections should not be made shortly before competition, because the therapeutic disturbance of tissues, together with the possible loss of natural pain inhibition, invites further injury, commonly increasing a partial ligament tear into a more drastic rupture.

Injections should not normally be made into weight-bearing joints of otherwise fit but impatient young sportsmen. There is controversy about the long-term consequences to cartilage of steroid injection and a possibility that some injected joints will disintegrate rapidly and unexpectedly. There is also a small chance of introducing infection. Injection of the joint may mean that inflammation has been temporarily suppressed but the surrounding joint capsule, lining and ligaments may not yet be ready to take up a full load.

The fitness test

The final step in treatment is the fitness test. This consists of full functional testing with particular attention being paid to the movements required for sport. It is no use seeing that a young man can jog happily out of the therapeutic gymnasium and declaring him fit for a game of football! Each relevant muscle, limb and movement pattern should be tested before training is allowed. There is no single fitness test but a series of progressive fitness assessments at each stage of recovery. Medical rehabilitation becomes training at a certain point of exercise intensity. Beyond that point it becomes progressive training. After the final assessment and survival of full training it becomes match fitness. Anything less than this increases the risk of further injury. It is utterly reprehensible to abuse the substitution rule, as for instance in soccer when a partly fit player is allowed to hobble on for part of the game just to see how he gets on. This still happens at international level.

20 Head and neck injuries

The head may suffer dramatic injuries from blows during contact sports or from balls or equipment. Neck injuries are most often caused by forcible strains such as diving or tackling with the head bent.

Knock-outs

Unconsciousness is usually very brief in sport but the concussion may cause confusion, disorientation and impaired judgement for some time afterwards. The classic example is of the rugby player who successfully completes the match after a knock without any subsequent recollection. Responsible medical opinion is unanimous that any loss of consciousness whatsoever should oblige a player to leave the field and abandon that game. Minor degrees of concussion without loss of consciousness may be acceptable for further play provided that the patient is not disorientated and has no headache, blurring of vision or amnesia.

Rarely, and extremely dangerously, temporary recovery may follow a blow to the head only to be followed after a 'lucid interval' by the onset of unconsciousness due to an extradural haemorrhage, usually from the middle meningeal artery in the temporal area over the ear. Any player suffering a knock-out should therefore be observed during the following hours.

A general consensus is that brief unconsciousness should disqualify from contact sport for a month and a more prolonged knock-out for perhaps 2 months.

Boxing is unique in that a major aim is to inflict brain damage, although in the amateur sport the risks of short- and long-term sequelae may be diminished by strict medical examinations and control.

In the past, boxers often developed the 'punch-drunk' syndrome of traumatic encephalopathy, with its characteristic slowness, aggressive behaviour, intellectual and behavioural deterioration, slurring and dementia. This is due to repeated subcortical haemorrhages in the brain and is associated not with the occasional knock-out but with many years of repeated lesser blows to the head. While the amateur regulations should do much to abolish this in future, compulsory headguards would do even more and, from a medical point of view, there is no reason why professional boxers should not also be entitled to long-term mental protection – whatever the blood lusts of the crowd may dictate. A similar 'punch drunk' syndrome can occur from any cause of repeated head blows such as heading of the ball at football, but while head- and neck ache are well known in this sport, there no clear descriptions of such long-term victims, because of the lesser decelerative forces in the more controlled head and neck movements.

Whenever loss of consciousness occurs, two actions are essential. First, the game must be stopped and the player cleared of all obstructions. Secondly, his airway must be secured.

The type of blow and duration of unconsciousness give some idea of the seriousness. The degree of amnesia, loss of memory, later elicited is a further indication of damage. During unconsciousness a dilated pupil indicates serious injury. Unconsciousness which lasts more than a few seconds, any deterioration in consciousness, or any change in condition such as dilatation of a pupil or any seizure or fit are extremely serious and need urgent hospital care.

The appropriate helmet or headgear should always be worn as a routine. There are circumstances where long hair can be undesirable, particularly where rapid blows or changes in direction of vision occur and a cap or hair restraint is an essential safety device. In cricket it is regarded as poor sportsmanship to use the ample supplies of hair grease in long hair for shining up the ball. On the other hand, in swimming total baldness has been exploited as a hydrodynamic aid.

Chewing gum

It cannot be too strongly emphasized that under no circumstances should chewing gum be used on any field of play. Whatever the popularity of this habit, it must be brought home to the playing public by constant education that several deaths occur each year because sports injuries are complicated by asphyxia due to inhaled chewing gum. The chewing gum kills in a possibly trivial injury or greatly complicates a serious one. This also applies to referees who have choked and suffocated without a tackle!

Eyes

Direct injury

The eyes are well protected by the overhanging bones of the orbit. Despite spectacular bruising, serious injuries are relatively infrequent. The most dangerous ones occur if a small ball fits into the orbit to put pressure on the whole eye socket. Squash balls are notorious for this because of their compressibility. A 'blow out' injury is caused when the ball pushes the eyeball inwards, with explosive displacement downwards of some of the fat padding the floor of the orbit (*Figure 20.1*). This leaves the eye looking retracted (enophthalmic) and the patient may complain of double vision. Scratches from fingernails or more major objects such as racquets may seriously damage the surface of the eye and cause rupture.

If there is any major blow, or any sudden failure of vision, apply a clean pad and seek urgent hospital help.

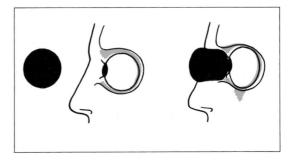

Figure 20.1
Impact of squash ball on orbit. The eyeball is compressed and fat forced through the floor of the orbit, rupturing it

Conjunctivitis

'Pink eye' or conjunctivitis may be due to infection, allergy or chemical irritation, particularly in swimmers. Allergy may be associated with other signs of hay fever such as seasonal catarrh and may need medication. Infective 'pink eye' may be due to skin infection elsewhere, or the spread of infected matter, for example on towels, and usually responds quickly to antibiotic eye drops. Chemical irritation may be due to unacceptable treatment of the swimming pool and the best remedy is to wear protective goggles.

Lenses

While most games can be played by people of widely varying eyesight, any vigorous sport should call for the wearing of unbreakable glasses and lenses. In the body contact sports this is not practicable and soft contact lenses should be considered, although these will obviously be expensive.

It is not wise for people with particularly short sight (myopia) to risk further eye trauma as this predisposes to detachment of the retina with further serious risk to vision.

Nose

Nose-bleed is stopped in an upright position by firm nasal pressure from pinching and with the application of cold. Nasal fractures, which may be caused by relatively light blows, are diagnosed by displacement of the central bone. Gentle manipulation of the nose back to the midline is permissible but there is seldom much to be done in the sports arena. Prolonged nose-bleeding can be staunched by packing the nostril with clean dressings.

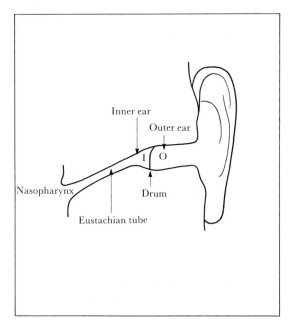

Figure 20.2
Normal ear; the drum separates the pressures of the inner ear (I) from those of the outer ear (O). Normally I = O

Ear

'Cauliflower ear'

'Cauliflower ear' is caused by the rapid formation of a bruise in the loose tissue between the cartilage and the skin of the ear. A direct hit or a grinding impact such as in a rugby scrum has this effect. The rapid swelling is trapped in the soft tissue and, unless it is surgically evacuated, scars to give the characteristic deformity. Early aspiration with needle or knife is simple and should be followed by firm compression bandaging.

Pressure damage

The ear is more seriously threatened by pressure damage, or barotrauma. The ear consists of an ear drum attached to the hearing apparatus with air at equal pressure on each side of the drum. Externally lies the atmosphere; internally the Eustachian tube leads to the back of the nasopharynx (*Figure 20.2*). Normally, any change in pressure such as moving in a lift or landing in an aeroplane is rapidly equalized by chewing, swallowing, yawning or similar actions by which the Eustachian mechanism matches the external air pressure on the ear drum.

Under some circumstances, the free exchange of air is impaired with pressure differences liable to cause injury, or barotrauma. In outer-ear barotrauma, a tightly worn diving hood, for example, causes artificial restriction of air movement and pressure in the outer ear. This may cause discomfort and blood blistering in the ear canal. Although this is not serious, it would be wise to insert a hole or a valve in the ear hood so that the pressure on the ear could be neutralized (*Figure 20.3*).

In otitic barotrauma ('the squeeze'), the outside air pressure rises, as in an aeroplane descent, and if the Eustachian tube does not allow equalization of pressure, earache results (*Figure 20.4*). If this pressure increases, small haemorrhages occur into the middle ear and the drum may burst as may also happen in diving at only about 3 m depth. Eustachian block is usually due to catarrh and decongestant medication may be necessary. In severe colds it is unwise to dive because of the associated Eustachian block.

Inner-ear barotrauma may occur in scuba divers or in marksmen where the positioning of the gun near the ear may create deafness due to sudden noise impact. Effective ear-muffs are available.

While it is uncommon for wax, which is a normal protective secretion in the ears, to give rise to hearing difficulties, sportsmen in the stress of competition sometimes become anxious about this. Simple syringing or solvent drops may be required.

Chronic external otitis is a common infection in swimmers. Antibiotics and ear drops may be necessary. Protective ear-plugs may be helpful in preventing recurrences.

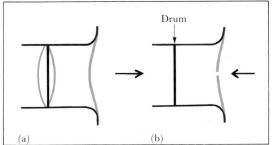

Figure 20.3
Outer ear barotrauma. (a) Tight membrane of diving hood stops free pressure equalization. (b) Prevention by perforation of hood

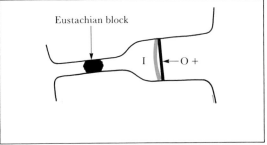

Figure 20.4
Otitic barotrauma: 'the squeeze'. Outside air pressure rises but a blocked Eustachian tube prevents free equalization of pressure, O>I

Teeth

Teeth may be broken by direct blows which may also cause adjacent jaw fracture. A dislodged tooth may occasionally be replaced intact in the socket and survive but, in the event of contact with the ground, tetanus toxoid should be given. Serious facial or dental injury needs specialist medical help as soon as possible. The healing power of the facial bones is good and contact sport can usually be resumed after healing, even though complex surgery and wiring may be required.

Spectacular reductions were made in the incidence of injury and cost of dental treatment in American football after the introduction of dental guards. These have the dual advantages of preserving teeth and acting as shock-absorbers of concussive blows to the jaw. Various gum-shields can be bought but the best fit and protection is gained when the shield is custom-moulded by a dental surgeon for the individual player. As a considerable number of schoolboy teeth are lost each year at rugby and soccer, dental shields should be more widely appreciated and used at all levels of contact sport by players of all ages and in all positions.

Neck

The neck is particularly vulnerable to injury because of its extreme mobility. It can be sprained by vigorous pulls to the side or when forced sharply forwards or backwards into flexion or extension. Notorious causes of severe neck injury include diving into shallow (or no) water, rugby tackling and having the neck forcefully bent in the middle of a scrum which is being collapsed. In this case the player's shoulders are fixed while his head is forcibly bent against his control. For this reason, the ploy of deliberately 'collapsing the scrum' has been outlawed in rugby.

Paraplegia

Because the entire nerve supply to the body passes down the neck, this area is uniquely vulnerable to spinal cord trauma which may lead to complete paralysis, or paraplegia. If the player has been felled, possibly unconscious, it may be difficult to assess accurately the full extent of tissue damage. The general alignment of the neck may be bizarre and indicate major fracture or dislocation.

The inability to feel or move any part of the body draws attention immediately to neck injury. If there is any doubt about this possibility, two steps are essential. First, the game must be removed from the player and, if necessary, abandoned. Secondly, the player should not be moved inexpertly. While the ambulance is awaited, the player's neck should be immobilized, if necessary with clothes or blankets, and any movement onto a stretcher should be effected only in the most gentle manner with an adequate number of people taking the body and limbs together, while the most expert person gently supports and slightly pulls on the head. In this way any tendency to aggravate an unstable fracture or dislocation with tissue damage in the neck is minimized.

The veteran club-rugby player becomes generally less fit and more stiff with age and is thus particularly vulnerable to neck sprains. Such sprains cause considerable local tissue damage with arm symptoms due to spinal cord or brachial plexus injury. Because the risks of recurrence remain high, it is a wise precaution for such a player to abandon active rugby for he is unprotected by satisfactory flexibility in his upper trunk and neck.

Low neck pain in the sportsman may be due to structural abnormality of the cervical spine which may lead to asymmetry and poor mobility which, in turn, predispose to ligamentous strains in the neck. Occasionally, an extra rudimentary rib or band of fibrous tissue may be present and press upon some of the soft-tissue structures including the nerves as they leave the cervical spine to make up the brachial plexus supplying the arm. Symptoms may be felt as a tingling or discomfort in the upper limb rather than simply as neck pain and may be reproduced by gentle traction downwards on the arm. Symptoms are more likely in older people but poor upper-body posture at any age allows sagging of the soft tisues with traction on the nerves. Remedial exercises are highly effective.

21 Arm injuries

Shoulder

The shoulder is a ball and socket joint between the shallow glenoid of the scapula and the round upper head of the humerus (*Figure 21.1*); it is inherently unstable. The joint is supported by the many overlying muscles and tendons.

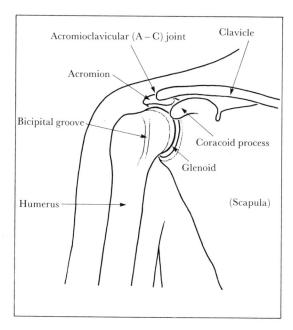

Acromioclavicular (A – C) joint

Clavicle

Acromion

Bicipital groove

Coracoid process

Glenoid

Humerus

(Scapula)

Acromioclavicular (A–C) joint

The A–C joint is easily sprained by direct blows such as rugby tackles or a fall on to the point of the shoulder. While the majority are minor, a few sprains disrupt the joint which, if it fails to heal rapidly, leaves the sportsman with a painful and unstable joint with the characteristic 'step' deformity (*Figure 21.2*). For this reason, the sprained A–C joint should be taken seriously, especially in contact sport or weight-lifting where future stability is required. Firm strapping or bracing should be applied early and sport should be avoided until the pain has subsided. An unstable A–C joint may prevent full weight-training and tends to suffer recurrent painful sprains. Therefore, if function remains impaired after several weeks, surgical fixation of an unstable A–C joint is highly desirable.

Clavicle

The clavicle, or collar bone, is commonly broken in falls onto the shoulder. Rarely, there are serious complications if a fragment either pierces the subclavian artery (*Figure 21.3*) and causes haemorrhage or causes brachial plexus nerve damage. Usually a firm strapping is applied to the broken clavicle to brace the shoulders back and achieve a position of comfort as well as sound healing, but this is discarded as soon as pain permits.

Dislocation of shoulder

Shoulder dislocation is common. Forced movements, particularly when the arm is in an unstable position rotated or held out sideways, are likely to dislodge the head of the humerus. Recurrent dislocation can also be due to a slight fault in formation of the top of the humerus or glenoid rim. If its contour is a little flatter than usual, the top is less likely to stay in the glenoid socket of the scapula whose firm cartilage rim reaches out beyond the inner bony portion.

With a dislocation there is, in most cases, pain and obvious distortion of the shoulder shape, although pain and inability to move may sometimes be the only signs. It is difficult to diagnose a fracture of the head or neck of the humerus without X-rays. Unskilled attempts to manipulate the joint should not be tried in case a broken bone is displaced onto adjacent nerves or arteries.

In non-contact or recurrent dislocation, however, prompt reduction is often possible, even by the patient. The arm is lifted sideways 20 degrees and rotated outwards before being brought back to the trunk and rotated inwards (Kocher's manoeuvre). Alternatively, traction can be applied to the arm with the patient lying down. The arm is gently pulled against counter-pressure in the axilla. A sling is worn for about 3 weeks to secure healing of the glenoid rim before exercising.

Circumflex nerve damage is a complication of shoulder dislocation (*Figure 21.4*) and the deltoid muscle should be checked on injury and before and after any attempt at reduction.

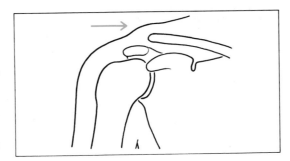

Figure 21.2
Sprained A–C joint

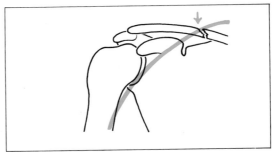

Figure 21.3
Fractured clavicle showing underlying subclavian artery

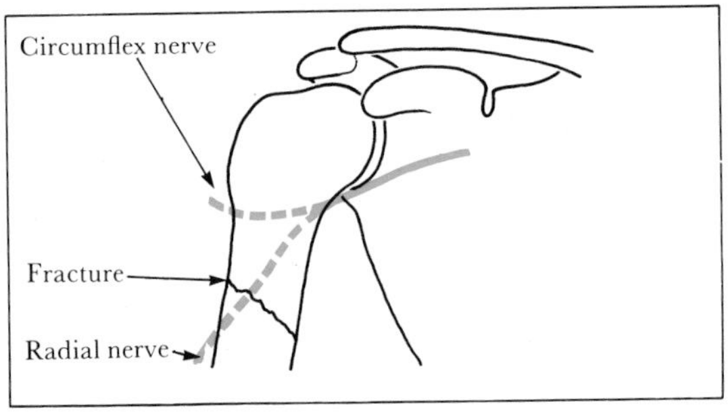

Figure 21.4
Relationship of radial and circumflex nerves to the shoulder and the shaft of the humerus

Epiphyseal damage

This is common in children where fracture-displacement of the epiphysis, or bone end, of the upper humerus occurs rather than dislocation of the shoulder joint. Epiphysitis can be caused by repeated throwing movements in the young, as in American 'Little League shoulder' from baseball pitching.

Upper-arm fractures

The humerus is normally broken by falling onto the outstretched arm. It may be difficult to distinguish between a fracture and a dislocation, hence the need for X-rays. Fractures can occur at different levels (*see Figures 21.2, 21.3 and 21.4*).

At the head of the humerus, a chip or crack may be

one of the causes of 'painful arc' but no special treatment is needed.

Fractures at the neck, just below the head, are often impacted without further displacement. A sling for comfort and early mobilization prevent stiffness. Mid-shaft fractures are difficult to immobilize with slings and splints and are potentially dangerous if spikes of bone cause damage to the radial nerve or the vessels on the inner side of the arm. These vessels supply the muscles which extend the wrist and their paralysis stops the ability to cock the wrist up, leaving wrist-drop.

Fractures at the elbow and the lower condyles of the humerus are often unstable and difficult to treat. Some, in fact, may be impossible to rehabilitate fully due to myositis ossificans (*see* Chapter 16) and/or malalignment of the fracture. In adolescents, this type of injury can involve the epiphyses, or growth plates, at the lower end of the humerus with danger to the brachial artery and ulnar nerve from displaced bone ends. Accurate surgical fixation is commonly needed.

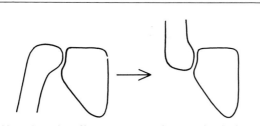

Normal rotation of humerus on scapula as arm is raised

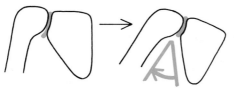

'Frozen shoulder'. No movement between humerus and scapula.
Apparent arc of movement due to rotation of both together with fixed joint

Figure 21.5
'Frozen shoulder' mechanism

Stiffness or permanent loss of some elbow movement may make full rehabilitation difficult after serious injury.

Soft-tissue injuries

A systematic examination puts the arm through its full range of movements – upwards, downwards, inwards, outwards, forwards and backwards, plus rotation – and the two sides are compared. Anatomical diagnosis depends upon the demonstration of pain related to the movements tested with or without resistance.

'Frozen shoulder' (capsulitis)

Abduction, or lifting the arm out sideways, is initiated by the supraspinatus muscle which is promptly superseded by the deltoid. This muscle takes the humerus up through the full arc of movement to the perpendicular during which the scapula stays behind (*Figure 21.5*). In the inflammatory condition of 'frozen shoulder' full movement is not possible because the scapula, fixed to the humerus, is unable to rotate fully upwards. At first the shoulder is painful and the arm cannot be lifted or rotated properly. Eventually some patients learn a 'trick movement' and can raise the arm by first swinging it forwards. This device involves the full mobilization of the scapula so that the fixed humerus and scapula move as one unit instead of separately as usual. Capsulitis may be due to falls onto the outstretched arm, or shoulder, or referred pain from neck or chest conditions, which are particularly common after coronary thrombosis. Some cases follow obvious lifting, reaching or throwing strains but many occur spontaneously.

Treatment consists of vigorous physiotherapy with the aim of mobilizing the shoulder. Anti-inflammatories and steroid injections are also widely used. However, despite such active treatment, which is often prolonged, results are uncertain and many cases remain fixed for a year or more. It is particularly important, therefore, to prevent capsulitis by mobilizing all shoulder injuries as soon as possible before secondary fixation can occur.

Even if a full range of movement cannot be regained quickly, active mobilization of the scapula and the shoulder muscles will relieve pain and restore sleep. Full movement usually returns eventually and patients should be encouraged to move the arm as much as possible.

'Painful arc' *(Figures 21.6 and 21.7)*

The 'painful arc' gives pain only through the middle part of the full arc of abduction of the humerus up to its perpendicular position. The pain is due to a limited number of conditions between the humeral head and the acromion, including supraspinatus tendinitis, calcific tendinitis, subacromial bursitis and a fine fracture at the head of the humerus.

Biceps tendinitis

At the front of the shoulder the commonest cause of pain is inflammation of the long head of the biceps tendon, or biceps tendinitis (*Figure 21.8*). The biceps tendon runs through the shoulder joint and down the bicipital groove of the humerus and is thus particularly vulnerable to fraying on vigorous rotation such as throwing or swimming. Pain is felt especially on externally rotating the abducted arm, and the so-called 'coat' pain on trying to reach back to put the arm into the coat sleeve: with females, it is painful to reach for the bra strap. Throwing and weight lifting often cause multiple strains which combine a generally sore shoulder with several different arcs of painful movement more closely related to the throwing style than to the simple anatomy. In addition, difficulty in identifying the deeper structures may be experienced because of the large overhanging deltoid muscle. Further examination may be necessary using an assistant to resist specified athletic movements from the patient, for example, throwing.

Accurate localization of diagnosis often allows

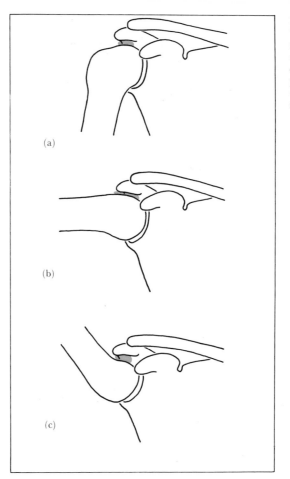

(a)

(b)

(c)

Figure 21.6
'Painful arc' mechanism. As the arm is raised from (a) to (b) the inflammation is compressed and becomes painful. Full raising from (b) to (c) decompresses with relief

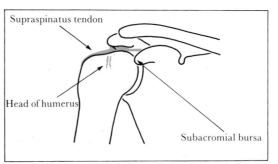

Supraspinatus tendon

Head of humerus

Subacromial bursa

Figure 21.7
Causes of 'painful arc'

Figure 21.8
Biceps muscle. (a) Normal.
(b) Long head rupture. (c)
'Popeye' deformity after
rupture

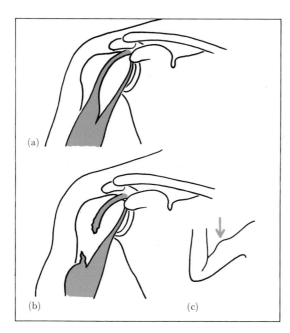

successful steroid injection but if a satisfactory anatomical diagnosis cannot be made, general treatment is indicated. Such treatment can include rest, heat or ultrasound with the use of anti-inflammatories before re-examination followed by more specific management.

Muscle injuries

'Fibrositis' is common, especially in shoulder muscles which are often stressed by violent effort. Also the pectoral muscles connecting the upper chest to the humerus can be strained during violent movement of the braced upper arm against the trunk, as for example in weight-lifting.

'Fibrositis'

This is a painful localized soft-tissue condition which is as common as it is unexplained. Small areas of painful muscle suddenly develop, most commonly in the neck, shoulder-girdle or back, often after cold exposure or unaccustomed effort. There are no biochemical findings and biopsy is negative. Like the related problem of 'stiffness', it awaits explanation.

Examination shows well-localized harder areas in muscles which are tender, and which often are very painful on pressure. Effective remedies include heat, exercise, aspirin, injections of local anaesthetic (with or without steroid), pressure and friction massage.

Biceps

The long head of the biceps can be ruptured by vigorous lifting, gymnastic movements or canoeing. Such ruptures produce the spectacular 'Popeye' deformity where subsequent contraction of the biceps raises a blob of muscle halfway down the upper arm (*Figure 21.8c*). Physiotherapy usually gives excellent results despite the alarming appearance and only rarely is surgical repair needed. (For the treatment of muscle injuries *see* Chapter 16.)

Weight-lifting and throwing strain each end of the biceps and rotation of the long head tendon in the bicipital groove of the humerus chafes the tendon against the bony trough to cause tendinitis. At the insertion of the biceps in front of the elbow into the radius and adjacent fascia, strain is often localized to the gristly tendon when bending the elbow against resistance (*Figure 21.10*).

The upper biceps is easily strained in several weight-lifting moves, particularly as the barbell is moved through the horizontal plane, for example, during the snatch or moving from the clean to the press, in which the tendon moves most against its groove.

The lower biceps insertion is stressed on initiating any lift or similar movement as in, for example, wrestling or judo.

During rehabilitation of strains it is important to reduce the weights normally handled. Gradual and small increases in training loads allow the tissues to recover and to be reconditioned.

The elbow and forearm

The elbow is a hinge joint between the humerus and the ulna with a further strut, the radius, meeting the front of the humerus adjacent to the ulna and permitting the forearm to rotate as well as hinge. This arrangement allows all the complexity of throwing and turning movements which could not have been made possible by means of one simple hinge movement (*Figure 21.9*).

The forearm is flexed mainly by the biceps at the front and extended by the triceps at the back. Rotation is controlled by the intrinsic muscles within the forearm (the supinator and pronators) together with the overlying extensors on the outer side of the elbow and flexors on the inner side.

The extensor muscles which raise the wrist and hand into extension originate from the lateral epicondyle on the outer side of the humerus in a common bulk before separating gradually into component muscles and tendons to the wrist and hand.

'Tennis elbow'

'Tennis elbow', or lateral epicondylitis, is usually an overuse injury in which the common extensor muscle origins are overstretched and become inflamed (*see Figure 21.10*). The vicious circle of pain, inflammation and further irritation continues and a wider area of tissue becomes involved and eventually becomes scarred and tethered down in contractures. Symptoms include pain over the outer side of the elbow on gripping, lifting or controlling any object such as a saucepan, suitcase or racquet handle. Forcing the down-turned hand upward at the wrist against resistance causes pain over the outer side of the elbow.

Causes of 'tennis elbow' are often obvious and include carpentry, screwdriving, painting, stripping wallpaper, and lifting or carrying suitcases. Causes may also be less than clear but unaccustomed

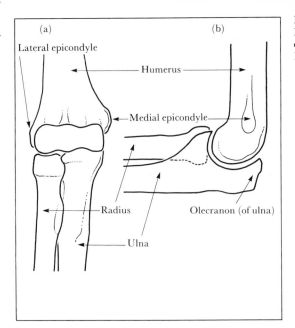

Figure 21.9
Basic anatomy of right elbow. (a) Front view. (b) Inner (medial) side view

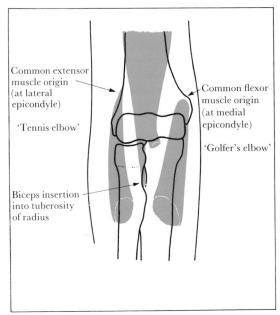

Figure 21.10
Front of elbow showing 'tennis' (extensor) and 'golfer's' (flexor) lesions and insertion of biceps tendon

exposure to play or practice often precedes symptoms. Equipment, too, is often at fault and the cumulative stresses of play with a heavy bat or racquet may cause pain, especially after prolonged sessions. 'Tennis elbow' is often due to use of uncomfortable equipment. If the club or racquet handle is too big or too small, extra effort has to go into gripping and this prevents free and efficient stroke play. A racquet which feels unbalanced or too heavy causes tension of the holding muscles with consequent strains. The remedy is often obvious and handles can be comfortably rebound to individual needs.

Because most minor lesions are rapidly reversible once pressure is taken off the affected muscle origin, early rest for a few days is effective. Should this not work, physiotherapy or injection is indicated – physiotherapists favour ultrasonic therapy and deep friction treatments. Other counter-irritants may also help and local steroid injections often are quickly effective but may need to be repeated several times for full effect.

A firm strapping, 1 inch (2.5 cm) wide, around the upper forearm is often effective and even with this or sophisticated splinting play may still be possible. A strap at the wrist for example, attached by a firm plastic splint to another around the common extensor origin restricts unnecessary rotations of the whole forearm while still allowing adequate movements for stroke play.

In resistant cases surgery is necessary because the muscle origins have become inflamed, scarred and tethered, causing pain and thus preventing the muscle working efficiently over its full range. If the muscle origins can be slightly lengthened by releasing the constricting scar, original alignment is restored and pain relieved. Recovery after operation is sometimes disappointing and may take several months – especially if there is much periostitis, or bone lining inflammation, at the epicondyle. Symptoms similar to 'tennis elbow' may be relieved, on rare occasions, by decompression of the radial nerve or soft-tissue bands in the upper forearm.

'Golfer's elbow'

'Golfer's elbow', or medial epicondylitis, is the equivalent condition which affects the common flexor muscle origin on the inner (medial) side of the elbow (*see Figures 21.10* and *21.11*). Pain is reproduced by pushing the open palm upwards against resistance and is also caused by forming an incorrect grip. More often the pain is due to overuse strains from repetitive movements such as golfing shots with poor style or sudden strain. A case in point is pain on the right elbow of a right-handed golfer when hitting a divot. 'Golfer's elbow' usually responds to all therapy much more quickly and satisfactorily than does 'tennis elbow'. Lack of adequate rest in the initial stages, however, too often makes for a chronic problem.

Triceps strain

At the back of the elbow the insertion of the triceps tendon is often strained and occasionally ruptured; this is particularly so with throwers of balls or javelins (*see Figure 21.11*). Poor stylists tend to get the most elbow pain. Apart from medical treatment, particular attention should be paid to the correction of style by coaching or, better still, to the early teaching of good throwing styles to children.

Medial ligament strain

Throwing, especially round-arm, may sprain the medial ligament on the inner side of the elbow often causing great pain (*see Figure 21.11*). Such pain settles promptly with treatment but, as with other injuries, any fault in style must then be corrected in order to prevent recurrence.

Arthritis

Arthritis is rare in the elbow. It is seen in those who repeatedly and violently wrench the elbow, as in some wrestlers or throwers. Arthritis, or synovitis, of the elbow is a serious condition, unfortunately needing prolonged rest. As distinct from 'tennis' or 'golfer's elbow', synovitis or arthritis of the elbow is characterized by a generally sore joint which may feel particularly limp, tired or weak – swelling may also be present and firm movements painful. Because of preceding mixed heavy training loads there are often present associated injuries such as biceps insertion strain or 'tennis elbow'. In addition, X-ray may show degenerative changes in the joint. It is essential, therefore, that this condition be fully rested and early resumption of full activity is never safe. Unfortunately, by the time players come to the clinic, degenerative changes may be well established causing uncertainty about their sporting future. With further sprains, the progress of arthritis is accelerated.

Fractures and dislocations

Fractures at the elbow are often extremely disabling and may leave permanently restricted movement. Also, the elbow is a common site of myositis ossificans (*see* Chapter 16). Fractures of the lower humerus, including adolescent supracondylar fractures, are mentioned above (page 161).

Heavy landings on the outstretched arm can crush the head of the radius (*Figure 21.12*) or knock chips out of the joint with similar damage to the corresponding end of the humerus. These loose fragments do not necessarily cause symptoms but may cause pain and a partial block to movement which must be relieved by their surgical removal.

Chips may be broken from the medial epicondyle of the humerus, the 'funny bone' (*Figure 21.13*), and such injury causes tingling and numbness down the distribution of the ulnar nerve from its groove under

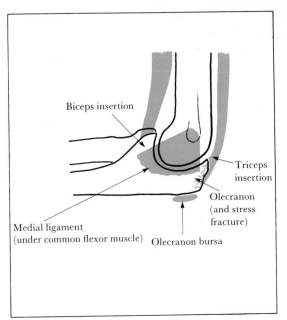

Figure 21.11
Inner (medial) side of right elbow

Biceps insertion

Triceps insertion

Olecranon (and stress fracture)

Medial ligament (under common flexor muscle)   Olecranon bursa

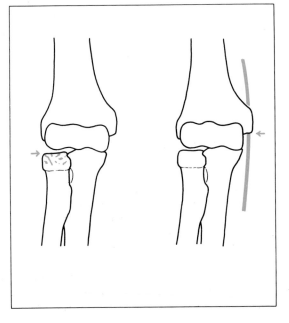

Figure 21.12 (left)
Head of radius may fracture, chip or dislocate
Figure 21.13 (right)
Medial epicondyle showing ulnar nerve passing under groove

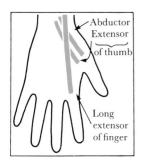

Figure 21.14
Right wrist showing site of
extensor tenosynovitis and
possible pressure on
underlying muscles

the epicondyle down the outer side of the forearm to
the little finger.

The tip of the olecranon (*see Figure 21.11*) may be
broken by direct impact or by stress fracture from
repeated throwing movements which, at the elbow,
can force the tip into contact with the groove at the
back of the humerus. In adolescents, similar
movements may cause olecranon epiphysitis with
pain at the tip of the elbow. In the first instance, rest
for 3 or 4 weeks is essential and style correction must
be applied to prevent recurrence. In prevention,
young players should be coached not to overtrain in
fast throwing or flinging actions.

In children, the head of the radius is sometimes
dislocated through wrenching movements. Pain and
reduced movement are the results. The displacement
is usually easily reduced by forearm rotations in
flexion.

Olecranon bursitis

This condition is a painful inflammation of a
soft-tissue sac which underlies the olecranon at the
back of the elbow but does not connect with the joint
(*see Figure 21.11*). Its usual cause is either a direct blow
or sustained pressure resting on the elbow; however,
unexplained bursitis can be a sign of gout (*see* Chapter
11).

Tenosynovitis

Tenosynovitis of the forearm extensor muscles is
common and caused by repetitive movements such as
canoeing, racquet playing or screwdriving. The line of
the tendon becomes swollen and crepitant, and,
although painful to move and tender to the touch is,
nevertheless, painless at rest and this gives the clue to
treatment. Rest usually relieves tenosynovitis rapidly.
As in normal daily activities it is awkward to rest the
wrist and forearm, a light strapping or crepe bandage
can be applied. In extreme cases, a light splint of

plaster-of-paris, plastic, plastazote or even a stiff or
rolled newspaper may be effective. Steroid injection of
the tendon sheath is often rapidly curative.
Resumption of activity must be gradual and should
not start until symptoms have subsided. If this rule is
not observed, symptoms can intensify and become
chronic with occasional progression to severe fibrosis
– the tendon sheath then needs surgical
decompression.

Sometimes hypertrophy, or overdevelopment, of
some of the forearm muscles impinges upon adjacent
tendons and causes pain and weakness, for instance,
as a result of the long extensors being overdeveloped
and 'nipped' by the thumb extensors (*Figure 21.14*).
Surgical decompression of these obstructions is often
rapidly effective and training can be resumed within
days.

Wrist and hand

Wrist

Wrist sprains are common in contact sports and falls.
Because of pain and swelling, it may be difficult to
know whether there is a fracture and X-ray is then
necessary. Marked restriction of movement with pain,
crepitus or deep grating in the wrist suggests a
fracture. Mild sprains, however, settle uneventfully
with a simple crepe bandage. Provided that there is
no fracture, exercise is encouraged from the outset
and should initially consist of isometric exercises such
as gripping and squeezing a ball without moving the
wrist up and down.

Wrist fractures

These are common as a result of falling on the hand or
wrist. Young children tend to get greenstick fractures
of the radius or ulna, with one side of the bone
bending to snap while the other side remains intact.
In adults, low forearm fractures of both the radius

and ulna are usual, often with displacement. When adjacent ligaments of the wrist are also ruptured they have to be repaired. All these conditions require reduction to correct positions and plaster immobilization for about 6 weeks (3 weeks for greenstick fractures) followed by active mobilization by exercises.

The scaphoid bone of the wrist lies at the base of the thumb and localized tenderness at this point after a fall is always suggestive of a scaphoid fracture. An initial X-ray may be normal but, if pain persists, it is occasionally found that the scaphoid has developed degenerative changes which may lead to chronic pain and disability due to non-union. In this case surgery may be necessary.

Carpal tunnel syndrome

Carpal tunnel syndrome (CTS) is caused by compression of the median nerve as it crosses the wrist, under the carpal ligament, with the flexor tendons (*Figure 21.15*). The space in this tunnel is often limited and congestion from posture, constriction by tight arm bands or heavy hand work causes pressure neuritis. There is weakness of grip, aching at the palmar side of the wrist, which may extend up the forearm or down into the hand, with tingling or numbness of the middle three finger-tips. Also, there are often minor variations in symptoms due to individual anatomical differences. Symptoms are usually troublesome at night, waking the patient in the small hours after a day of hand work.

Treatment is by simple rest splints, successful within a month in over 80 per cent of cases, often with no further recurrence. Steroid injection of the carpal tunnel, without anaesthetic, is often permanently effective. Persistent symptoms need surgical cure by a small incision of the carpal ligament which then gives permanent relief. It is inadvisable to postpone surgery if symptoms persist because wasting and weakness of thumb and finger muscles will increase the disability.

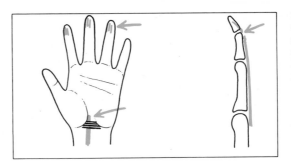

Figure 21.15 (left) Carpal tunnel syndrome showing median nerve compression by carpal ligament and typical finger-tip numbness
Figure 21.16 (right) Mallet finger showing rupture of extensor tendon at terminal phalanx at finger-tip

Hand

Fractures

Fractures of the hands and fingers are usually obvious because of pain and deformity following injury. Many minor fractures are treated simply by taping two adjacent fingers together and trying to continue movement. This clearly excludes contact sport but allows considerable activity and continuation of general training. Some hand fractures require complex surgical wiring, however, and all suspected fractures should be X-rayed and medically assessed.

Sprained thumb

Sprained thumbs are common in sport. The thumb may be forced back during a rugby hand off or during a mistimed basketball catch. A firm strapping is required to support the thumb base but it may be modified on return to play thus allowing some degree of movement and protection without necessarily permitting full abduction.

A severe sprain may rupture the ulnar collateral ligament rendering the joint lax and liable to further damage. Surgical repair gives good results.

Sprained finger

Finger sprains, which may be extremely painful and persist up to a year, do not preclude safe participation in sporting activity. In contact sports, protective strapping may be required, as much for confidence as for healing, and in cricket, for instance, extra padding inside the glove might be desirable. As a general principle, after injury hand and finger movements are encouraged and there have to be strong medical reasons for immobilizing any part of the hand for long periods. In any event, only the affected finger should be immobilized.

Stiffness of the fingers may persist after sprains or fractures and can cause considerable disability. The patient should make every attempt to move the hand. Passive movement and stretching during convalescence are essential and specific techniques of oil massage by a physiotherapist may also be helpful. Sometimes, the gripping of an implement, for example a discus, is compromised by finger injury and if surgical correction is impossible the event will have to be abandoned or drastically modified to accommodate the altered grip.

Mallet finger

A blow on the finger-tip, such as may occur in cricket, baseball or goal-keeping, may simply sprain the interphalangeal joints or, more seriously, rupture the extensor tendon insertion into the terminal phalanx. If this happens, the end of the finger is left hanging downwards in the so-called Mallet deformity (*Figure 21.16*). A straight finger splint worn for about 4–6 weeks and followed by persistent exercise ensures recovery with minimal loss of movement.

Blisters

Blistering and local skin tears of the hands are common problems with bowlers, racquet players, pole vaulters and fencers. Problems are made worse by a hot climate or humid indoor arenas. Skin breakdown can be prevented by the use of skin creams and hardening solutions such as surgical spirit; but if the skin is broken, care must be taken to avoid secondary infection. Regular cleansing of the wound and clean dressings are essential. The rules of a particular sport may dictate the limits of strapping, for instance, a bowler cannot strap his spinning finger because of the unfair advantage thus gained in imparting spin to the ball.

Occasionally, as in the pole vault, it may be necessary to apply resin to the hands to ensure a firm grip of the implement.

Subungual haematoma

Bruising under the nail is painful because of the pressure of the enclosed blood. Treatment is similar to that of toenail bruises – a sterile blade or hot pin is used to make a small hole in the nail letting out the haematoma with dramatic relief of pain.

22 Spinal injuries

The spine consists of a column of bony vertebrae, separated by cartilage discs which allow both compression and flexibility (*Figure 22.1*). These bones are secured by ligaments and muscles which allow limited movement – forward, backward, sideways and in rotation. Each vertebra has joints with those adjacent thus forming a long and complex system of interconnected joints and making possible a co-ordinated range of movements throughout the spine. Normal mobility varies considerably between individuals, from the stiff and unathletic to the highly mobile young gymnast. Mobility is mostly determined by inheritance and there are limits to the amount of extra movement which can be acquired, even with conscientious practice. If spinal ligaments or bones break, as in spondylolisthesis, there is danger that the instability and extra movement thus given to the vertebrae may cause them to slip and press on surrounding structures, including the spinal cord and nerves. Because the whole spine is interconnected, injury or damage at one level tends to lead to compensatory realignments elsewhere. The spinal arch contains the spinal cord from which arise the nerves supplying the rest of the body. Spinal injury, for example, in the neck during rugby scrum collapse, may cause pressure damage to the cord.

Scheuermann's disease

The spinal bones, or vertebrae, develop in stages. The initial cartilage is gradually calcified and the full strength and final configuration is attained only after adolescence. Scheuermann's disease, or adolescent osteochondritis, occurs when there is imperfect fusion of the centres of ossification in the vertebral bodies. This leaves one or more vertebrae irregularly shaped and potentially weak or unstable instead of being firmly squared off (*see Figure 22.2*).

Because Scheuermann's disease is usually symptomless, its occurrence is often detected only by chance on a chest X-ray. It may, however, cause chronic backache during the teens and if there is painful restriction of movement at this age it is wise to avoid heavy spinal loading throughout adolescence subject to regular review in the light of clinical and X-ray progress. This condition is usually self-limiting but occasionally leaves an irregularly shaped spine which may not stand up well to heavy weight-training or sport.

Spinal anomalies

The spine is often imperfectly or incompletely formed. It is normal for the spine and spinal cord to be laid down in the embryo as a long tube which gradually closes off. Occasionally, this closure fails and the spina bifida deformity occurs in the newborn (*Figure 22.3*).

Lesser degrees of this failure to close fully are seen in spina bifida occulta. In this case, there is partial failure of the arch to fuse in a complete circle at the end of development. This does not matter for normal

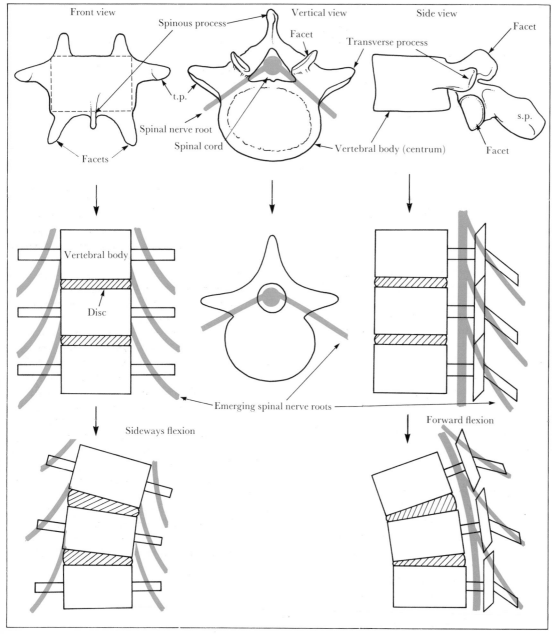

Figure 22.1
Diagram of normal spine.
Note emerging spinal nerve
roots and changes on spinal
flexion

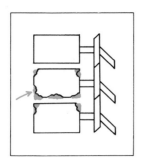

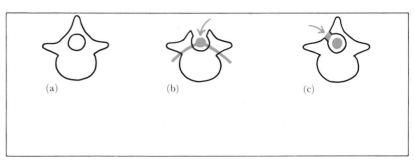

Figure 22.2 (left) Scheuermann's disease – adolescent osteochondritis
Figure 22.3 (right) Spinal arch malformations (a) Normal. (b) Spina bifida. Open arch with possible open sinus to skin exposing original neural tube. (c) Spina bifida occulta. Incomplete bony fusion of spinal arch, usually bridged by cartilage. Cord not exposed, but potential weakness due to asymmetrical bone and supporting ligaments

purposes but may be associated with other congenital anomalies which tend to be associated with backache under heavy loading. Similar imperfections of early-life development can cause considerable asymmetry of the spinal bones so that there may be a very large transverse process on one side of the vertebra but not the other or, more commonly, there may be considerable asymmetries at the pelvic junction (*Figure 22.4*). While these anomalies do not usually matter for normal living purposes, they represent an asymmetry not only of bone but of supporting ligaments so that with heavy loading, such as weight-training, lifting or throwing, the asymmetry of mechanical support in the lower back may cause disc or ligament breakdown and backache. This is not always appreciated by doctors whose non-sports practice rarely presents this particular problem. Persistent back pain in association with congenital anomalies tends to carry a poor prognosis in heavy stress events.

Lifting and back strain

The back is capable of supporting considerable weights but is liable to break down if the weight becomes too heavy or if the angles of movement are mechanically unsound. If the spine is kept straight during lifting, the joints are held fixed by the vertebral shape and supporting muscles and ligaments. If weights are lifted with a bent back, however, much more stress is put on each of the

spinal joints and a rapid slip or change of momentum may cause a sudden strain on one part of the spine with collapse of the whole supporting system with pain and spasm. The most serious lifting injuries damage the disc structures and occasionally the bone. Ligament and muscle strains are incurred which may also persist as 'lumbago', or backache. Every effort should be made to practice weight-lifting techniques smoothly and symmetrically. Coaching is as important as for any other technique event in which self-observation is impossible.

The spine is supported while lifting by muscular and hydrostatic systems. Muscles pull on the spine both to support and move it, and also to support the weights. The hydrostatic pressure in the body cavities – the thorax and the abdomen – serves to hold the spine straight under stress. Hence the importance of strong abdominal muscles in helping to regulate the hydrostatic support of the spine in all lifting, bending and straining movements. When weight-lifters wear a body belt, this is not to hold up or strengthen the bones, but to enhance the hydrostatic pressure in the abdominal cavity (*Figure 22.5*). Occasionally, heavy weight-lifting leads to ruptures because the pressure in the abdominal cavity may become great enough to force open a weakness in the tissues at the groin where inguinal hernia may occur (*Figure 22.5*). Surgical repair is then required because of the danger that the hernia will become stuck.

173

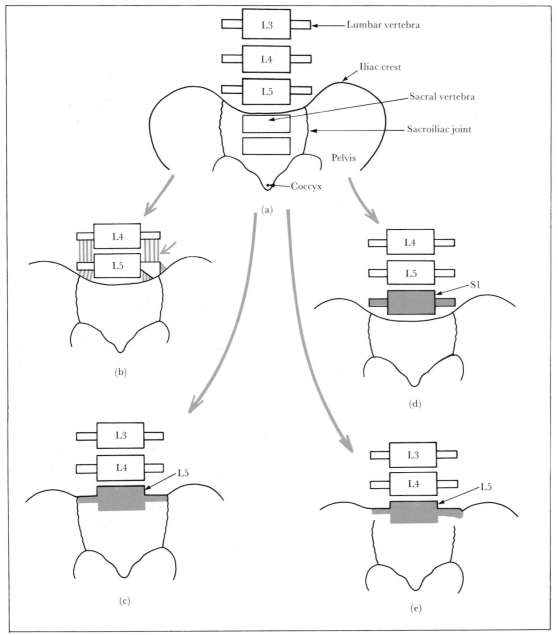

Figure 22.4
Some common anomalies of the lower spine
(a) Normal
(b) Asymmetrical transverse process of L5. Note asymmetry of supporting ligaments
(c) Sacralization of L5; leaves shorter, less mobile lumbar spine
(d) Lumbarization of S1; longer, more mobile lumbar spine
(e) Combination of anomalies, e.g. sacralized L5 with asymmetrical transverse processes

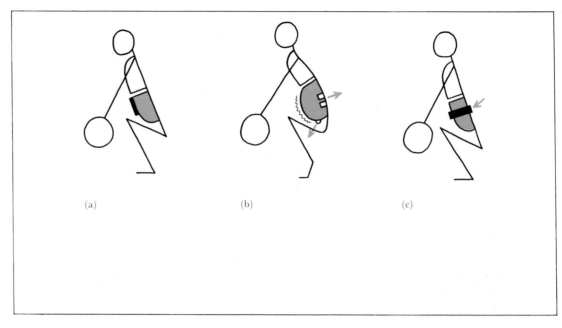

Figure 22.5
Lifting and hydrostatic pressure. (a) Basic position with good abdominal muscles. (b) Poor lifting posture, lax abdomen, ineffective use of hydrostatic mechanism. Risks include disc prolapse and hernia. (c) Use of belt to enhance hydrostatic pressure

(a)

(b)

(c)

Intervertebral discs

Heavy loading of the spine may cause weakening, strain or rupture of the intervertebral discs (*Figure 22.6*). These discs consist of an inner gelatinous core – the nucleus pulposus – and a tough outer fibrous ring – the annulus fibrosus. Discs slowly stiffen with age, lose their resilience and shrink due to gradual dehydration. Thus the disc gradually becomes more brittle and likely to rupture. *Figure 22.6* shows the forces which cause disc prolapse.

The hydrostatic pressure in the discs is least when lying flat. It rises on standing and yet again on sitting. Extra strain such as lifting adds further pressure. This explains why backache is so often caused or worsened by sitting, especially in poor sagging postures, or by lifting with a bent back.

When pressure rises, the healthy disc absorbs the extra stress. Later, when the disc deteriorates or if excessive straining occurs, the nuclear pulp is squeezed through the fibrous ring gradually or suddenly. Slow seepage of nuclear fluid into the surrounding tissues causes pain and stiffness a day or two later. Sudden rupture is often felt as a 'snap' with acute backache. There are no nerves in the discs themselves so pain is due to irritation of adjacent tissues, including spinal nerve roots.

Figure 22.6 shows how a prolapsed disc pulp can press either on the spinal cord or nerve roots or between the two without causing nerve damage. Fragments of disc may be unstable enough to shift and cause changing or frequently recurring symptoms.

Initial treatment by traction or manipulation may squeeze the pulp back into place or displace it from symptomatic positions. Rest allows gradual healing by the formation of a firm scar. In reality, most patients are inadequately rehabilitated and suffer inevitable recurrences due to poorly healed discs and avoidable careless backstrain.

Prolapsed discs press upon adjacent structures to cause backache. Pressure on nerves coming out of the

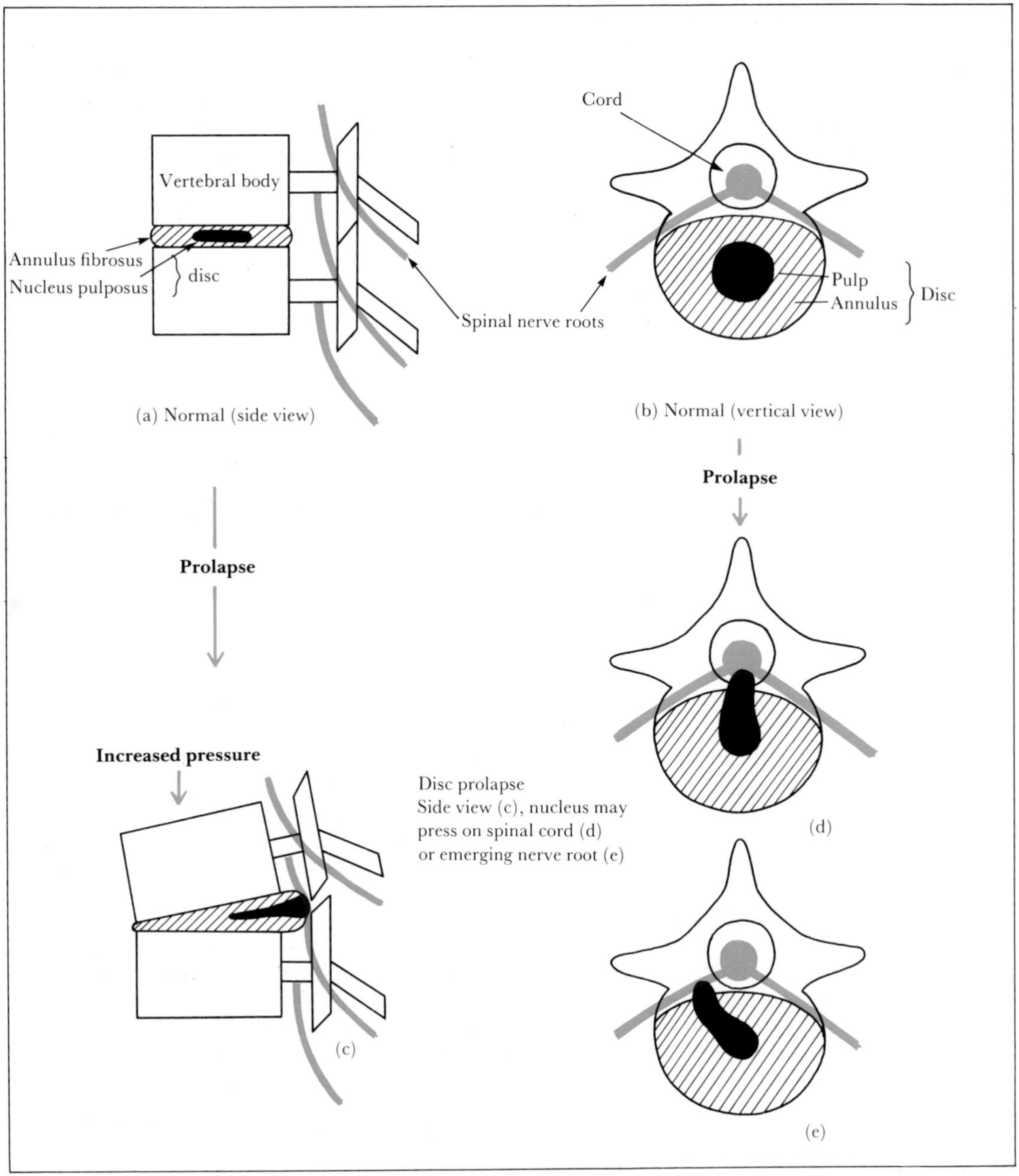

Figure 22.6
Intervertebral discs, normal and prolapsed ('slipped')

spinal canal causes pain, numbness or weakness in the area supplied by the nerve concerned. Thus in the neck, disc pressure on one of the low cervical nerves may give rise to arm or hand pain and weakness; in the lumbar region, pressure causes sciatica with symptoms radiating down the leg. Symptoms are made worse by pressure and movement. It usually takes some weeks of careful therapy to recover from a disc lesion and premature return to training usually leads to relapse and chronic symptoms.

If traction or manipulation is not available, complete bed rest is standard effective treatment for slipped discs and all other acute backache. The vast majority of backaches will settle in about a week with strict bed rest. This means lying flat with no more than a thin pillow, not sitting half-propped in bed which causes an increase in disc pressure. It is permissible to rise only for toilet purposes as this is much more comfortable out of bed than using bedpans in back-straining positions.

Full doses of soluble aspirin or soluble aspirin with codeine are helpful for pain relief and warmth helps by relieving spasm. A simple hot-water bottle is adequate.

Following this advice would reduce considerably the overall disability thus lessening industrial time loss as well as personal distress. As the pain subsides, gradual resumption of activity is essential but with very careful attention to posture (*Figure 22.7*).

It is essential to respect the back at all times. One injudicious movement can ruin a whole sports career. A good warm-up and stretching exercises are important, followed by graduated loading with weights or exercises. Warming-down afterwards and avoidance of sitting around and getting chilled are essential as chilling often causes backache after a successful session. After any episode of backache, resumption of training must be gradual. It is always dangerous to go straight back to heavy loading because the muscles and soft tissues will have lost tone and not be as strong as previously. As a means of continuing in training or building up again, swimming is hard to beat because it offers

well-supported symmetrical and mobile exercising of any required degree without the jarring or movement stresses associated with jumping, running or lifting on dry land. By its partial relief of gravity, it enables a far wider range of movements than on land and this enhances spinal and pelvic mobility.

Most sportsmen are woefully stiff outside the narrow requirements of their event, and as the player gets older, he may find that, for no very good reason, he is perpetually stiff and sore in the back. There is no specific injury, but deliberate attention to mobility exercises may completely relieve the limiting symptoms. A proportion of these pains represents chronic minor disc damage. In fact, many middle-aged runners have found to their advantage that a slight diversification of their training effort to spend 1 day in 4 or 5 swimming instead of running and to do back and hip mobility exercises, not only makes them more mobile and comfortable but often improves their running as well.

Spondylolisthesis

Heavy stress on the back may sometimes cause fractures of the spinal arch rather than disc or ligament rupture. *Figure 22.8* shows how sudden traumatic fracture or slower onset stress fractures can break part of the supporting arch of the vertebra (spondylolysis). This may persist with or without chronic backache or healing. In a proportion of cases, particularly if both sides of the arch break, there is displacement of the vertebrae as lack of arch support lets body weight drag one over the other. The associated disc, or discs is/are also displaced possibly to cause new symptoms of spinal cord or nerve compression.

Despite the alarming X-ray appearance of spondylolisthesis when the bones have slipped, many patients are hardly inconvenienced and some settle with basic physiotherapy or a corset for support. Persisting unrelieved backache or nerve compression are the two frequent reasons for operations to stabilize

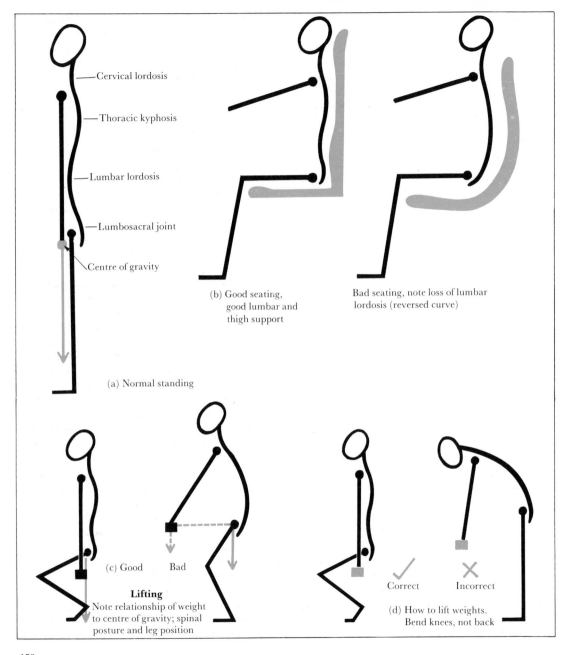

Figure 22.7
Posture

—Cervical lordosis

—Thoracic kyphosis

—Lumbar lordosis

—Lumbosacral joint

Centre of gravity

(a) Normal standing

(b) Good seating,
good lumbar and
thigh support

Bad seating, note loss of lumbar
lordosis (reversed curve)

(c) Good   Bad

Lifting
Note relationship of weight
to centre of gravity; spinal
posture and leg position

Correct   Incorrect

(d) How to lift weights.
Bend knees, not back

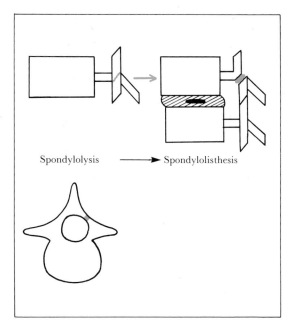

Figure 22.8
Spinal arch fracture

Spondylolysis ⟶ Spondylolisthesis

the bones. Either bone grafting or screwing up of the broken arches is effective, the latter procedure having returned many sportsmen to full performance. Even in older patients with considerable slip, the operation may be effective in relieving pain. However, surgery may stabilize the back and relieve pain at the expense of some loss of mobility, thus possibly affecting sports techniques.

Backache in sport

No part of the body has attracted more mythology and pseudoscience than the back. Doctors, physiotherapists, osteopaths, chiropractors and many others all have their views and therapeutic habits; however, much of the science remains uncertain because of the technical difficulties in gaining access to the tissues. It may therefore be simpler to suggest some fairly straightforward guidelines for the sportsman who gets backache.

Acute backache during sport is usually due to wrenching of soft tissues, including discs – rarely is a bone broken. Landing violently on the back or on straight legs may cause crushing of the vertebrae. Occasionally spinal arch fractures occur when there is repeated vigorous low-back movement as in gymnastics, weight-lifting, javelin throwing, hurdling or twisting and kicking. Pain may be sudden and severe, or develop more gradually.

The player with sudden backache must leave the game. Acute pain radiating across the lower back, buttock, thigh or leg suggests sciatica and, as with all backache, the victim should try to lie down as soon as possible. Armchairs, car seats and the like are uncomfortable, partly because they are poorly shaped for the spine's natural shape and partly because the sitting position greatly increases the pressure upon the discs.

If pain is extreme or unremitting or if there is numbness radiating down the leg or arm, medical help should be sought immediately.

Rest and careful attention to correct posture so as to avoid slouching should be standard treatment for backache. *Figure 22.7* shows the natural spinal curvature. There is a blend of curves which together compensate continuously for postural changes. The lumbar lordosis is the concave curve of the lower back in the strongest mechanical posture. The commonest postural fault is slouching into seating which does not support this lumbar lordosis. As a result the lower spine sags out into a reversed curve, or kyphosis, with a resultant increase in disc pressure and stretching of ligaments. It is common to get acute backache on getting up from poor seating.

Correct seating includes a firm lumbar support (*Figure 22.7b*) and a simple cushion can be an effective substitute.

Lifting stresses are increased by loss of lumbar lordosis (*Figure 22.7c*). The body's centre of gravity is in the pelvis and the poor lifting posture shown increases stress by placing the weights outside the line of the centre of gravity. Thus, extra work must be done by the spinal muscles to make up for this less efficient displacement of the weights from the best line of lift which is through the centre of gravity.

Bending often causes backache (*Figure 22.7d*). The safest way to lift objects is by keeping the spine straight but bending the knees – not the other way around.

Any form of exercise should be started cautiously. Gradual mobilization is achieved by putting the back through its full range of movements – forwards, backwards, sideways and in rotation from side to side. A warm-up and easy movement is the aim since sudden, violent or jerky movements may be painful. Often a particular movement or exercise is painful, especially backward extensions: such exercises should be abandoned and painless ones continued. It is worth remembering that exercises performed in water have the benefit of partial relief of gravity which allows better movement. The local heated swimming pool is usually suitable for such exercises.

Arthritis

Many older sportsmen have osteoarthritis in the spine. This may reflect damage from old injuries at work or play or simply the gradual changes associated with age. The rule is to be guided only by the symptoms and a certain amount of stiffness and immobility is to be expected with increasing age. Provided the player can warm up and play satisfactorily, the chance finding of osteoarthritic changes on an X-ray, perhaps taken for something quite different, should not be a deterrent to activity.

Ankylosing spondylitis.

Ankylosing spondylitis is a rheumatic inflammatory condition which usually afflicts younger men. It causes pain initially in the small of the back, which may spread up the spine and cause increasing stiffness of the whole back. The modern treatment of this condition is by continued vigorous exercise with anti-inflammatory medication – this method achieves better results than irradiation or immobilization. Ankylosing spondylitis may cause extremely painful episodes of generalized illness between much less active periods before it finally subsides. Medical guidance is essential throughout the course of this condition, but it is certainly consistent with considerable physical activity. For instance, in younger men there are usually periods of remission or minimal symptoms during which activity can be encouraged. Older sporting patients are sometimes found to have had previously undiagnosed ankylosing spondylitis throughout a career of sport and a few patients progress to considerable spinal fusion with apparently trivial symptoms and no curtailment of sporting effort.

Sacroiliac joints

Sacroiliac joint disease and strains are widely postulated as a cause of backache in athletes, but, apart from those few patients with proven ankylosing spondylitis, such assertions are almost totally unproven. The structure of the sacroiliac joint is such that disruption, short of the most violent external forces, is virtually impossible and the exact joint line of the sacroiliac surfaces is rarely particularly tender in athletes. It is likely that most back pain around the sacroiliac area is due either to disc prolapse or to soft-tissue strains in the profusion of criss-crossed ligaments overlying the whole of the sacral, sacroiliac and lumbosacral areas. Because of the connotations of 'slipped disc' or 'sacroiliac' disease, it seems much simpler to talk about 'lumbago' or 'strained back' and to treat empirically along the lines indicated above rather than to cause alarm or confusion by inappropriate use of unjustifiable technical terms.

Pregnancy and backache

Spinal changes associated with pregnancy may make women more liable to strain their backs at this time.

There are few contraindications to exercise in pregnancy or the puerperium (soon after childbirth) but, to facilitate childbirth, hormonal changes cause softening of the ligaments. After childbirth it takes some months for these ligaments to tense up again and resume their normal taut state ready for full athletic activity. Therefore, in later pregnancy and the puerperium, heavy weight-training and vigorous activity should be avoided and full training loads should be resumed in progressive steps rather than violently, to minimize the risk of injury.

23 Trunk injuries

Ribs

Bruised, cracked or fractured ribs are common in contact sport and cause pain which worsens with deep breathing. Also, there is crepitus at the tender area when the broken bone ends are rubbed together. It used to be standard practice to strap the chest wall thoroughly with adhesive tape on the affected side thereby in the early stages increasing the sufferer's comfort. Strapping is not strictly necessary, however, and need be tried only if the pain warrants it. Local anaesthetic can be injected into the fracture area for temporary relief if pain is particularly severe or, perhaps, if an awkward journey must be undertaken. Ribs heal quickly and simply but contact sport should be avoided until secure bony union is achieved, in 4–6 weeks.

Abdomen

Stitch

Stitch is a cramp-like muscular condition which usually occurs in the lower right quadrant of the abdomen (*Figure 23.1*), although it occasionally occurs elsewhere. It is strictly related to exercise and any similar pain which persists at rest requires full medical assessment. Despite numerous unproven theories the cause of stitch is unknown. It is characteristically relieved when effort is stopped and it tends to recur on resumption.

Well-known precipitants of stitch include eating too much or too soon before exercise, fizzy drinks, and lack of abdominal muscle tone. While the dietary faults are obvious, it is always worth strengthening the stomach muscles by simple step-up exercises combined with trunk curls and sit-ups, as this frequently prevents further symptoms. Stitch during running can often be overcome by breath-holding or by pulling in the abdomen and bending forward for a few strides.

Particularly persistent stitch should be carefully evaluated by the coach or doctor as it is a well-recognized stress symptom, for instance in students at exam time.

Other abdominal pain

Other abdominal pain may also trouble athletes. Dyspepsia, or indigestion, is fairly common where activity levels preclude regular meals, as for instance with P.E. teachers or highly stressed sportsmen in heavy training. The stress of intensive athletic training has led to peptic ulcers in a number of world-class sportsmen and such ulcers may be difficult to treat because of the conflicting pressures to which the victims are subjected. Dyspeptic pain occurs usually in the upper, epigastric portion of the abdomen (*Figure 23.1*). It may relate in time to meals and be relieved by milk or antacids; and it will probably feel sharper and qualitatively different from stitch pain.

Two muscular pains of separate origin low in the abdomen may simulate stitch or appendicitis. Chronic adductor muscle strain high in the groin may cause aching by referral deep in the lower quarter of the abdomen, as may also psoas muscle strain deep under the hip region. Appropriate muscle testing will locate the painful movement patterns and permit anatomical diagnosis. Appendicitis rarely causes a similar movement-related pain, however, and should not usually cause confusion on medical examination. Occasionally, female athletes may present with similar pain related to ovarian function, but this should also be distinguishable by careful history and examination.

Solar plexus

The solar plexus is an autonomic nerve centre deep in the epigastric part of the abdomen and a sharp blow on the upper stomach causes a temporary reflex paralysis of the diaphragm which winds and may, momentarily knock out the player. No treatment is required and recovery is prompt. The player, as in any case of collapse, should be left on the ground when stunned and not held upright as this exaggerates the temporarily diminished blood flow to the head.

Genitalia

A blow on the testicles may wind or knock out a player by a similar vagus nerve reflex. While painful, recovery is usually prompt. Because of the high risk of genital trauma, the wearing of suitable protective boxes is essential in certain games but a box made of metal should be worn rather than the flimsier plastic device which has been known to splinter and add to the casualty surgeon's, as well as the patient's, misery!

The male genitalia are liable to a number of insults by virtue of their exposure. Male fertility is partly dependent upon ambient temperature and the

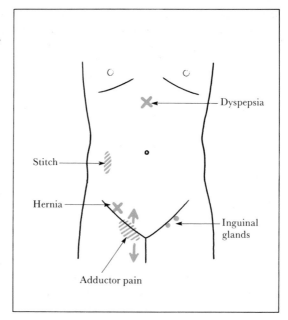

Figure 23.1
Abdominal pain

Dyspepsia

Stitch

Hernia

Inguinal glands

Adductor pain

constant wearing of jockstraps or similar tight clothing may, by raising the testicular temperature, diminish sperm formation in some individuals. This diminution is promptly reversible when required, but should not be regarded as a reliable form of birth control! Scrotal bruising may cause considerable pain and spectacular discoloration – ice packs offer the most effective immediate treatment.

Torsion of the testicle may occur in cycling, particularly in teenagers, and the appearance of pain in the testicles after riding calls for immediate medical examination with, if necessary, relief of the mechanical torsion. Under no circumstances must this procedure be attempted by amateurs for fear that the torsion may inadvertently be increased. A rare complication of cycling may be priapism, or persistent erection, due to vascular obstruction: this condition calls for urgent medical intervention.

The female genitalia are at risk of direct contusion from implements or falls, for instance on to gym apparatus which may also cause pubic fractures. Also well documented are the dangers of forced douching in water ski-ing which can give rise to serious internal lacerations of the genitalia. For this reason, water ski-ers should be adequately protected with waterproof clothing over the pudendal region.

Groin

Pain in the groin may be due to swollen lymph glands. Such pain may be caused by the spread of infection up from the foot accompanied by the red line of lymphangitis, or from local infection near the groin, including genital infection. It is common to find swollen and tender glands in the groin after unaccustomed exercise and the clear relation of symptoms to recent effort should make this clear. If there is no obvious cause for swollen glands in the groin, the feet should be carefully examined as fungal and secondary bacterial infection from athlete's foot or septic nails may provide the hidden focus. As with

hidden dental infection, there is an undermining effect on health and athletic performance.

In the front of the groin, pains related to effort are most often due to strains of the adductor muscles (*see Figures 23.1* and *23.2*). These muscles help stabilize the pelvis and connect it to the femur. Adductor muscle strains are particularly liable to occur in sprinters, footballers, hurdlers and riders. Sprinters tend to come out of the blocks with their feet out-turned so that during the initial part of the sprint, before the feet come into the straighter ahead alignment, there is an extra stress on the out-turned adductors. In hurdling, this effect is magnified by the extreme degree of hip rotation required to clear the hurdles and land as quickly as possible. With soccer players the tendency to kick with the inside of the foot means that the adductors are constantly stretched by turning forces as well as by the abrupt movements of kicking (*Figure 23.3*).

The adductor muscles may be tender at any point in their length and, particularly so, at their origin high in the groin. Careful examination of the adductor muscle complex will identify the affected area. The tenderness becomes worse on resisted movement of the muscle and often the same area experiences pain when the opposite thigh is moved against resistance. In addition, the psoas muscle may also be strained and occasionally the tendon pulled off its insertion into the tip of the lesser trochanter of the femur (*Figure 23.4*).

In any case of groin pain the hips should always be examined and it should not be forgotten that, especially in the young, hip pain is commonly referred to the knee so that a limp or an ache in the knee may be a sign solely of hip disease. Hip movements should be compared on each side and any restriction or difference noted. There is a wide variation in hip range between normal people, females being more flexible than males, the latter often having poor flexibility in lateral and rotational movements. As joints tend to be least mechanically efficient in the extremities of their range, it follows that the more flexible a player's joints, the better the power and

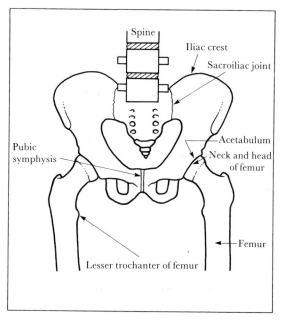

Figure 23.2
Pelvis

control during the middle range where skills are most frequently exercised.

Pubic pain is common in footballers, riders and some long-distance runners and may be due to chronic strain on the adductor magnus origin, producing general discomfort around the pubic area. However, with footballers especially, repeated adductor pulls, body checks, kicks and rotations, may tend to loosen the pubic symphysis, which consists of fibrocartilage set between the two wings of the pelvic ring. If this does happen, there may be persistent discomfort and, when the player stands on one leg, examination may show marked movement of the two halves of the pubic symphysis (*Figure 23.5*). X-rays may be used for confirmation. Treatment includes rest, steroid injections, physiotherapy or surgical fixation. Pain with inflammation but no displacement is recognized as osteitis pubis which probably originates as a chronic overuse strain.

Occasionally, pain at the pubic symphysis may be associated with Reiter's disease, an obscure condition associated with arthritis, eye inflammation, urethral discharge or dysentery. The venereal form, in association with urethritis, may also present in this way.

Hips

The structure of the ball and socket joint of the hip may also vary considerably between individuals and sometimes the socket, or acetabulum, is particularly shallow (*Figure 23.6*). This shallowness may lead to relative instability under stress but the precise relation of anatomy to symptoms is not always clear. What is more important is that there are conditions of adolescence which cause hip pain as well as damaging hip function. Serious impairment may be caused for later sports and premature adult osteoarthritis can follow. Perthes' disease occurs in growing children: over a period of 2 or 3 years, the bone at the head of the femur fragments and becomes compressed and thereby irregularly deformed. Any child with a limp

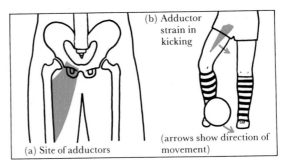

Figure 23.3
Adductor muscles

(b) Adductor strain in kicking

(arrows show direction of movement)

(a) Site of adductors

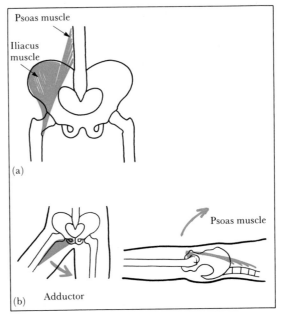

Figure 23.4
Psoas muscle. (a) Psoas muscle arises from the lumbar vertebrae, is joined by the iliacus from the pelvis and inserts into the lesser trochanter of the femur to flex the thigh.
(b) Comparison of actions of psoas and adductor

Psoas muscle

Iliacus muscle

(a)

(b) Adductor

Psoas muscle

should be sent for detailed medical examination without delay.

The growing head of the femur may slip off its shaft during adolescence (slipped upper femoral epiphysis) and, if untreated, may become detached and necrotic; urgent surgery is thus required. The point is made, again, that any adolescent player who develops a limp must receive urgent medical examination.

Occasionally, particularly in adolescence, violent

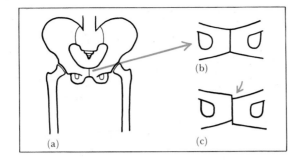

Figure 23.5
Instability of pubic symphysis.
(a) Normal. (b) Lying or standing on both legs. (c) Standing on one leg

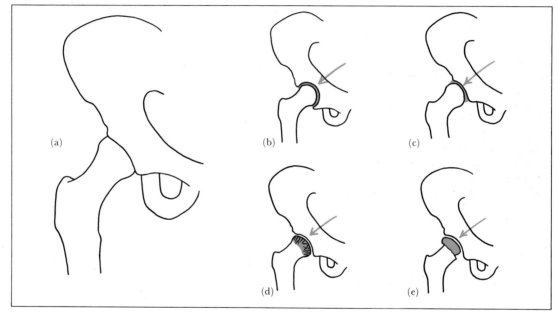

Figure 23.6
Hip disorders.
(a) Normal hip. (b) Normal hip – deep joint. (c) Normal hip – shallow joint. (d) Perthes' desease. (e) Slipped upper femoral epiphysis

blows cause avulsion of part of the pelvic bony structures, before the growing plates, or epiphyses, have fully fused into their final adult state (*Figure 23.7*). The iliac crest can be fractured, severely contused or avulsed, giving pain over the rim of the pelvis below the waistline. The anterior superior iliac spine may be avulsed, usually by a violent lunging or sprinting-type force, allowing the sartorius and tensor fascia lata muscle origins to pull off the bony attachment. A similar force on the thigh, caused by,

for example, sprinting or jumping, may cause avulsion by the iliopsoas tendon of the lesser trochanter of the femur.

Similar forceful avulsions of the adductor muscles at the pubic ramus may be caused. Posteriorly under the buttock, avulsion of the hamstring origins at the ischium may occur.

All these conditions need careful clinical and X-ray assessment and sometimes, but by no means invariably, early surgical repair. The long-term outlook is uniformly good, despite the rather alarming nature of the injury.

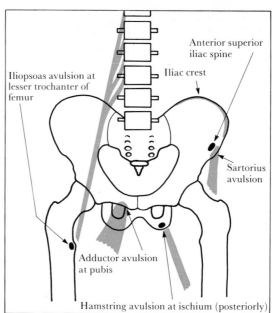

Figure 23.7
Disorders of pelvic epiphyses

Iliopsoas avulsion at lesser trochanter of femur

Anterior superior iliac spine

Iliac crest

Sartorius avulsion

Adductor avulsion at pubis

Hamstring avulsion at ischium (posteriorly)

24 Knee injuries

Anatomy

The knee is a relatively unstable hinge joint between the femur and the tibia. It is secured internally by two cruciate ligaments and a capsule and externally by closely adjacent ligaments, muscles and tendons (*Figure 24.1*). The normal range of hinge movement is from straight extension to about 145 degrees flexion. There is some rotation of the tibia on the femur at the knee joint and this can be seen when the knee is slowly straightened. The knee is internally cushioned by the two semilunar cartilages, or menisci, which by their semicircular shape help to track the rounded ends of the moving femur. Because of the extent of movement required at the front of the knee, the synovial lining is folded and sometimes liable to become nipped.

The third bone at the knee is the patella (knee-cap) which sits in the thick common tendon of the quadriceps muscle as it condenses into the patellar tendon leading to insertion into the top of the tibia. The patella is one of the body's sesamoid bones, the mechanical function of which is to lift the line of pull of a tendon up and away from the joint it serves so as to increase mechanical leverage. The knee joint is otherwise cushioned by fat pads and by extensions of the synovial joint space into bursae or pouches above, behind and below the joint.

In health there is minimal synovial fluid in the joint, but in many injuries the inflamed synovial lining secretes an effusion. This effusion is detectable by gently pressing the knee-cap up and down against the held upper knee (*Figure 24.2*) and is known as 'water on the knee'. An effusion always indicates inflammation and needs medical attention.

Below the knee, the fibula joins the top of the tibia in the superior tibiofibular joint.

There are some common congenital deformities of the knee (*Figure 24.3*) including genu valgum (knock-knee), genu varum (bow-leg) and genu recurvatum. All may present problems for sportsmen by causing abnormal alignment. Increased joint laxity in genu recurvatum predisposes to patellar dislocation and chondromalacia. Some people are born with rather higher, less well formed or loosely secured patellae; these increase the chance of knee pain or dislocation and may need to be stabilized surgically. The underside of the knee-cap is roughly wedge-shaped and slides up and down the groove between the two prominent condyles at the lower end of the femur as the knee bends and straightens.

Occasionally the patella fails to ossify fully and two or three separate components may be seen on an X-ray giving rise to a bi- or tripartite patella. This is not clinically significant unless associated with further injury or overuse strains.

Internal injuries

Damage to the knee usually causes effusion with painful restriction of movement. There may be bruising or yellowish discoloration if the joint capsule has been ruptured. The very rapid development of

189

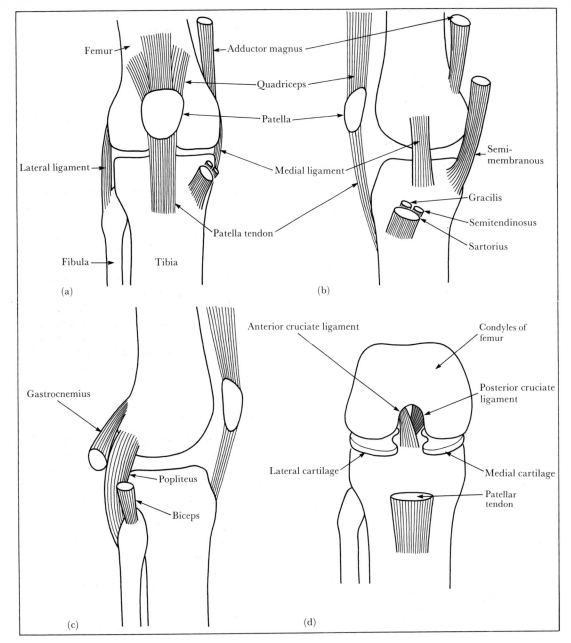

Figure 24.1
General anatomy of the
right knee
(a) Front view
(b) Medial (inner) side view
(c) Lateral (outer) side view
(d) Front view of flexed knee

Figure 24.2
Knee effusion ('patella tap' test).
On gripping the patella in the normal knee, (a), there is no fluid and finger pressure causes no movement. If there is an effusion, (b), the patella sits on the swollen joint and the patella can be 'tapped' up and down by the examining finger

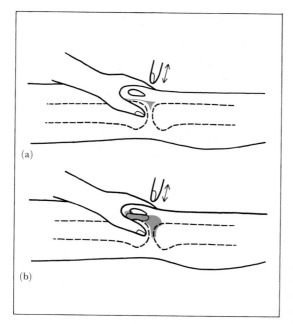

Figure 24.3
Variations in knee alignment

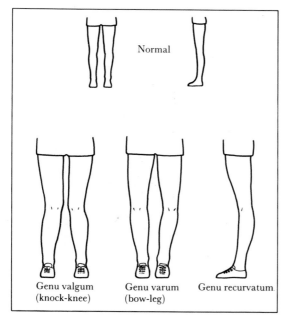

Normal

Genu valgum (knock-knee) Genu varum (bow-leg) Genu recurvatum

effusion indicates a cruciate ligament tear, whereas the slower formation of fluid over a day or more after injury suggests a more general synovitis in response to spraining of the joint capsule and lining.

Locking

If a cartilage is torn, usually by bending and rotating the knee, locking can occur. True locking is always due to a mechanical obstruction in the joint and should not be confused with false locking which is a failure to move freely because of painful inhibition of movement rather than actual mechanical blockage.

Mechanical block, usually by a torn cartilage or a loose body, causes the knee to lock somewhere in its arc of movement. It cannot either bend or straighten by voluntary effort. Usually the patient or an assistant can, by manipulating the leg, induce release as the obstruction is gently shifted aside. The joint should not be forced as this may create further damage. If the block is released, a firm bandage should be applied and medical help should be sought as soon as possible as many diagnoses can best be made as soon as possible after the acute injury and may become increasingly difficult as partial recovery proceeds.

Medial ligament sprain

The commonest knee injury is a sprain of the medial ligament (*Figure 24.4*) which, apart from a direct blow, is vulnerable to two injuries. First, an acute valgus force such as a hard tackle from the lateral side of the knee may spring open the inner side of the knee and stretch the medial ligament causing sprain or rupture. Secondly, rotation of the leg about a fixed foot puts the medial ligament on the stretch, as in a sudden turn at ski-ing or football, and often sprains it. The knee bending and rotating movement which causes medial meniscal tear often causes a simultaneous medial ligament sprain, and initial diagnosis between the two may be difficult. The patient presents simply with a painful inner side of the knee. As cartilage tears do not always cause locking, diagnosis of this part of the injury may have to await rehabilitation from the medial ligament injury. As time and strength progress, it may become evident that all is not well within the knee. There may be some conscious block to movement or a feeling of insecurity, especially on weight-bearing or vigorous movement which may draw attention to the likelihood of cartilage damage.

More violent injuries of this type may contain a third major component, the ruptured anterior cruciate ligament. This is overstretched as the tibia is wrenched violently against its anchorage to the femur, during the injury movement. This so-called 'triad' (*Figure 24.5*) causes severe damage which needs surgical repair.

Cartilage tears

The cartilages (*see Figure 24.1*) are semilunar-shaped shock-absorbing pads between the femoral condyles and the top of the tibia. Because the tibia rotates slightly during straightening, there is always the chance that forced rotation combined with weight-bearing will nip and tear a cartilage. Typically, the soccer player may catch his studs and be tackled over a fixed foot; this forced flexion and rotation shears the medial cartilage.

Cartilage tears can be partial or complete. They may cause minimal symptoms of aching only or the full syndrome of a suddenly painful locked knee. Locking and giving way are key symptoms and mechanical block to full knee range is an important sign.

Medial meniscal tears may be confused with – and combined with – medial ligament tears. Lateral tears are often difficult to diagnose, with some aching and vague instability on active training often being the only symptoms.

While normal X-rays are unhelpful, the acute major tear is clinically obvious. Lesser tears are often ignored but persisting instability, effusion, block or

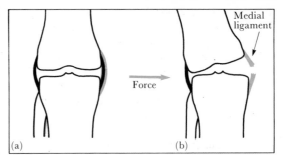

Figure 24.4
Medial ligament sprain. (a) Normal knee. (b) The medial ligament is commonly disrupted by the force of a tackle on the lateral side

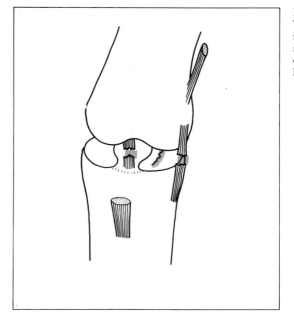

Figure 24.5
The 'unhappy triad' of knee injuries consisting of medial meniscal tear, and anterior cruciate and medial ligament ruptures

giving way (in addition to pain) are indications for expert consultation.

Arthroscopy, internal examination by illuminated instrument, has much improved accurate diagnosis. Contrast-dye X-ray, or arthrography, gives accurate information in experienced hands.

Unless there are major signs, no athlete should agree to an operation for cartilage removal unless he has fully developed his quadriceps muscles in the chondromalacia patellae (C.P.) regimen. In the past, up to 40 per cent of meniscectomy operations removed normal cartilages, probably mostly because of unrecognized C.P. (*see* page 196).

Meniscectomy increases the chances of arthritis later in life and should be performed only for removal of actual tears. There is a swing towards partial removal, that is removal of torn fragments only, and this can often be effected simply through the operating arthroscope, avoiding major joint surgery and speeding up postoperative recovery.

Rehabilitation after knee operations should in every case be strenuously completed. It is based on the usual principles of progressive resisted exercises under the physiotherapist's supervision. Failure to do this leaves a weak knee exposed to further injury. Recent research has shown that immediate active muscle rehabilitation prevents the otherwise inevitable muscle wasting and weakness caused by rest and immobilization. Cast braces permit a limited range of knee movement and early recovery in contrast to the traditional full-leg rigid plaster cast.

Cruciate tears

Certain violent injuries may tear one of the cruciate ligaments, with or without other damage. Anterior cruciate tear is part of 'O'Donoghue's triad' (*Figure 24.5*) with medial ligament and medial cartilage tears. *Figure 24.6* shows the way in which the cruciates stabilize the knee by linking the end of the femur with the tibia.

To test cruciate function the knee is bent and the tibia firmly grasped. The anterior cruciate attaches to the anterior part of the tibia and restrains anterior movement. If it is ruptured, the tibia can be pulled forward (anterior draw sign). Conversely, pressure on a torn posterior cruciate pushes the tibia posteriorly.

Cruciate laxity varies considerably. Some gymnasts and footballers have considerable tibial movement without injury. Most are fairly 'tight'. Without arthroscopy, or definite note of a change in knee stability it may be impossible to know if a cruciate has been stretched or torn, or is simply lax. Posterior

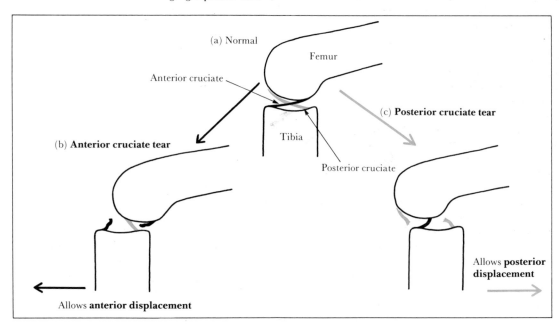

Figure 24.6
Cruciate ligament tears

cruciate tears are often associated with ruptures of the posterior joint capsule.

Ideally, cruciate repairs should be made because an unstable knee is very prone to further damage – especially cartilage tears. Surgery for this condition is not yet universally established however. Whenever cruciate function is impaired, intensive rehabilitation is required for the quadriceps which becomes the main stabilizing force on the knee. This follows the lines set out for C.P. (*see* page 196).

'Giving way'

Spontaneous giving way of the knee on weight-bearing is usually due to sudden relief of a mechanical obstruction, either a torn portion of cartilage or a loose body lying in the joint. The patient is walking or running along and finds that the knee has, without warning, or necessarily pain, given way under him. This condition must be distinguished from the less serious complaint of 'giving way', which after careful scrutiny turns out to be a rapid reflex causing the patient suddenly to withdraw voluntary support from the knee when pain is triggered, as for instance, by a painful knee-cap on certain movements in chondromalacia patellae. In this case there is no inherent instability but usually an easily cured inflammation inhibiting normal muscular action.

Loose bodies

The two common causes of knee locking or giving way in the athletic age group are a torn cartilage and loose bodies from osteochondritis dissecans (*Figure 24.7*). The latter is an obscure condition, usually of adolescence, where part of the cartilage lining a joint becomes impaired by an unknown disease process and may drop off the surface of the joint. It is obvious on X-ray and surgical removal or reattachment of the loose body may be successful. This condition occasionally recovers spontaneously but often gives rise to aching of the knee in a teenager, associated with occasional effusion, weakness and sometimes locking or giving way. Osteochondritis tends to cause

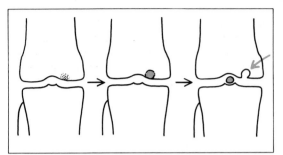

Figure 24.7
Osteochondritis dissecans showing formation of loose body

degenerative arthritis in later life and therefore does not carry a good prognosis for the sportsman.

Hip disease

Knee pain should always be remembered as a sign of hip disease with pain referred from the hip joint, particularly in adolescence.

Infection

Infection of the knee joint is rare and causes a warm red swollen joint in contrast to the effusion from a chronic sprain which is cool, with no overlying redness.

Cysts

There are three common cysts about the knee (*Figure 24.8*). Occasionally a cyst may form on one of the cartilages, usually the lateral cartilage in the front half of the knee joint. The cyst may present as a pea-sized lump which seems to pop in and out of the joint as it is moved. It cannot always be demonstrated but if a nuisance, it can be removed; however, its presence may not greatly trouble most people and no action is then needed.

At the back of the knee the 'Baker's cyst' is a pouch of the synovial lining of the knee joint. In general, this is harmless unless there is associated injury or disease present, such as rheumatoid arthritis, or unless the sheer size becomes mechanically obstructive in which case surgical dissection is necessary.

A cyst on the inner posterior aspect of the knee may be the semimembranosus bursa. This is a small extension of the synovial sac underlying the insertion of the semimembranosus tendon. Constant irritation or pressure may cause this to expand, for instance in horse-riders. Management depends on the size and awkwardness of the lump, rather than its presence.

Bursa

Tissue friction may enlarge the prepatellar bursa in the soft tissue in front of the knee and cause pain, swelling and redness ('housemaid's knee') which is relieved by rest and anti-inflammatory measures.

Adolescent conditions

There are occasional growth faults at the front of the knee (*Figure 24.9*). At the lower corner of the patella, the adolescent epiphysis may become deformed and inflamed, causing pain and limitation of movement (Sinding–Larsen–Johannson disease). This is closely similar to Osgood–Schlatter's disease, which is a traction epiphysitis or osteochondritis at the tibial tubercle at the lower end of the patellar tendon. Both conditions are usually self-limiting in adolescence and worsened by vigorous movements like kicking, rather than walking. Conservative treatment such as rest and heat may need to be prolonged. Local steroid injections tend to give temporary relief, and the main problem is to decide whether surgery is necessary in a condition which will in any case tend to limit itself by

the age of about 16. If it is particularly painful despite rest, then surgical excision of the bone fragments at the end of the tendon may be helpful.

Age and arthritis

The young knee is surprisingly elastic and, compared with the examination of the adult knee, often shows almost alarming degrees of movement. Adolescence sees ossification and tightening up of the musculoskeletal structures and increasing age brings gradual loss of tissue elasticity. At the same time, the general tendency to develop osteoarthritis (osteoarthrosis or degenerative arthritis) is increased in sportsmen who have had injuries to joints. Age and degenerative arthritis give rise to small bony excrescences called osteophytes at the edges of joint margins and this, together with a gradual deterioration of the quality of the joint cartilages in the knee gives a characteristic X-ray appearance of joint space narrowing with fraying at the edges (*Figure 24.10*). Clinically, there may be no symptoms at all or simply some harmless creaking (crepitus) on bending and straightening the knee. This is particularly evident between the patella and the underlying femur.

The main clinical problem is that once degenerative changes have set in, particularly after previous injuries or meniscectomies (cartilage removals), further injury or strain of the knee joint may give rise to disproportionately serious symptoms. The appearance of 'Saturday night knee' is

Figure 24.8 (left) Cysts at the knee. (a) Cyst of lateral cartilage in lateral view. (b) Rear view of left knee with common cysts. (c) Prepatellar bursa (p.b.) and semimembranosus bursa (s.b.) in medial (inner side) view
Figure 24.9 (right) Epiphyseal disorders

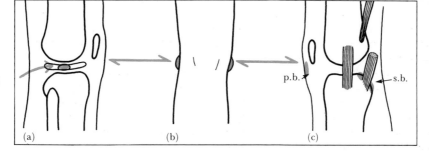

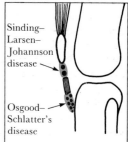

particularly daunting. This typically is suffered by a player who somehow gets through Saturday's game with discomfort in his knee, and then finds in the hours following the game that there is increasing pain and swelling of the joint. He may be unable to train or play for several days, hoping that the effusion and symptoms will settle sufficiently by next Saturday to permit him to play again. Once this pattern of symptoms is established, it is virtually impossible to get the player back to his accustomed level. This degree of joint inflammation and scarring is usually irreversible and further strenuous play only accelerates the slide into severe osteoarthritis.

Every effort must therefore be made to treat thoroughly and immediately all knee injuries in sport because the late sequels are disabling as well as potentially avoidable.

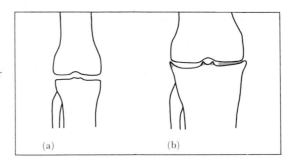

Figure 24.10
Osteoarthritis of the knee
(a) Normal
(b) Degenerative changes include narrowing of the joint space and formation of osteophytes

Chondromalacia patellae (C.P.) ('Sportsman's knee')

Causes

Chondromalacia patellae has numerous eponyms such as jogger's knee, jumper's knee, runner's knee, cyclist's knee and so on. The condition is usually due to a functional distortion of the muscles acting on the patella; this in turn often reflects underlying abnormalities of leg alignment.

The main pull of the powerful quadriceps muscle comes obliquely down the thigh (*Figure 24.11*) to the patella where, in the general meeting of tendons, its line of pull turns a slight angle through the knee-cap into the patellar tendon where the extending pull is transmitted to the attachment into the tibial tubercle.

This line of pull exerts a bow-string effect, tending to pull the patella out to the side. This happens in chondromalacia and a painful irritation of the undersurface of the patella is set up by its rubbing on the lateral condyle of the femur. In normal health and anatomy, however, this bow-stringing tendency is

countered by the pull of vastus medialis, the smallest component of the quadriceps which comes into the knee-cap from the inner side. Thus there is a balanced set of forces which acts on the knee-cap and keeps it correctly aligned.

Why do these mechanisms break down so commonly to cause 'sportsman's knee'? Most importantly, vastus medialis contracts fully only in the last 10–15 degrees of straight leg extension, thus it is a muscle of straight-leg, rather than of bent-leg, function. A moment's reflection will recall that the majority of sporting actions as well as training stresses concern the bent leg, whether in cycling, running, exercising at gym, weight-lifting from the squat position, diving, jumping or landing. Furthermore, the movements of daily living tend to stress the bent knee rather than hold the straight-leg position. For instance, sitting, driving, cycling or climbing stairs are all dependent on bent-knee function. It happens, therefore, that the leg is relatively underexercised in the firmly held straight position. This may not matter for most people most of the time.

If the heavy stresses of sport are repeated sufficiently, however, there arises a state of relative overdevelopment of the obliquely acting part of the quadriceps muscles relative to vastus medialis. It must be realized that fully 'normal' muscle is involved and that the crucial factor is not the absolute strength of any part of the muscle, but the relative strength of one portion to another. Thus sportsmen who

Figure 24.11
Chondromalacia patellae
(C.P.), 'Sportsman's knee'
(a) Normal alignment of
right knee with forces on
patella
(b) Lateral distraction of
patella in response to
weakness of vastus medialis
or other mechanical factors
(*see* text)
(c) Lateral displacement of
patella causes friction on
side of femoral groove

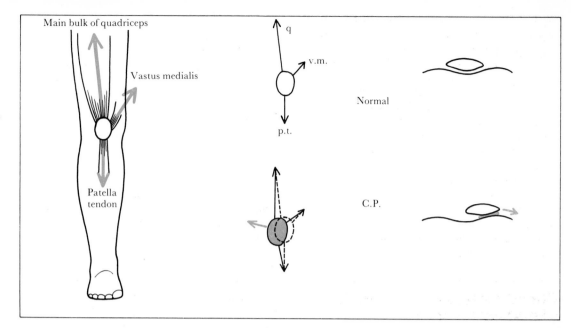

repeatedly and intensively train their bent knee run the risk of muscular imbalance at the patella.

Symptoms

The symptoms of C.P. are of aching around the knee-cap and may be caused by any unaccustomed exercise including a run on a hard surface. Within hours there is a reflex inhibition of vastus medialis and an aching which may relate particularly to climbing or descending stairs, cycling, or getting up from sitting in a bent-knee position, as well as while running. A typical story is of a runner who sets out on his training run to find that at a fixed point of, say, 5 min or half a mile into his run he starts aching and seizes up, being forced to stop – whereupon the pain disappears. After a pause, he resumes his activity only to find that the pain recurs, and so on. At this point most doctors will find nothing wrong on examination and a frequent fault is to prescribe vigorous knee exercises in flexion, for instance the well-known

extension exercises of the bent knee against a resisted pulley. In this way, symptoms are almost always worsened because the bent knee is being further stressed while insufficient attention is being paid to the held, straight-leg position.

This vicious circle tends to continue indefinitely and many surgeons have been forced to perform meniscectomies almost in despair because of prolonged unrelieved symptoms, only to find the removed cartilages to be normal. The sportsman then makes a rapid recovery because for the first time his rehabilitation programme has offered him an intensive straight-leg development programme!

Diagnosis

The cardinal steps in the diagnosis of C.P. are, first, the history, as above. Secondly, if the two legs are compared side by side and fully contracted into a static quadriceps bracing exercise, the weakness and wasting of vastus medialis is apparent. Often an examining finger can be dug well into the weak medialis compared with the fit side or, if both sides are affected, there is an obvious discrepancy between the two weak vasti mediales and the more tensely muscled main quadriceps bulk. Thirdly, if the patella is gently held by one hand and the quadriceps strongly contracted against it, there is severe pain and crepitus on the affected side.

X-rays may be normal, show lower pole demineralization of the patella, or eventually, but rarely, cystic erosions and arthritic changes on the underside of the patella. Direct examination shows a shaggy fibrinous exudate on the underneath of the patella.

Treatment

The primary treatment for most C.P. is therefore obvious. A simple mechanical defect, i.e. vastus medialis weakness, is simply remedied by the repeated performance of strongly held, straight-leg static quadriceps contractions. The straight-leg position with the foot at the right angle is adopted and the athlete holds his quadriceps in a 'stats' for as long as possible and as hard as possible. Usually the first few contractions are held for perhaps 10–15 seconds before medialis starts flickering weakly.

An effective plan is to hold 10 maximal contractions every hour, counting 15–20 seconds each, with 5-second relaxations between holds. A common fault is to do repeated quick twitches. Both legs must be exercised.

Failure to get satisfactory relief is usually due to one of the following causes:

- Failure to do the exercises.
- Performing the exercises correctly but also carrying out intensive knee bending exercises such as resisted leg extensions or squats. In this case, stop the latter and concentrate entirely on straight leg work.
- Performing the exercises, omitting those for flexion but sabotaging the attempt to re-educate the

straight-leg musculature by such daily repetitive action as stair or ladder climbing, cycling, and so on, thus involving an unrecognized component of knee flexion. The answer is obvious. The patient should remember that C.P. reflects a balance between extension and flexion of the knee. The key to understanding and controlling C.P. is to understand the mechanism of that balance.

- A small proportion of patients seem to lose the automatic neuromuscular control of a well-co-ordinated quadriceps contraction and make an unco-ordinated contraction of its different components. They usually respond to one or more treatments of faradism, which seems to re-educate the nervous control mechanisms.
- Many patients have complex anatomical malalignment and need correction, usually of foot posture, by corrective orthotic devices (*see* Podiatry, below).

Total failure to respond to the C.P. regimen may, in some people, be due to an undeveloped or misplaced patella which may need to be anchored surgically. Also, in some people the patella can be permanently pulled over laterally. In recent years identification of this group of athletes has led to the development of the operation of lateral retinacular release, in which some of the patella's lateral retaining tendons are slit subcutaneously with a very fine blade, which allows the patella to slip towards the midline into a more effective anatomical position between the femoral condyles.

Occasionally in major knee reconstructive surgery realignment of the soft tissues is performed to enhance the stability of the joint. The patellar tendon is brought further towards the inside of the knee and a lateral retinacular release is performed.

British experience of major knee reconstruction of this sort is relatively limited because of the much safer nature of British soccer and rugby compared with American football which permits massive blind-side tackling causing horrific anatomical disruption of the knee. Despite injuries of this nature and almost equally heroic surgical reconstruction, many players resume the game but, remembering the high risk of further injury and major disability in middle life, the wisdom of this intention must be questioned very carefully with the patient.

Podiatry

Many disorders of leg anatomy have been shown to cause pain by forcing the foot to tread abnormally during gait. Correction of many such structural discrepancies is possible, after detailed clinical assessment, by the construction of corrective insoles known as orthoses or orthotics. These will be further discussed in the chapter on the foot (Chapter 27).

The cumulative stresses of sport, especially longer-distance running on hard surfaces, cause symptoms of overuse injuries not seen frequently in normal medical practice and for this reason many sportsmen gain little help from orthodox medicine.

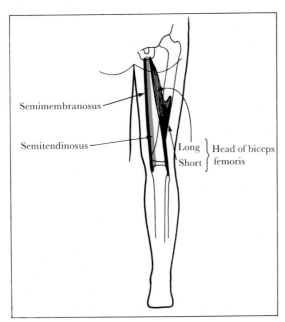

Figure 24.12
Hamstring muscles

Semimembranosus

Semitendinosus

Long
Short } Head of biceps femoris

Foot malalignments are commmonly associated with C.P. and appropriate orthotic correction is often dramatically successful.

Soft-tissue injuries at the knee

Soft-tissue injuries occur around the knee but independently of the joint itself. Hamstring tendon insertions are often strained in sprinting, kicking or dancing. The semimembranosus and semitendinosus tendons insert on the inner side of the back of the knee and the biceps on the outer side (*Figure 24.12*). Strain is particularly likely to occur after running on slippery or hilly surfaces where the hamstring mechanism is put on a slightly fuller stretch than usual and tends to claw the body forward over the ground. Accurate history and detailed palpation of the back and side of the knee usually makes this diagnosis obvious. Rest, thorough stretching and warm-up, graduated acceleration and running all help in rehabilitation. Occasionally physiotherapy or, very rarely, steroid injections may be required.

Pain and clicking on the outer aspect of the knee joint may be due to sprain of the lateral ligament, a less significant structure than its medial counterpart already described. This condition may be caused by twisting strains, direct blows or springing of the joint from a blow on the inner side.

A clicking discomfort occasionally felt over the outer side of the knee near the lateral hamstring insertion may be due to slipping of the iliotibial tract of tendon over a bony outcrop of the lateral femoral condyle with repeated stereotyped running movements (*Figure 24.13*). This may occur in long-distance runners and skiers, with painful 'clicking' at about 30 degrees of knee flexion during movement. Once this condition is firmly established, inflammatory and fibrotic tissue continues to rub against the adjacent tract. If rest and local steroid injections are not effective, surgery may be required.

The patella may be dislocated by a blow or twisting force, especially if the patello-femoral groove is shallow, the patella small or highly placed, or the patient's tissue lax. Recurrent dislocation may need surgical fixation.

Conclusions

General indications for medical help in knee injury

- Any severe injury with instability, locking or giving way.
- Any effusion.
- Any instability or pain persisting after thorough quadriceps exercise regimen as outlined under C.P.

Methods of investigation

A detailed clinical history and thorough physical examination go a long way to making a diagnosis in the injured knee. It is true to say, however, that injured knees are, for most doctors, either straightforward or extremely difficult! If initial examination does not conclude a diagnosis then consultation with a specialist is imperative.

Further techniques available include: *arthrography*, in which dye is injected into the knee (often with gas) to obtain a more detailed contrast picture of the cartilages, ligaments and lining; *arthroscopy*, in which a fibrescopic torch is introduced and direct visual examination can be made of different internal structures; and *arthrotomy*, or open operation, at which even more detailed assessment of damage can be made.

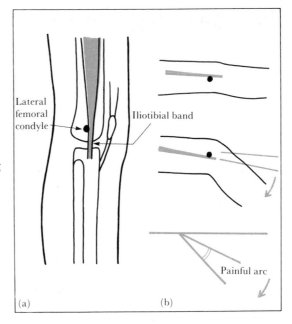

Figure 24.13
Iliotibial band friction syndrome.
(a) Normal position of iliotibial band and lateral femoral condyle. (b) Movement of i.t.b. over l.f.c. in partial knee flexion showing arc of painful movement often associated with 'clicking' sensation

The advantage of the arthroscope is that its compact size allows a thorough examination of most parts of the knee – often without a general anaesthetic and on an out-patient basis. Performance of a full open operation is thus avoided unless the preliminary arthroscopy findings justify it.

It is true that there is no area of orthopaedic surgery as full of controversy and variable results as knee surgery. It is also strangely true that a vast number of injured knees defy a full and satisfactory diagnosis but may nevertheless be carefully rehabilitated to a satisfactory functional result.

25 Lower-leg injuries

In Osgood–Schlatter's disease of adolescence, pain at the insertion of the patellar tendon into the tibial tubercle at the top of the shin is usually exacerbated by violent movements such as kicking or jumping. Trial and error will determine whether cycling and jogging or even faster running can be tolerated – usually after an initial 2–4 weeks' rest while the inflammation settles.

Tibial fractures occur in contact sport and may be simple or compound (*see* Chapter 18). On average, 6–8 weeks in plaster are followed by another month of rehabilitation. Direct blows to the shin cause painful periosteal haematomas on the tibia and can be prevented or minimized by proper shin guards – guards which, surprisingly, are often discarded during the course of a game just as reflexes and defence mechanisms become tired and injury risk increases. Cold compresses and early movement are effective early treatment.

Shin soreness (shin splints) and shin fractures

Cortical bone thickening is one of the normal reactions to repeated stress and is sometimes seen to a remarkable degree in a runner's tibia, although most people do not respond in this way.

Surprisingly, there are no nationally or internationally agreed definitions of the expressions 'shin splints' or 'shin soreness'. For practical purposes it may be simplest to consider pains in relation to the tibia, the fibula, the anterior compartment of soft tissue in front of these bones and the posterior compartment of soft tissue behind them (*Figure 25.1*). The tibia and fibula are joined by a sheet of connective tissue or fascia from which mucles to the foot originate posteriorly and anteriorly. This fascia is occasionally calcified, not necessarily from injury, but the X-ray appearances may be alarming to the unwary.

Shin soreness usually presents as pain on, or next to, the tibia during active weight-bearing (*Figure 25.2*). It may be caused by unaccustomed footwear or changes in training habits, such as longer-distance or faster speed runs, or harder or softer surfaces than usual.

Careful examination of the shin, preferably with the knee bent and the patient thoroughly relaxed, will show whether the surface of the tibia itself is tender to touch. Rarely, in the presence of a stress fracture there is a localized painful lump on the bone which indicates this diagnosis, confirmed by X-ray. The key feature of the athlete's story is the 'crescendo' history (*see* page 144) and this should always make the coach suspicious. A general mild tenderness on firm palpation of the tibia would not necessarily indicate fracture however. It may in some cases indicate the 'pre-stress fracture state' where the bone is beginning to become structurally distorted in response to repetitive mechanical stresses but has not actually cracked. Radioisotope studies may indicate increased metabolic activity of the bone in this area but it is usual only to employ normal X-ray techniques and these may show no abnormalities.

Further examination proceeds down the full length of each tibia in turn, comparing sides. In a high proportion of cases tenderness will be found bilaterally even if there is only complaint of running pain on one side.

Knotty fibrotic areas of tender tissue may be felt up against the margin of the tibia on its inner aspect, and these often extend into the muscles leading away from the bone down towards the ankle. These are the deep flexors of the foot and ankle. Their repeated strainings at their origins on the back of the tibia may be responsible for most cases of shin soreness. However, *see also* Chapter 28 for discussion of shin soreness in relation to running style.

Often the tibial shaft and lining is neither tender nor lumpy but there is a distinctly separated area of painful lumpy tissue, perhaps half a finger-breadth away in the muscular tissue. In these cases there need be absolutely no doubt about the soft-tissue nature of the shin soreness. Unfortunately, if there is bony tenderness or a tender lump up against the bone lining, or periosteum, there is always some doubt about the possibility of early stress fracture. As it is plainly not feasible to X-ray every patient with shin soreness, a reasonable compromise is to note carefully the quality of the pain (thinking of the typical 'crescendo' of the stress fracture) and if there is doubt training should be stopped for a few days and resumed at a slightly lower level.

Lower down the tibial shaft, tenosynovitis of the long flexor tendons causes pain on moving the foot up and down, and swelling and crepitus over the tendon up against the inner edge of the tibia confirms this diagnosis. Rest is needed for up to 2 weeks while the exudate subsides. Physiotherapy and steroid injections may, in skilled hands, be effective in accelerating recovery.

Tibial stress fractures are frequently seen in military recruits who are required to undertake strenuous exercise in heavy boots. They are far less common in civilian athletes but possibly more

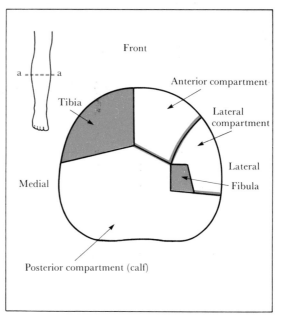

Figure 25.1
Shin. Cross-sectional view of right shin at level a/a, showing division of soft tissues by tibia, fibula and fibrous sheet

frequent in adolescents. It should be emphasized that a stress fracture can be gained despite a relatively small amount of running. Stress fractures are by no means confined to very-long-distance road runners, and the occasional adolescent athlete may become a victim on a mere 10 miles (16 km) per week of training on a hard surface, although this is unusual.

Fibular stress fractures are more frequent than tibial lesions in runners, commonly occurring in the lower third of the fibula at or just above the lateral malleolus of the ankle (*Figure 25.3*). The 'crescendo' history may be characteristic and, if initial X-rays are unhelpful, bone scans and follow up X-rays may be required. A trial spell of rest is indicated by the history alone and accompanying tenderness on palpating the fibula – even if an X-ray is not available.

The problem with stress fractures is that they are liable to proceed in one stride from a crack to complete fragmentation without warning. Occasionally, this causes considerable swelling,

Figure 25.2 (left)
Causes of shin soreness
Figure 25.3 (centre)
Sites of tibial and fibular
stress fractures
Figure 25.4 (right)
Fibular subperiosteal
haematoma

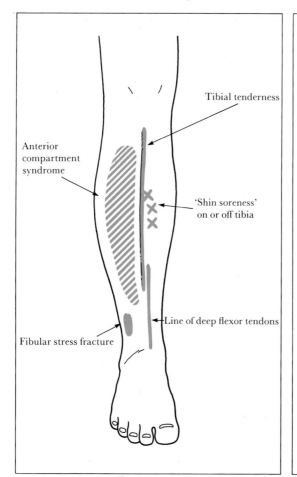

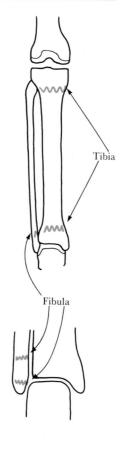

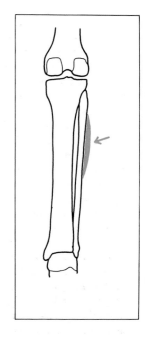

bruising and discomfort of the lower leg, and in the female athlete may give rise to clinical doubt about deep vein thrombosis perhaps related to taking the contraceptive pill. Occasionally a similar, but more acute, history is obtained in which case the X-ray shows a subperiosteal haematoma to have stripped the periosteum of the upper fibula shaft (*Figure 25.4*). This painful condition requires no special treatment other than avoidance of running and responds over the same 4–6 weeks as a true stress fracture. While

some sportsmen have repeated stress fractures, there is no need for pessimism about recurrence provided that the original lesion is soundly healed.

As the initial pain subsides, the temptation to resume running within 10–14 days must be firmly resisted because complete healing clearly needs at least 4–8 weeks and some cases are particularly slow to heal. Premature resumption of training merely invites recurrence. No special treatment is needed for most stress fractures. They are well-defined responses to stereotyped mechanical pressures and a relief of these movements alone brings full recovery.

Compartment syndromes

Potentially serious and painful variants of shin soreness are the 'compartment syndromes'. The anterior compartment of soft tissue is firmly bound in by the tibia, fibula, connecting fascia, and the tight fascia at the front of the shin (*Figure 25.1*). Occasionally, if an unaccustomed and drastic amount of exercise such as marching in heavy boots or a particularly hard run is undertaken, there may be so much swelling and congestion of the tissues in the anterior compartment that it blocks off its own blood supply. This leads to the classic anterior compartment syndrome of congestion leading to gangrene and requires immediate surgical decompression of the restraining fascia. Why this syndrome occurs so infrequently is not known – it probably needs a combination of activity and restricted anatomy, and most soft-tissue compartments are large enough to accommodate extra tissue swelling and congestion after exercise. The essential first aid measures are elevation of the lower leg and ice packing.

The posterior compartment syndrome is less easy to define and probably a more chronic entity than the dangerous, if unusual, anterior syndrome. With posterior compartment syndrome, a sportsman who has been much troubled over a long time by soft-tissue inflammation of the deep flexor muscle origins on the inner aspect of the tibia eventually arrives at a state where the soft tissues are so inflamed, scarred and tethered that he can no longer stretch them back into action with each training run. He suffers chronic shin soreness on the inner and posterior aspect of the tibia.

Causes of shin soreness

A major factor in shin soreness is the hardness of playing surfaces; increasing hardness increases the shock-absorptive stresses on the tissues. For the same reason, hard-soled shoes, boots or running spikes aggravate this condition. Running on slopes often increases the stresses by altering the angle of the foot and ankle, and similar anatomical malalignments of the foot and lower leg can predispose to shin soreness. Many cases remain obscure except in simple terms of overuse.

Danger times for every sportsman are the changes of season, particularly when a holiday lay-off leads to a quick return to overintensive training. Changes of surface from cross country to track or *vice versa* for the runner, or the rugby player's return from the sandy beaches of summer to hard-studded boots on hard-baked autumn surfaces, can cause shin soreness as well as most of the other overuse sports injuries of the lower limb.

Treatment of shin soreness

The cause must be sought and corrected. For instance, slight reduction in running with a change to a softer surface, such as from road onto grass, is often all that is required. Footwear is often faulty and can be simply remedied (*see* Chapter 29) – a change of shoes often alters the landing angle of the foot and may thus relieve the original stress. A useful tip is to rotate two or three pairs of sports shoes over two or three different types of training and surface during a 3- or 4-day rota. Many cases of shin soreness are related to highly repetitive movements and if these can be varied even slightly, much of the stress can be removed from the strained tissues. Further, careful attention should be paid to the runner's gait (Chapter 28), orthotic correction of which may have an important part to play in many cases of shin soreness.

Physiotherapy, particularly ultrasound and ice applied before and after training, is often very effective. Resistant cases often respond well to local steroid injections. Very rarely surgical decompression may be required in chronic cases of tenosynovitis or compartment syndromes.

Calf strains

Calf strains, or 'tennis leg', (*Figure 25.5*) are relatively common, particularly in the older player of either sex. The calf muscle works in a complex manner which both braces the lower leg against the forces of landing and at the same time launches the foot into the take-off thrust. This complex double mechanism, achieved by the gastrocnemius and soleus muscles, through the final pathway of the Achilles tendon, is more than a simple pull on the lever of the heel bone, or calcaneum.

The calf and Achilles mechanism is often strained if there is a sudden change of movement such as tripping over an obstruction or treading awkwardly on to a step. The sudden tear of the calf muscle, for instance at tennis, is alarming but not always serious, despite much bruising. Surgical repair of a major tear is performed if severe disability persists.

It may be difficult to make a clear anatomical diagnosis at the heel because there is much anatomical variation in the low calf musculature and its insertion into the Achilles tendon which may even present as a double or treble structure. The small plantaris muscle may run its long thin tendon the entire length of the calf muscles and Achilles tendon, and it may sometimes rupture causing pain and much diagnostic confusion with calf or Achilles lesions.

The deep flexor tendons run part of their course from the back of the tibia and fibula round and under the back of the ankle to their insertion on the underneath of the foot and may develop overuse tenosynovitis. Because these tendons are particularly well hidden from view and deeply tucked under the back of the ankle, they do not always give rise to such characteristic pain or examination findings as do more superficial tendons. The sportsman, usually a runner, complains of either very low shin soreness on the inner aspect of the tibia, deep posterior ankle soreness or even a discomfort apparently associated with the Achilles tendon. Crepitus may be felt by the patient – reappearing on manipulation of the ankle gently up and down. Occasionally the soft-tissue X-ray reveals considerable shadowing associated with thickening and inflammation of the deep flexor tendons. This area is difficult to inject with accuracy, although injection sometimes is effective as is surgical decompression in chronic cases.

Achilles tendon

This major tendon does not have a synovial sheath. The general characteristics of tendon injury are described in Chapter 17 (pages 139–141). The Achilles tendon is particularly stressed in sport because of its dual functions of shock absorption and foot leverage. Hard surfaces and insufficiently

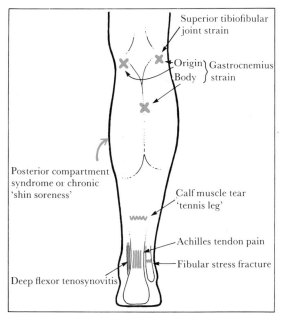

Figure 25.5 Causes of calf pain; rear view of right leg

Superior tibiofibular joint strain

Origin } Gastrocnemius
Body } strain

Posterior compartment syndrome or chronic 'shin soreness'

Calf muscle tear 'tennis leg'

Achilles tendon pain

Fibular stress fracture

Deep flexor tenosynovitis

cushioned shoes increase the ground impact and injury risk. A lower-than-normal heel-raise increases the range of movement of the tendon and is often a crucial factor causing pain.

The notorious Achilles heel-tab on shoes (*see Figure 17.1*) is a potent source of Achilles tendon injury. The remedy – shoe adjustment – is described on page 242 (*see Figure 29.3*).

Achilles tendon lesions are summarized as follows.

Achilles tendinitis

Pain is experienced on or following exercise. There is no swelling, but the tendon is painful on touch/squeeze.

Treatment is by heel pad and rest; the condition usually settles within a few days.
If neglected, tendinitis usually progresses to peritendinitis.

Achilles peritendinitis (*Figure 25.6b*)

Pain is experienced on or following exercise. There is stiffness after rest, especially first thing in the morning. Swelling occurs around the tendon, with palpable creaking.

Treatment is by heel pad and rest; or rarely by injection.

If neglected, peritendinitis gradually worsens to constrict the tendon and this may need surgical clearance. Physiotherapy results vary because some cases are made worse by physical contact. As this lesion is due to tissue friction, it is not logical to apply therapeutic friction massage. This treatment is sometimes successful, however, presumably because it breaks loose some unstable fibrous tissue. Unfortunately, it is impossible to predict which cases will be made worse by the friction's causing an increase in inflammation and forming more scar tissue.

Injections may cure early lesions but must be aimed into the soft tissue around the tendon, never into the tendon itself!

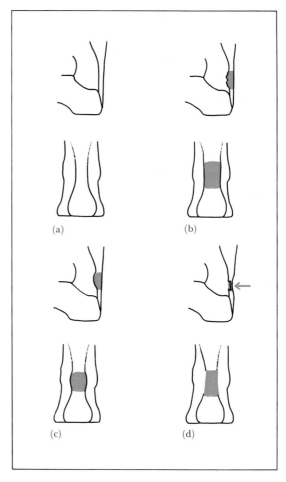

Figure 25.6
Achilles tendon lesions
(a) Normal
(b) Peritendinitis
(c) Partial rupture or focal degeneration
(d) Total rupture

Partial rupture and focal degeneration (*Figure 25.6c*)

Under heavy loading the tendon may form micro-ruptures which lead to small, enclosed lesions which cause localized pain on exercise, possibly due to increased pressure. The differentiation is partly one of degree. A considerable proportion of the Achilles tendon may rupture. A characteristic feature is the 'snapping' sensation felt by the athlete. Later findings are weakness of foot thrust and calf muscle wasting.

The Achilles is tender and locally swollen.

Treatment is ideally by surgical correction. Alternatively up to 6–12 months rest, followed by cautious return to training may allow full recovery. Walking, cycling and swimming are encouraged but jumping, dancing or running eliminated. A heel pad is used initialy.

Total rupture (*Figure 25.6d*)

The victim feels a sudden 'snap' or 'impact' in the tendon or may hear a 'snap'. Loss of Achilles function leads to calf wasting, inability to stand on the toes and some or total loss of foot plantarflexion. Squeezing the calf muscle of a patient who is lying in the prone position does not move his foot because the tendon no longer transmits the contraction.

The tendon cannot be felt clearly. There is a gap in the tissues and later there may be considerable bruising.

Treatment is ideally by immediate surgical repair; prolonged immobilization by plaster casting gives sound but slower results and may leave residual muscle wasting and weakness sufficient to impair full athletic movement.

26 Ankle injuries

The ankle joint acts in two ways in connecting the lower leg with the foot. First, it is a hinge allowing simple leverage up and down and, secondly, it allows rotational movement above the ankle to be converted to simple leverage to the foot (torque conversion). In the foot itself, complex buffering of movements of the small joints accommodates constant shifts of posture. The foot and ankle thus serve as a balancing mechanism which constantly adapts to changes in stride, speed and surface by internal posture adjustments.

The ankle joint itself consists of the lower end of the tibia and fibula, bound together by the firm talofibular ligaments forming a receiving mortice into which the upper surface of the talus articulates (*Figure 26.1*). The adjacent surfaces are smooth and arc-shaped, so that the rounded surface of the talus can slide smoothly to allow the foot to point upwards (dorsiflexion) and downwards (plantarflexion). The whole joint is bound by its capsule and firm ligaments on all sides, particularly reinforced on the inner and outer sides as the medial and lateral ligament complexes, respectively (*Figure 26.2*).

Os trigonum

Occasionally, a congenital anomaly arises at the back of the talus with the formation of an extra ossicle, the os trigonum. This can be a separate bone or an excrescence on the back of the talus (*Figure 26.3*). Its presence may not matter but occasionally it causes a mechanical block to full and free movement of one or both ankles which is shown by comparing the range of movement at each ankle. A difference between the two sides suggests a mechanical block at the front or back of the ankle joint. Sometimes a player may have limited movement on both sides which can be due to similar mechanical obstruction. This restriction of ankle movement is shown by X-rays of both joints taken laterally in full dorsi- and plantarflexion. If there is not already too much other joint injury due to chronic sprains, mechanical block usually responds well to surgery.

Ankle sprains

Ankle sprains are usually caused by a forced inversion or eversion of the ankle joint, for instance, while being tackled or from tripping while running. The ligaments and/or joint capsule may be stretched or torn (*Figure 26.4*) and may bleed internally or externally. Internal bleeding into the ankle joint leads to joint effusion, with considerable disability and swelling on both sides of the joint. In contrast, external bleeding leads to more extravagant bruising, usually on one side only of the joint but with considerable localized unilateral swelling. Ankle joint swelling is best seen from behind where the fullness of the normal hollow on one side of the Achilles tendon suggests external sprain whereas a fullness of both hollows is more likely to be due to an effusion within the joint.

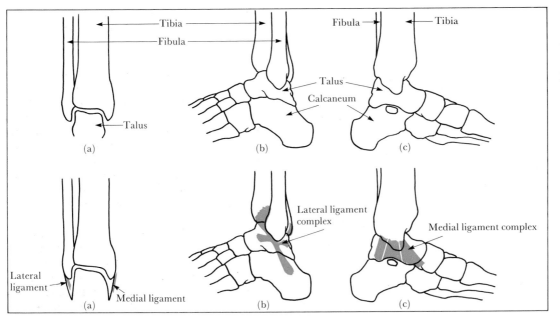

Figure 26.1 (top) Ankle, basic anatomy. (a) Front view. (b) Lateral view. (c) Medial view
Figure 26.2 (bottom) Ankle ligaments. (a) Front view. (b) Lateral view. (c) Medial view

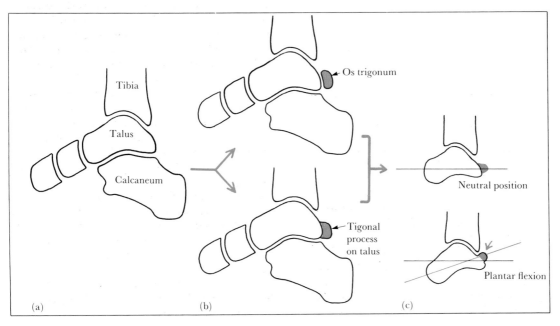

Figure 26.3
Os trigonum.
(a) Normal. (b) Frequent variants. (c) Block to movement by prominent os trigonum impingeing on back of tibia in ankle plantarflexion

Figure 26.4
Sprain of ankle lateral
ligament

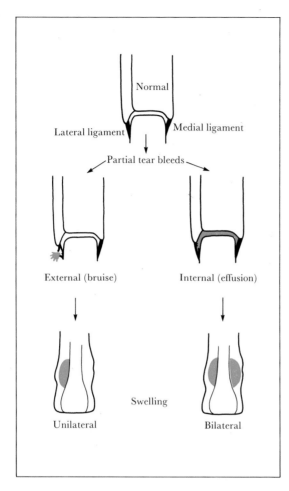

Many ankle sprains are very slight and the player may safely continue his game after a momentary break. Any more substantial injury cannot be accurately diagnosed on the field, however, as it is impossible, without X-ray, to determine the full extent of tissue rupture and possible fracture of any of the ankle bones. First aid treatment is to remove the player from the game, to rest the affected ankle and to apply cold compresses followed by firm strapping, or splinting with care being taken not to make the strapping too tight. Ice applications and ultrasonic therapy can start immediately and frequent intensive treatments, several times daily, secure the best and fastest results.

In practice, for most sportsmen the first decision is whether or not to seek medical help. The miserable sequels of neglected ankle sprains are such a burden to the sportsman that it is worth erring on the side of caution. The commonest fault with ankle sprains is to undertreat them. The standard management often is to be dismissed from the Casualty Department with a crepe bandage after a simple X-ray which shows no fracture. Nature may take care of many sprains but this management is inadequate and encourages the development of chronic pain and instability.

If there is effusion in the joint, it must be rested. Many sportsmen have learnt the hard way that weight-bearing on an injured major joint simply prolongs the inflammation and disability time.

Firm strapping or temporary immobilization with a plaster cast or back-slab is effective and ultrasound with ice treatment can continue. The ankle usually settles in 1–3 weeks and training can gradually be resumed. The main complication is ligament rupture which, by removing one of the natural bindings of the ankle, introduces instability whenever the ankle turns. Rupture of the lateral ligament allows the joint to spring open when the foot is turned into inversion on forceful movement (*Figure 26.5*). This opening is felt by the player as a momentary instability, with or without pain; often with ankle sprains a feeling of insecurity or instability follows. Examination shows that the injured ankle can be inverted far more than normal which then can be confirmed with forced inversion X-rays, taken first with the foot in the neutral position and then with the foot being inverted under firm manual pressure. This pressure opens up the mortice of the ankle joint. Both sides should be compared because some people have enough normal joint laxity to open the ankle mortice without injury.

Instability is due to rupture of both the joint capsule and the ligament and also to damage to some of the nerve fibres responsible for proprioception, or natural position sense. The ankle is temporarily deprived of its automatic sensory awareness of its position in space, especially on movement.

Fortunately, this awareness can quickly be regained with strengthening and balancing exercises, particularly on the 'wobble board' – a circular wooden platform underneath which is a simple hemisphere (*Figure 26.6*) – which allows the player to stand on the platform and literally wobble about on one or both legs. These exercises re-educate positional sense and usually cure instability. Wobble boards are easily made and are so effective that all sports clubs and gymnasia should possess them for conditioning and rehabilitation. If there is significant damage to the capsule or ligament, however, satisfactory results are unlikely until the torn structures have been surgically repaired. It is notable that British medical practice is more conservative in respect of surgical repair of ligaments than is that of the Americans.

For simpler ankle sprains, initial pain relief with cold therapy followed by progressive resisted exercises and early weight-bearing, later accompanied by some form of heat or cold treatment, should produce a satisfactory result within 2–4 weeks. A careful final fitness test of any player is always essential before exposure to full training or contact sport and, as usual, full training should be resumed only by stages.

Strapping

Strapping has an important part to play in ankle sprains. While American practice suggests that no one should take the field without protection, European practice is much more conservative. There are two purposes of strapping: first, protective support of a vulnerable joint and secondly, to increase proprioceptive, or positional, awareness.

The conventional figure-of-eight strapping is cumbersome and restricts straight up-and-down movement. It also occupies a disproportionate amount of boot. If strapping is desired, then a simpler technique is to apply a simple 'U'-shaped stirrup

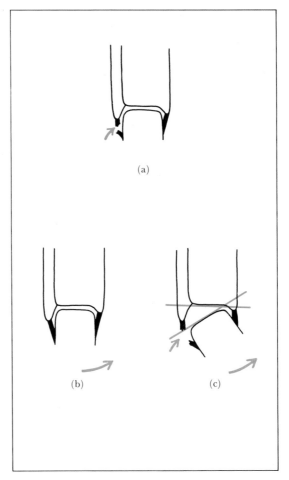

Figure 26.5
Ankle, lateral ligament rupture.
(a) Resting position. (b) Inversion pressure on normal ankle – no displacement. (c) Inversion pressure on ruptured ligament – opening of joint mortice, demonstrable instability

(*Figure 26.7*). The lower leg should be shaved and Friar's Balsam applied for ease of application and removal. Adhesive elastic strapping is then applied under the heel and up on each side to form the 'U'. The strapping is reinforced by a few simple rounds of similar strapping above the ankle. This method has the advantage of offering a modicum of mechanical support to the weak collateral ligaments of the ankle while not prejudicing foot movement in the way that the figure-of-eight bandage does.

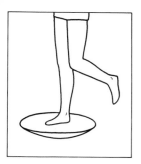

Figure 26.6
The wobble board

If strapping is effective, it restricts movement and this will be prejudicial to the player's safety. If it is ineffective, then the question is begged. However, the application of some sort of strapping around the ankle increases the rate at which the proprioceptive, or positional sense, nerve fibres fire impulses just before the foot lands during walking or running. Thus, while there may be no direct mechanical support to weak structures, the enhanced proprioceptive response ensures that the correct neuromuscular preparations for landing are reinforced. It is suggested by research that prophylactic strapping may not alter the primary injury rate but nevertheless lowers the chance of recurrent sprains in those who have already been injured.

Older style football and rugger boots with high sides tend to restrict ankle movement and provide useful protection. The more modern low-cut slipper styles obviously expose the ankle more to instability and sprains. However, the higher up the boot comes, the higher the injury, so that a given violent tackle may cause either a severely sprained ankle in the player wearing the shoe or a broken tibia in the high-booted player. Experts may prefer an ankle sprain rather than a damaged knee, so the debate on footwear style is likely to continue!

Soft-tissue pains

Other pains around the ankle may sometimes cause difficulty in diagnosis and management (*Figure 26.8*). The surface of the talus may be chipped in osteochondritis and occasionally form a loose body in the joint. This may not show up on routine X-ray but causes discomfort and restriction of movement.

Soft-tissue inflammations adjacent to the ankle may masquerade as ankle damage. For instance, tenosynovitis of the deep flexors has been referred to in Chapter 25. Sportsmen may present at the clinic complaining of 'ankle pain' when in fact they are suffering from Achilles tendon lesions only. Stress

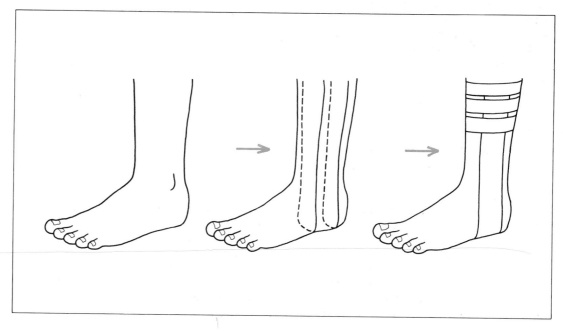

Figure 26.7
Simple 'U'-strapping for ankle sprain

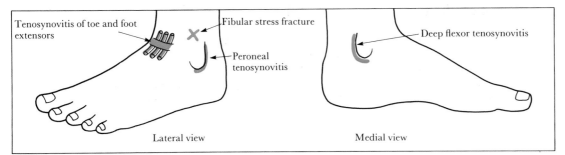

Tenosynovitis of toe and foot extensors

Fibular stress fracture

Peroneal tenosynovitis

Deep flexor tenosynovitis

Lateral view

Medial view

Figure 26.8
Common ankle pains

fractures of the lower parts of the tibia and especially at the fibular malleolus are sometimes treated by the unskilled as ankle sprains. At the front of the foot the fibrous retinaculum, or retaining band, of the anterior tibial tendon and toe extensor tendons may become constricted and cause tenosynovitis just in front of the ankle joint. Many of these lesions are mild overuse strains, often with little to find on examination, particularly if the player has rested recently. They therefore create much doubt in the doctor's mind about the possibility of complex ankle pathology. Gout and some rheumatic diseases occasionally present as unexplained ankle pain.

'Saturday night ankle'

'Saturday night ankle' is similar to the knee condition (*see* Chapter 24). The player, usually after many injuries, slides into a state of more or less permanent capsulitis or arthritis, with swelling and pain after vigorous sporting activity, and finds it difficult to do any training between games which themselves become harder to play and survive. The outlook by this time is poor in terms of further play, although by no means necessarily bad for daily living purposes provided that contact sport is abandoned and a full course of rehabilitation undertaken. Further damage accelerates the progress of arthritis.

'Footballer's ankle'

'Footballer's ankle' (*Figure 26.9*) is a condition not of ankle joint damage but of adjacent capsular strain and inflammation, which causes small bony outgrowths, or osteophytes, at the edge of the joint capsule at the front of the ankle joint on the top of the foot. This condition is due to repeated downward stretching and kicking impacts on the front of the ankle. As these osteophytes develop they may cause pain and obstruction to full movement and the footballer's range of ankle movement slowly diminishes. He has discomfort, usually at the front of the ankle, especially after vigorous activity. If a short spell of rest and rehabilitation does not prove effective, the bony and inflammatory tissue at the edge of the ankle capsule can often be dissected away, often with full functional recovery.

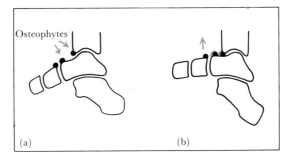

Osteophytes

(a)   (b)

Figure 26.9
'Footballer's ankle'. Development of anterior osteophytes, (a), may obstruct full upward dorsiflexion of ankle, (b)

Combined injury

The outlook is bad if 'Saturday night ankle' is combined with 'footballer's ankle' changes, because there is widespread capsulitis, ligament strain and arthritis. Surgery may not relieve the anterior mechanical block because of the poor general state of the joint and capsule.

The player should be told that continued play and injury will only cause more pain and arthritis and that future comfort in daily walking is at risk. It may be possible, as a compromise, to change to refereeing and remain active without further sprains.

27 Foot injuries

The foot supports the body in static and active postures. The splayed-out toes and metatarsal bones towards the front allow postural variation on different surfaces and permit vigorous leverage for the take-off thrusts of walking and running. The mid-foot is a complex interconnection of small bones and joints which transmit the various rotations and leverages during locomotion from the forefoot to the rear foot and also play a major part in the shock absorption of landing stresses. The rear foot includes the ankle bones and the heel bone (calcaneum) which extends backwards to provide leverage for the whole of the calf muscles through the Achilles tendon, which by pulling the heel up, forces the front part of the foot down into the thrusting movements of take-off (*Figure 27.1*).

There is a wide variation of normal anatomy in the foot bones and this, together with possible differences in the lengths of the two legs, makes for a corresponding variation in individual gait. While the majority of anatomical variations are unimportant for normal living purposes, they become important at higher levels of activity. For instance, a simple leg-length discrepancy of perhaps a quarter of an inch (5 mm) is normally neither noticed nor corrected in everyday medical practice. A marathon runner, however, may get various foot, leg, hip or even back pains as a result of prolonged road running during which each 100 miles (160 km) of weekly training adds between 3 and 4 million extra strides annually to his everyday load. It is thus important to study the alignment of the sportsman's legs and the pattern of his foot movements as well as the design of his shoes, whenever there is a complaint of foot pain.

In recent years, much attention has been paid to the application of biomechanical principles to gait study. Mechanical discrepancies, such as limb-length differences, limb-bone torsions and joint malfunctions are sought for, and corrected, by custom-made orthoses (orthotics) which are corrective shoe inserts. The complexity of biomechanical theory may seem daunting but the proven success of much simple therapy should see the correction of common disorders brought gradually within the range of most doctors and physical therapists. The limited number of podiatrists would then be available for more complex cases.

The heel

Sever's disease

Pain at the back of the heel, usually fairly low under the curve of the calcaneum, is often due to simple bruising, as with jumpers or hurdlers. During adolescence, however, this pain may be due to Sever's disease, in which the immature apophysis, or bony plate, which is about to seal firmly on to the rest of the calcaneum becomes faulty (*Figure 27.2*). This, like adolescent epiphyseal disturbances elsewhere, is a self-limiting condition and rarely leads to any long-term harm. The pain is usually too great to permit continued training or competition and rest together with simple heel padding at all times is the

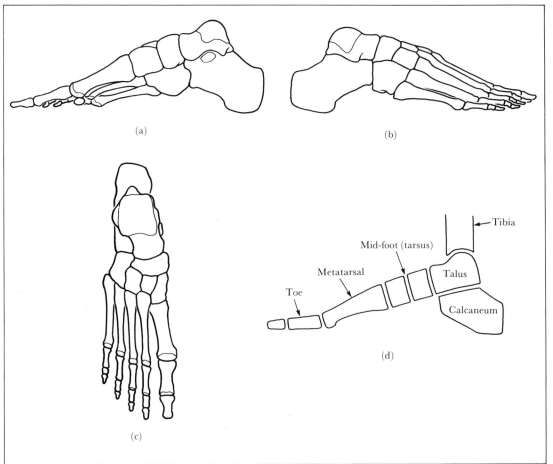

Figure 27.1
Foot, bony structure.
(a) Medial view. (b) Lateral
view. (c) Superior view. (d)
Diagrammatic
representation

essential treatment. Thereafter, cautious return to sport may be tried at intervals but should not be persisted with if pain recurs.

This condition may be partly due to traction by the Achilles tendon on the apophysis ('traction apophysitis') and might suggest an adjustment of sporting activities away from vigorous jumping or heel-thrusting. It usually settles satisfactorily with up to 6 months of avoidance of heel impacts and, in any case, will come to an end later in adolescence when

the two areas of bone finally fuse firmly into strong adult bone.

Bursitis

Calcaneal bursitis is common. At the Achilles tendon insertion into the back of the calcaneum, a bursa, or sac of connective tissue, may swell either deeply between the tendon and the calcaneum or superficially between the tendon and the skin (*Figure*

27.2). In either case, the pressure of movement and shoe-backs rubbing on the heel causes gradual enlargement and often a bluish discoloration. Bursae often fluctuate considerably in size between an obvious lump after a long run and a minimal swelling a few days later.

Immediate treatment is to remove any tight shoe-back which may be pressing on the heel, to apply a circular pressure-relieving pad to the back of the heel so that the bursa is no longer pressed-upon directly and to rest from training while there is pain and swelling (*Figure 27.3*).

Aspiration of the bursa and injection with steroid may provide relief for a while but, once bursae get to a certain size, they tend to progress relentlessly until they are dissected out surgically, with excellent results.

Blisters

Heel blisters are often a problem, especially on wearing in new boots or shoes. The most effective treatment, which permits continued training, is to clean the blister and adjacent skin thoroughly with soap or antiseptic, then to pierce the blister top with a clean pin, scalpel or scissors, releasing the fluid and cutting off some of the roof of the blister. After drainage, the raw skin may be hardened, although painfully, with spirit or Friar's Balsam and a length of zinc oxide plaster then applied directly to the raw wound. Although there is initial pain with this procedure it does guarantee continuation of sport. All

other methods of treating blisters involving padding and strapping merely add further layers which can continue to rub but do nothing to accelerate the formation of new hardened skin layers under the blister.

It is simpler to try to avoid the formation of blisters and sportsmen should give more attention to their shoes and socks. Intelligent choice of socks so as to fill out the sports shoe comfortably and absorb sweat can often prevent blisters altogether. The habit of using brand-new footwear for too long a session is the quickest way of inviting blisters, yet such practice is frequent, even among international athletes.

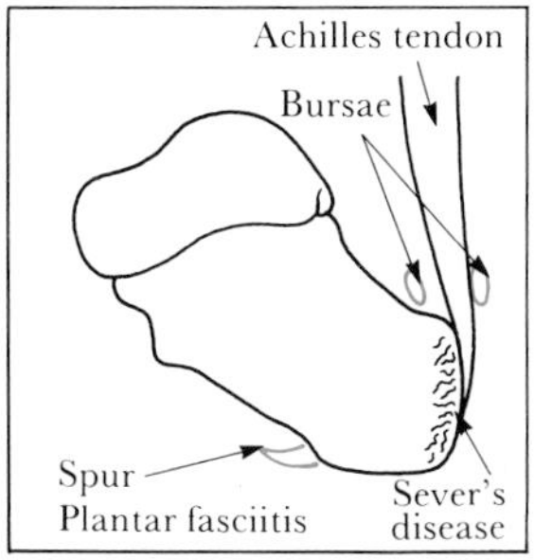

Bruising

With road runners heel bruising often occurs around the edge of the calcaneum and is probably due to jamming of the heel into the corner of the shoe on hard surfaces (*Figure 27.4*). Initially simple padding should be tried together with a change to a softer surface, and footwear should be carefully reviewed for good fit and sufficient heel padding. Further treatment includes physiotherapy or steroid injection and possibly shoe or podiatric correction.

The foot
Plantar fasciitis

Pain is felt on the sole of the foot just in front of the forward edge of the calcaneum. The plantar fascia connects the calcaneum to the metatarsal arch at the front of the foot and has to yield with each foot-landing impact, as well as serve a general function of supporting the underneath of the foot (*Figure 27.5*). Plantar fasciitis is common in non-athletes with flat feet and poor posture and also in active athletes, particularly those running or training on hard surfaces in too stiffly soled footwear. In either case, undue stress is put on the plantar fascia in respect of shock absorption and overuse strain develops at its origin.

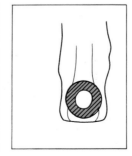

Figure 27.2 (left)
Heel disorders (side view)
Figure 27.3 (right)
Circular cut-out pad to relieve pressure on bursa

Hallux rigidus

Whenever a sportsman suffers from plantar fasciitis, a check should be made of big toe (hallux) mobility. Hallus rigidus is a premature arthritic fixation of the big-toe joint, not usually related to exercise or injury (*Figure 27.6*). The toe cannot bend up to its normal extent during the take-off movement of running and the middle and back of the foot have to overcompensate for this stiffness. The available structure for this purpose is the plantar fascia, hence the frequency of plantar fasciitis in association with hallux rigidus. This condition may occur in teenagers.

Correction of hallux rigidus is essential and consists initially of physiotherapy to increase mobility and settle down any inflammation of the toe joint. Long-distance runners who have been doing heavy mileage in thin shoes and are suffering inflammation of the big-toe joint will benefit from a short rest, anti-inflammatory treatment or physiotherapy to the toe, a change to better-produced running shoes and use of softer training surfaces. These measures may contain the problem satisfactorily for some years, although hallux rigidus tends slowly to progress. Alternative management consists of providing a metatarsal bar under the ball of the foot or line of the metatarsal heads inside the shoe, or a shoe sole adjustment to restore some of the leverage missing from the rigid toe (*Figure 27.6d(i)*). A simple method for the runner is to glue a suitable leather or felt bar on to a shoe insole.

A further possibility is to use adhesive felt (orthopaedic felt) and to stick a strip of this under the line of the metatarsal heads regularly before activity. In some cases an orthosis may help, especially in early cases. Finally, if all else fails, surgical procedures are available which either excise part of the rigid joints or perform an osteotomy which angulates one or other of the forefoot bones to build in some extra leverage (*Figure 27.6d(ii)*). All these treatments and procedures are consistent with the resumption of sport but are often difficult to come by through orthodox medical channels.

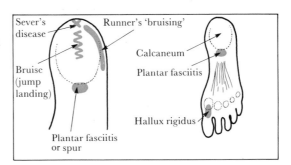

Figure 27.4 (left) Heel pain, from below
Figure 27.5 (right) Plantar fascia

'Foot strain'

Ligament overuse strains cause aching under the arch of the foot forward of the area of plantar fasciitis (*Figure 27.7*). This may be helped by an arch support but is much better treated by strengthening exercises for the intrinsic foot muscles (*Figure 27.8*). These are performed by sitting with the foot comfortably placed on the floor at a neutral angle and the toes then curled as if to pull the rest of the foot forward. Variations include rolling a pencil or rolled bandage with the toes and squeezing the toes firmly down on the floor while keeping the rest of the foot still. Another simple exercise is to invert the foot so as to turn it on to its outer border while keeping the ankle as straight as possible and then curling the toes in as far as possible towards the heel. It may be difficult to get the hang of intrinsic foot exercises and a short course of faradic stimulation is useful to re-educate neglected movement patterns.

Metatarsalgia

Metatarsalgia is pain under the ball of the foot where the supporting ligaments of the metatarsal heads become strained in the line of the toe joints (*Figure 27.9*). This condition is common in people who stand a lot at work and is also caused by activity on hard surfaces, for example, running in thin-soled shoes or hard-studded boots.

Treatment is simple and consists of footwear correction, intrinsic foot exercises (*see* above) and a

Figure 27.6
Hallux rigidus, 'stiff big toe'
(a) Normal hallux range
(b) Reduced movement in
H.R.
(c) (i) Normal resting
position of plantar fascia.
(ii) Normal response on toe
movement. (iii) H.R.–fixed
toe forces fascia to stretch as
whole foot compensates.
(d) Cures. (i) Metatarsal
bar, inside or outside shoe,
restores leverage.
Operations may alter the
joint (ii) or the metatarsal
angle (iii) to restore leverage

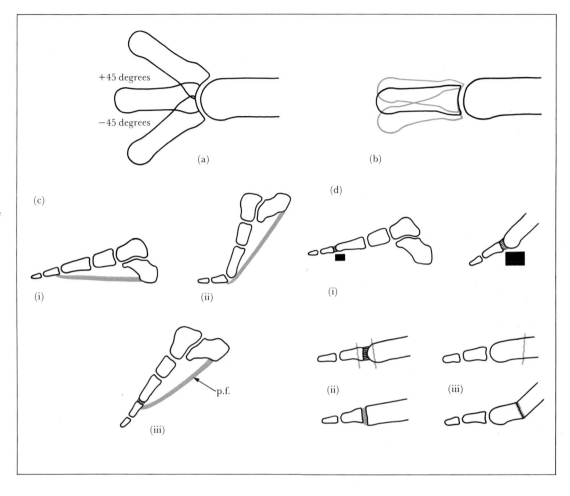

simple metatarsal support under the middle of the ball of the foot. Many metatarsal supports are available commercially but the simplest and most satisfactory for the highly mobile sportsman's foot can be made by cutting out a roughly oval or circular piece of sticky-backed orthopaedic foam or felt and sticking this under the ball of the foot, using trial and error to find the smallest amount of padding required and its optimum site. This method has the advantage of being entirely specific for the wearer and uses only

the minimum space in the already tight sports footwear. It also leaves the sportsman's foot unencumbered by elastic bands or extra fastenings which often slip awkwardly and cause blisters.

Hallux valgus

Pain in the big-toe joint is common, particularly in the older sportsman. Hallux rigidus has been described above. At this joint, the stresses of heavy use and tight footwear combine over the years to form bunions and calluses with the gradual diversion of the joint from its original straight alignment towards the outer side of the foot in the deformity of hallux valgus (H.V., *Figure 27.10*).

Bunions are the gradual bony thickening of the metatarsal bone at this joint and calluses are the soft-tissue thickening usually found over them. Hallux valgus causes difficulty in finding comfortable footwear and increasingly exposes the joint to even more stresses from landing and kicking impacts. It is associated with a tendency of the small sesamoid bones in the tendons underneath the big-toe joint to become painful and slightly diverted towards the outer side of the joint. In the early stages of this gradual progression of bony deformity, intrinsic foot exercises (*see* above), really wide and comfortable footwear and, occasionally, corrective padding may be beneficial. There is no doubt, however, that many people progress to these deformities regardless of

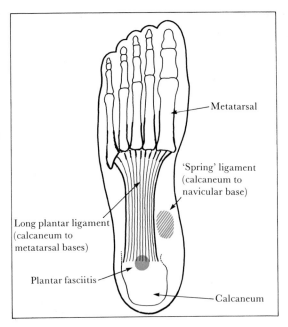

Figure 27.7
Foot, deeper structure of sole

Metatarsal

'Spring' ligament (calcaneum to navicular base)

Long plantar ligament (calcaneum to metatarsal bases)

Plantar fasciitis

Calcaneum

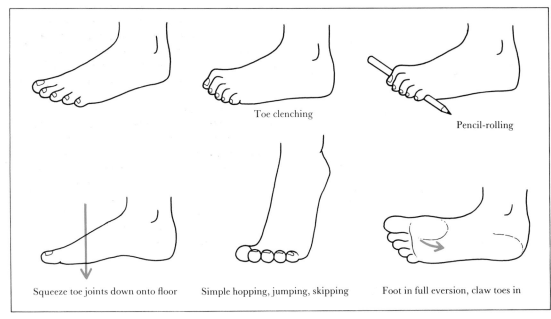

Figure 27.8
Intrinsic foot muscle strengthening exercises

Toe clenching

Pencil-rolling

Squeeze toe joints down onto floor

Simple hopping, jumping, skipping

Foot in full eversion, claw toes in

222

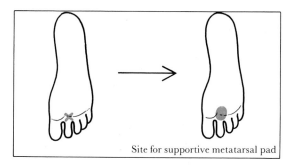

Figure 27.9
Metatarsalgia

Site for supportive metatarsal pad

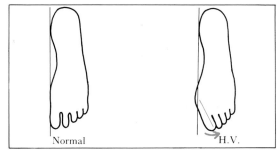

Figure 27.10
Hallux valgus

Normal   H.V.

preventive measures once the original sequence has been started.

A look at, say, Indian feet will show how rare the hallux valgus deformity is in the well-used bare foot. Unfortunately, European footwear is in general far too narrow-fronted for the feet it purports to fit and there is little doubt that the years of wearing narrow pointed sport and daily shoes cumulatively distort the anatomical line of the forefoot.

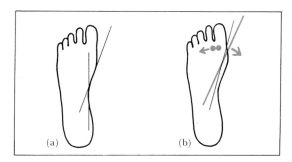

Figure 27.11
Metatarsus adductus primus.
(a) Normal. (b) Increasing angulation of first metatarsal medially with corresponding sesamoid shift laterally

(a)   (b)

Metatarsus adductus

At the other end of the scale, some people are born with an abnormally diverted first metatarsal bone (metatarsus adductus primus) which may lead to a teenager's presenting with a considerable degree of secondary hallux valgus and sesamoid pain which may resist all treatments except surgical correction (*Figure 27.11*). In others, this condition presents as uni- or bilateral hallux valgus during early or mid-adulthood.

Sesamoid bones

The sesamoid bones may cause considerable pain under the big-toe joint. These bones are sometimes painful after unprotected or unaccustomed hard-surface effort but settle down within a few days. If pain becomes persistent, however, they may prove very difficult to treat. Rest from impact, sorbo padding and revised footwear, physiotherapy and steroid injection may all succeed or fail.

In pathological terms, the condition of sesamoiditis is identical to that of chondromalacia patellae (*see* page 196) and it is worth trying a really intensive course of strengthening exercises for the intrinsic foot muscles (*see* above) before embarking on more drastic measures. Surgery may be used to excise the sesamoids but this is undesirable as they protect the underlying big-toe joint and increase the leverage of the flexor tendon pull on the toe. Thus, no more than one sesamoid should be removed if surgery really is necessary. Success has been claimed for the replacement of an excised sesamoid with a silastic substitute allowing successful resumption of full training. Metatarsus adductus primus must be treated where present in order to reverse the secondary effect on the sesamoids. Occasionally sesamoid fracture occurs.

223

Podiatry

In all cases of foot pain, hallux valgus and adducted metatarsals, the foot posture and gait should be examined. Callus formation is always secondary to pressure on the skin internally by bone or externally by shoes. Orthotic correction and footwear changes are important preventive as well as curative steps. (*See* Chapter 28 for fuller discussion.)

Minor foot deformity

Various common minor foot problems, such as hammer toe or the common overriding deformities of the smaller toes, become important for the sportsman because of the high degree of activity required and the general tendency of sports shoes to be rather tight-fitting which, in turn, leads to further pressure and callus formation over any misplaced toe. This may mean that a number of relatively minor deformities need surgical correction, not because of medical problems but because there may be no other way in which satisfactory shoes can be found and worn.

Infections

In-growing toenails, septic nails and athlete's foot, the common fungal infection of tinea pedis, are all common results of neglect. These conditions may be due to poor personal hygiene or dirty changing rooms where infection may spread easily. Toenails should be scrupulously trimmed and any serious sportsman should recruit the help of a chiropodist if there is any difficulty whatever about a tendency for nails to in-grow. The quite incredible degrees of self-neglect in simple foot hygiene, shown even by international sportsmen, are amazing. It is worthwhile for any serious sports team to institute regular foot inspections rather than risking the loss of key players in vital competitions. Warts and verrucae (plantar warts) should be actively treated (*see* page 104).

Subungual haematomas, painful bruises under the nails, are quickly relieved by puncture with a sterile blade or needle pressed through the nail. This releases the tense underlying blood..

Stress fractures

Stress fractures frequently occur at the middle of the foot in the metatarsal bones (*Figure 27.12*). These fractures were originally called 'march fractures' because of their high incidence in army recruits forced to march in heavy rigid boots. They may also occur in runners or other heavy foot-users and the typical 'crescendo' history of the stress fracture (*see* page 144) should be sought. The metatarsal shafts usually involved are the second, third or fourth, and localized pain on running is confirmed by tenderness over the metatarsal shaft and, occasionally, the tender bony lump of the newly formed callus can be felt.

Stress fractures need 4–6 weeks of rest from sport and no further treatment is usually required. Return to training must be gradual after the end of the recovery period and should depend on satisfactory X-ray evidence of healing.

Osteochondritis

Rarely, foot pain in the sporting adolescent may be due to osteochondritis of the navicular bone in the mid-foot or at the head of the second or third metatarsal bone at the ball of the foot (Freiberg's disease) (*Figure 27.13*). Aching, particularly on

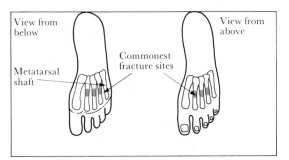

Figure 27.12
Metatarsal stress fractures

weight-bearing and exertion, tenderness on palpating the affected area and X-rays confirm the diagnosis. Many cases settle with a few weeks' rest and surgical removal of part of the disrupted metatarsal head is rarely necessary. These conditions are self-limiting within the course of adolescence.

Mid-tarsal pain

Mid-tarsal pain is common with athletes in all sports. Apart from extensor retinaculum inflammation or dorsal tenosynovitis (*see* page 213 and *Figure 26.8*) sportsmen often feel pain on the top of the mid-foot immediately in front of the ankle (*Figure 27.14*). This is often precipitated by hard-surface play or training and may be felt only after a long session of walking barefoot or in different shoes, rather than during exertion.

Much mid-tarsal pain is probably due to minor jarring of the many mid-tarsal joints with consequent painful stretching of the overlying joint capsules and supporting ligaments. Gait and posture examinations may reveal malalignments or functional faults such as excessive tarsal pronation or flat footedness which may precipitate tarsal strain. A drastic change of footwear or surface may also precipitate this syndrome. Unduly tight lacing of shoes or boots may, by adding an artificial degree of restriction to the foot movement, cause acute tarsal discomfort.

This condition should not be confused either with 'footballer's ankle' (*see* page 214) or a simple insertion strain of the tibialis anterior tendon into the mid-foot near the base of the first metatarsal bone which is easily strained on kicking vigorously with the foot pointing fully downwards. Rest usually settles this quickly; occasionally physiotherapy or local steroid injection may be required.

Mid-tarsal pain may be difficult to treat unless a satisfactory explanation is found for symptoms. Adjustment of footwear and padding will prove more effective than purely medical treatment, although symptomatic physiotherapy may be necessary in severe cases. Intrinsic foot exercises are strongly recommended to improve muscular tone throughout the foot, including the important arch structures. In chronic cases, manipulative treatment may be effective in breaking down adhesions but manipulations will not hold new positions unless the appropriate strengthening exercises are also performed. Gait and biomechanical examination is important and orthoses often necessary.

Tenosynovitis

Tenosynovitis on the top of the foot is commonly due to constriction of the toe extensors by tight lacing or footwear. On the inner side of the ankle it is due to swelling of the tendon of tibialis posterior because of overuse or direct pressure from friction against the shoe-collar. On the outer side of the ankle the peroneal tendons may become inflamed from overuse or footwear pressure (*Figure 27.15*). Treatment includes symptomatic physiotherapy, rest initially, and footwear and lacing adjustment.

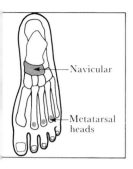

Figure 27.13
Sites of adolescent osteochondritis

Figure 27.14
Tarsal pain

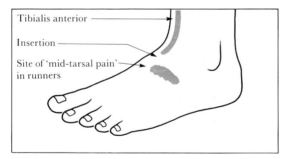

Tibialis anterior
Insertion
Site of 'mid-tarsal pain' in runners

Figure 27.15
Pain at fifth metatarsal base

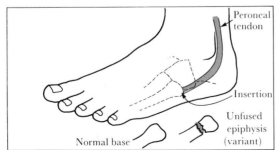

Peroneal tendon
Insertion
Unfused epiphysis (variant)
Normal base

Clicking tendons

Occasionally the tendons on either side of the ankle may be congenitally slightly misplaced in a way which allows them to click out of their usual grooves and cause discomfort and inflammation on their way to insertion in the foot. Careful examination and the patient's history will reveal this problem and surgical anchoring of the aberrant tendons in a more secure manner can be very effective.

Fifth metatarsal

The base of the fifth metatarsal bone on the outer border of the foot may be painful due to overuse strains of the peroneal tendon insertion, landing impacts, direct blows or, possibly, to an inflamed unfused bone present as a variant of normal anatomy (*Figure 27.15*). This abnormality may cause confusion on X-ray, especially during adolescence, but is not usually similar in appearance to typical stress fractures. Symptomatic treatment only is required, including an initial spell of rest while inflammation settles.

28 Running injuries

Style and injury

There are two styles of running and these are illustrated in *Figure 28.1*. The classic sprinter has a vigorous upper arm and leg movement, thrusting himself forward with powerful upper-leg muscular drive involving particularly the quadriceps, adductor and hamstring groups of muscles. Knee lift in front and heel kick-back behind are both high. Arm drive is vigorous throughout.

In contrast, the long-distance runner moves with much lower arm and leg carriage. So redundant may the arms often seem to be, that serious arm weakness may even be consistent with world record performance; witness Murray Halberg's world records and Olympic gold medal at 5000 metres with a partly paralysed left arm. Also, leg carriage is lower with less knee lift and kick-back than in sprinting.

Typically, the sprinter suffers injuries which relate to his most active muscles – particularly the hamstrings and adductors – while the longer-distance runner is plagued by foot and lower-leg injuries below the knee.

Sprinting injuries

Back strain is due to excesses of weight-training or callisthenics but both these types of training are rarely adopted conscientiously by long-distance runners.

Adductor strains (*see* page 185 and *Figure 28.2*) are liable to occur in the early stages of a sprint race and particularly from the starting blocks where the legs tend to be turned out. This turned position puts the adductor muscles under greater strain than usual – the strain gradually diminishing as the legs rotate to a more forward-facing position as the race proceeds.

Hamstring tears are especially liable to occur with failure properly to warm up and to use suppling exercises. The sprinter remains unprepared for the sudden violent strains on the hamstrings during acceleration.

Obviously, a sprinter may sustain other sports injuries but this chapter presents the most typical event-related problems which illustrate the relation between style and breakdown.

Long-distance running injuries

Style

Studies of injuries and styles suggest that the average 800-metre runner is usually a long-distance runner by innate style – a fact not really evident to the grandstand crowd appreciating, say, a 52-second lap when it seems that the whole field is 'sprinting' flat out. Slow-motion or still pictures will reveal that most members of the half-mile field present the lower-leg-carriage style outlined above.

There are, of course, exceptions and it is interesting to note that many of the more dramatically successful distance runners have, in fact, shown styles more appropriate to that of classic sprinters. This anomaly becomes even more pronounced during their final sprints in longer races when remarkable turns of speed are produced with the style of the classic high knee lift. In contrast, more rangily built runners with a lower carriage have difficulty in mustering such 'electric' changes of pace and must, therefore, rely on a more ferociously sustained pace over a longer part of the race. The biological division into 'sprinter' or 'strider' is complex and depends partly upon the individual composition of the runner's muscle fibres (*see* Chapter 5) and partly on the mechanical limb leverages, i.e., the ratios of trunk to leg, and thigh to lower-leg, lengths. The lucky man in the middle-distance races is probably an inherently fast, high strider who has disproportionate stamina. There is not much that the natural low strider can do to acquire basic speed or acceleration but he must learn to develop his maximum endurance potential and then to run tactically.

The middle- and long-distance runner presents a well-defined range of injuries which he shares with the typical jogger (*see Figure 28.3*).

Backache

Backache is common in long-distance runners (*see also* Chapter 22). It is usually non-specific 'lumbago' but may develop into a full-blown lumbar disc syndrome with sciatica. The latter condition may masquerade as 'hamstring strain' or leg weakness and it may be possible to continue running even with considerable nerve root pressure impairing the knee reflexes.

Hard-surface running, hurdling and steeplechase landings all cause backache. Limb-length discrepancies lead to pelvic tilting and scoliosis, or curvature, as compensatory mechanisms and these in turn create uneven traction on the lumbar ligaments, joints and muscles. Such discrepancies should be corrected by a shoe-raise (*Figure 28.4*). Congenital anomalies (page 171) may also be underlying causes.

The backache is usually a dull, mid-lumbar ache but may extend over the lumbosacral and sacroiliac areas and may be associated with spasm over the

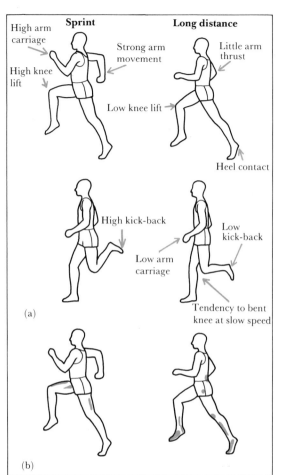

(a)

(b)

Figure 28.1
Running style and injury
(a) Style differences in sprinting and longer-distance running
(b) Characteristic injuries related to different types of running

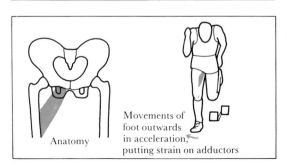

Figure 28.2
Adductor strain in sprinters

Figure 28.3
Injuries – long-distance
running and jogging

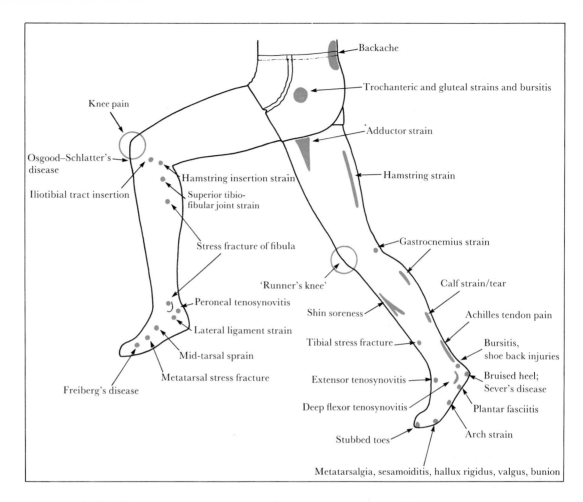

Backache

Trochanteric and gluteal strains and bursitis

Adductor strain

Hamstring strain

Knee pain

Osgood–Schlatter's disease

Iliotibial tract insertion

Hamstring insertion strain

Superior tibio-fibular joint strain

Stress fracture of fibula

Gastrocnemius strain

'Runner's knee'

Calf strain/tear

Peroneal tenosynovitis

Shin soreness

Achilles tendon pain

Lateral ligament strain

Tibial stress fracture

Bursitis, shoe back injuries

Mid-tarsal sprain

Bruised heel; Sever's disease

Metatarsal stress fracture

Extensor tenosynovitis

Plantar fasciitis

Freiberg's disease

Deep flexor tenosynovitis

Arch strain

Stubbed toes

Metatarsalgia, sesamoiditis, hallux rigidus, valgus, bunion

buttocks and thigh (*Figure 28.5*). In sciatica, the pain may shoot down the back and side of the leg and foot. Prolonged standing or sitting in a slouched position may exacerbate symptoms. Leg-length differences can lead to unequal stride length and pelvic rotation, leading to strain of the lumbosacral or sacroiliac joint and unilateral low back pain.

Hip and thigh pain

True hip-joint pain (page 186) may be due to overtraining on hard surfaces. Pain around the hip is frequent in road runners and is usually due to trochanteric bursitis or overuse strain of the gluteal muscles (*Figure 28.6*). The pain is felt, often after a long, hard-surface run, around the bony upper arc of the hip with tenderness over, above, in front of, or behind the bone.

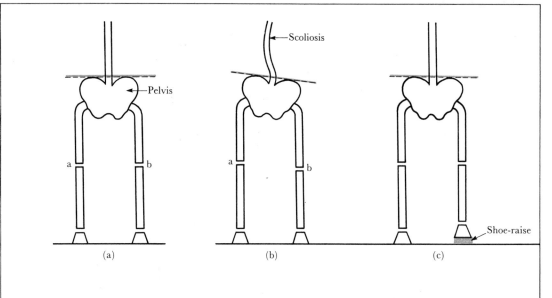

Figure 28.4
Leg-length difference
(a) Normal. a = b. Pelvis
parallel to ground. (b) Short
leg. a > b. Pelvic tilt leads to
compensatory lumbar curve
(scoliosis) to keep head
level. (c) Correction with
shoe-raise

Rarely, discrepant limb length or femoral rotation may be responsible for hip pain by consequent unequal hip movements. The same effect may be caused by excessive running on one part of a cambered road which tilts the hip and pelvis and causes pelvic pain.

Adductor strains are usually caused by unaccustomed runs on uneven or slippery surfaces where, in order to preserve pelvic and leg stability, the adductor muscles connecting the two are forced to work excessively, rather than explosively as with accelerating sprinters.

Hamstring strains usually follow from the same circumstances, particularly when hill running is added to an unstable surface since the tendency to 'claw' the body up the slope leads to overuse strain (*Figure 28.7*). Occasionally, adductor and hamstring strains are a direct consequence of the long-distance runner's trying to acquire basic speed through overenthusiastic sprinting. Pain down the back of the

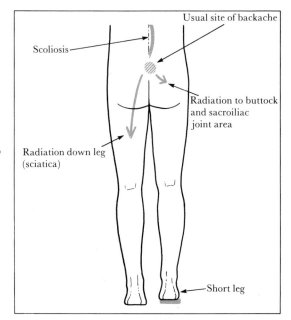

Figure 28.5
Low back pain in runners – causes

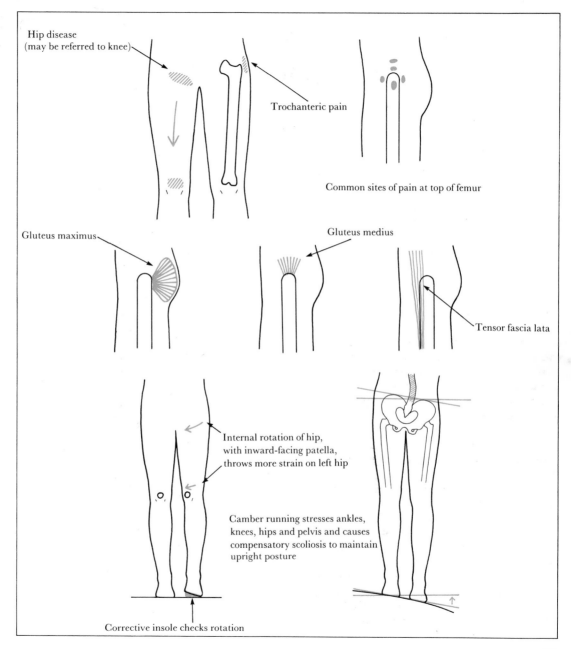

Figure 28.6
Hip pain in runners – sites
and mechanisms

Hip disease
(may be referred to knee)

Trochanteric pain

Common sites of pain at top of femur

Gluteus maximus

Gluteus medius

Tensor fascia lata

Internal rotation of hip,
with inward-facing patella,
throws more strain on left hip

Camber running stresses ankles,
knees, hips and pelvis and causes
compensatory scoliosis to maintain
upright posture

Corrective insole checks rotation

thigh should be remembered as a symptom of sciatica (*see above*).

Knee pain

At the knee, chondromalacia (runner's or jogger's knee), medial ligament strain, patellar tendinitis, hamstring insertion strain and iliotibial tract inflammation are all characteristic injuries (*see* Chapter 24).

Lower-leg pain

Shin soreness may be due to tibial stress fracture, periostitis, overuse strain or tenosynovitis of the long flexor muscles, as well as anterior or posterior compartment syndromes (Chapter 25). The tibia may show marked degrees of cortical thickening in response to chronic distance running and stress fractures may sometimes be difficult to identify.

The fibula may suffer stress fractures or periosteal haematoma (page 203). The superior tibiofibular joint may become painful after hard-surface running due to irritation by repeated jarring of a fairly rigid joint which nonetheless allows some springing movement on impact. This pain may cause diagnostic confusion with lateral ligament sprain, biceps insertion pain or even knee damage (*see Figure 28.8*).

Calf muscle tears are more frequent in older runners, especially veterans seeking a turn of speed on hard surfaces. These tears are probably due to the gradual increase in body weight and shift of the runner's centre of gravity with age so that he is effectively shuffling his lower legs harder as he forces his progressively inelastic muscles to shift an increasing forwardly placed body mass!

Achilles tendon pain

See Chapters 17 (tendon injury) and page 205.

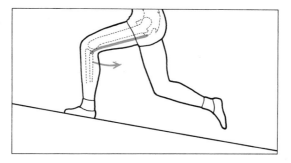

Figure 28.7
Hamstring strains from 'clawing' up slope

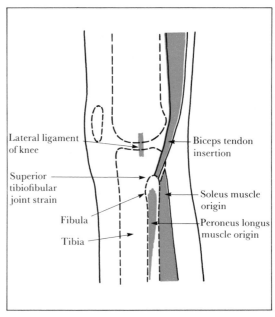

Figure 28.8
Pain near the superior tibiofibular joint

Lateral ligament of knee

Biceps tendon insertion

Superior tibiofibular joint strain

Fibula

Tibia

Soleus muscle origin

Peroneus longus muscle origin

Ankle pain

Ankle sprains from running almost always cause pain on the outer side of the ankle because the foot naturally lands upon its outer border at all speeds of running (*Figure 28.9*). This being so, chronic overstrain involves mainly the lateral ligament complex and, should the runner actually fall, then the chances are in favour of his falling with the ankle inverted, thus spraining the lateral ligament more

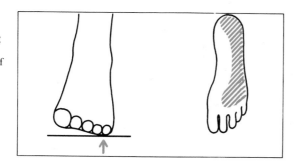

Figure 28.9
Ankle, lateral ligament
sprain. The normal running
action with landing area
(shaded) on the outer side of
the foot, at all speeds, puts
the lateral side of ankle at a
greater 'stretch' than the
medial side

severely. In fact, the runner will only sprain his
medial ligament if he actually falls over something
accidentally in an abnormal way.

Camber running is often neglected as a cause of leg
ache but repeated stressing of the feet in exactly the
same way on the same curve of road or hill leads to a
tendency to stretch and overstrain the lowermost
lateral ligament and the uppermost medial ligament
(*see Figure 28.10*). Runners often follow one camber to
the point of injury without appreciating that this

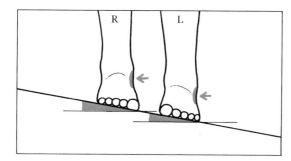

Figure 28.10
Camber running. This
camber persistently
stretches the lowermost
ankle ligaments, i.e. right
medial and left lateral
ligaments, as marked

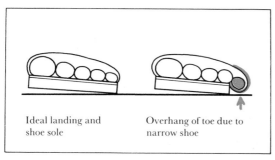

Figure 28.11
Outer border foot pain

Ideal landing and
shoe sole

Overhang of toe due to
narrow shoe

mechanism can be reversed by remaining on the same
side of the road for the return journey! It has been
shown to be safer to run facing the oncoming traffic,
however.

Foot pain

The outer border of the foot may be painful from
repeated landing impacts particularly if the running
shoe is thin soled and narrow so that the foot
overhangs laterally to strike directly against the road
surface at each landing (*Figure 28.11*).

Heel bruising, plantar fasciitis, arch strain,
metatarsalgia, big-toe pain and mid-tarsal pain are
all discussed in Chapter 27.

General management of runners' overuse strains

Mileage

First, the training schedule should be thoroughly
assessed. Many runners follow a 'blind' routine and
are not sufficiently sensitive to critical inquiry. Why,
for instance, must a runner do 'x' miles/week?
Athletes' clinics are full of runners who say that they
do, say, 100 miles (160 km) a week. Upon enquiry, it
transpires that they have done only 30 or 40 miles for
the previous 2 or 3 weeks because of injury and they
may only have reached 100 for a week or two before
that owing to recovery from previous injury. They are
now going to spend several weeks at a lower level
recovering from the present injury so that the true
average through the year may well be only, say, 50
miles/week – and all this during a year full of tedious
overuse injuries! Why not, for instance, settle for a
target of 50 or 60 miles/week and aim to remain
uninjured and in continuous training?

Shoes and surfaces

Footwear and surfaces must be matched; footwear is
the subject of the next chapter, but we shall here
consider surfaces. Climate probably governs training

environment more than anything else but there is no doubt about the fact that the harder the surface, the more frequent the injuries. It is often possible to keep an athlete running by halving his mileage and transferring him from road to sand, gravel or grass, and selecting better, more protective shoes. There is a myth among distance runners that the cumulative weight of running shoes impairs performance. While this is true in theory, in practice, what all too often happens is that the runner exposes himself to hard surfaces and long distances in grossly unprotective thin shoes. He would survive far better if he remained uninjured thanks to the extra protection afforded by a few extra grams of padding in a more substantial shoe. However, myths die hard!

Age

The older runner often finds that he cannot cope with increasing stiffness of the lower back and legs caused by hard-surface running. He is often unsupple and probably extremely stiff in lateral and rotational movements. He may well not be able to touch his ankles on bending forward.

With increasing age, sportsmen tend to take longer to get stiffer after each major effort but this stiffness takes a little longer to subside. Many athletes cannot manage daily hard-surface running at the age of 40 or 50 in the way that they could at 20 or even 30.

Unfortunately, many runners become fairly obsessional about their habit but, if they can be persuaded to invest, say, one or two days a week in rest and one or two in an alternative exercise, such as swimming, together with a deliberate effort at mobility exercises, they will often become notably fitter, more mobile, symptom-free and, as an incidental by-product, faster runners.

One of the doctor's most important functions is to try to dispel the obsessional belief that a single missed training session will have disastrous consequences! Intelligent interspersion of rest with light runs as well as severe training sessions will benefit most athletes and prevent much overuse injury.

Podiatry

Podiatry includes the correction of abnormal gait by means of corrective appliances, usually individually moulded and balanced insoles or orthoses ('orthotics').

While the mechanical complexities of the foot at rest and in motion are difficult to understand without a comprehensive knowledge of anatomy and biomechanics, much simple podiatry should be widely known to all medical and coaching practitioners. So many foot, leg and back symptoms are caused by simple biomechanical disorders that an awareness of this field is essential.

Gait analysis

Full analysis of walking and running is performed in specially equipped Gait Laboratories. The subject walks along a strip of flooring which contains pressure-sensitive plates. A complete profile of the gait cycle can be compiled in terms of overall body–ground interaction. With more detailed apparatus, including shoes containing multiple pressure-sensitive transducers, a picture of the entire foot–ground contact cycle can be drawn. This is already leading to new mechanically based improvements in sports shoe design. Ciné-film, video and computer recordings are widely used in gait studies.

Visual examination of gait With practice the observer can become skilled at simple clinical gait analysis. The subject can be observed walking, jogging or running from the front or side. The observer must sit or lie low enough to get a good view of the foot movements on the ground. Patience is essential. Each feature should be looked at in turn as long as necessary before going on to the next one.

Sideways (Figure 28.12a–e) This is the commonest way of watching runners on the track. Arm and knee action should be studied, together with foot landings. The arms should be compared for symmetry of movement, power of thrust and degree of relaxation. The knees may be vigorously straightened during running, as in sprinters, or may remain slightly flexed, especially in slower, older or heavier subjects. Relatively bent-knee running is an important factor in the causation of knee pain ('runner's knee', or chondromalacia patellae, page 196).

From the front (Figure 28.12f–j) Look for symmetry or asymmetry of the whole leg or one part. Some runners 'flick' out one or both thighs, others show considerable asymmetry of lower-leg movements. Such movements are a clue to leg-length difference and marked degrees of rotation of the limb(s).

The knee cap should face straight ahead. Some people show a marked deviation from the midline so that the patella faces outwards. Sometimes inward deviation is so obvious that the whole thigh appears

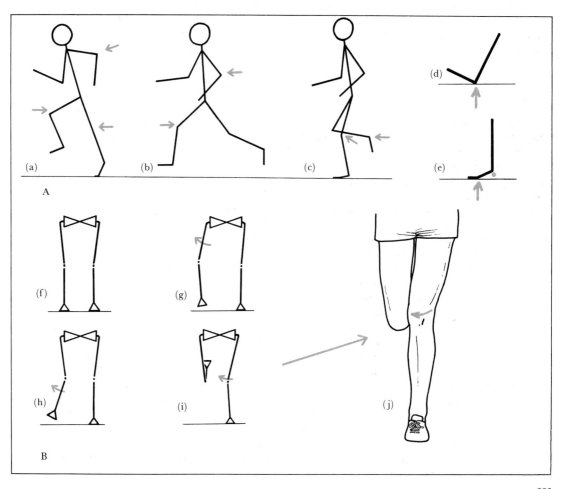

Figure 28.12
Some features of running gait
A Side views, showing different arm and leg positions in sprint (a) and longer-distance (b and c) striding. Foot landings on the heel (d) or ball of foot (e). Note that the heel may not be grounded during the gait cycle
B Front views, showing normal (f) leg alignment, outward rotation of thigh (g), rotation of lower leg (h) and internal rotation of the femur on landing (i), with patellar movement (j) in close-up

to rotate inwards as the foot lands and the knee straightens. This is frequently associated with chondromalacia patellae.

The general alignment of the leg may be curved (*Figure 24.3*, page 191) to give genu valgum (knock-knee) common in females, or genu varum (bow-leg). Bowing of the shin, tibial varus, is particularly common in runners with leg symptoms. It is not necessarily symmetrical and may be associated with leg-length difference or effectively create a functional length difference – hence difference in stride length. Tibial varus is also associated with excessive mid-foot pronation – an essential compensatory mechanism.

From the back Mid-foot pronation is best seen from behind as is pelvic tilt which is often due to leg-length differences and scoliosis.

Leg length In conventional medical practice, considerable leg-length discrepancies are usually disregarded and differences of over an inch (2.5 cm) may not give rise to symptoms in non-active persons. It is imperative, however, to realize that the tendency to cumulative tissue stress in sports training and competition may lead to symptoms in the active athlete in the presence of leg-length differences of no more than 1 cm. Extremely accurate radiological studies have shown that leg-length differences of as little as 3 mm are correlated with leg symptoms in active subjects. It is often difficult in clinical practice to measure leg length with great accuracy because of the mobile soft tissue over the bony reference points; also some subjects have poorly defined bony edges at the iliac spines. Leg-length measurement by X-rays will only give valid results if the subject's posture is carefully standardized. Unnecessary X-ray exposure is always contraindicated.

To measure leg length (*Figure 28.13*), lie the patient flat with the legs straight, heels on the surface (not hanging over the edge). The bony iliac crest can be traced from the side of the pelvis round to the prominent knob of the anterior superior iliac spine

(ASIS) above the mid-groin. This is the upper reference point for the tape measure. At the ankle the medial, or tibial, malleolus or inner bony prominence is used as the surface landmark. A steel tape is preferable to cloth which may stretch. Several measurements should be taken of each leg and, if possible, by two observers to secure a reliable result.

Discrepancies in tape measurements, or between the tape and the gait pattern, or difficulty in identifying bony landmarks call for X-ray grid measurement by a standardized technique.

Leg-length difference may be evenly distributed throughout the leg, or may be confined to the portion above, or below, the knee. Extreme degrees of bowing (tibial varus) may give apparent discrepancies, although the actual length of bone may be equal on both sides. The functional result is the same as for true shortening.

Effects of limb-length difference Differences are common, only rarely being due to disorders such as polio or hip disease, or the end result of fractures. It is emphasized that length differences should not automatically be treated unless relevant symptoms are present.

Leg-length differences lead to unequal stride lengths and correspondingly asymmetrical movements of the hips, pelvis, sacroiliac structures and lower spine. Pelvic tilt is common and this leads to scoliosis, or compensatory spinal curvature. Thus, any athlete presenting with backache, hip ache or leg symptoms should have his leg length checked.

In more upright running styles, the 'longer' knee may not straighten as fully as the 'shorter' side and chondromalacia may result. In long-distance runners the 'shorter' Achilles tendon may be more prone to pressure from a high or firm shoe-back, because the foot is more plantarflexed or down-turned to make up for the overall shortness of the leg. The 'longer' leg may show excessive pronation in gait.

Pronation (Figure 28.14) The foot acts as a rigid lever in landing and take-off and as a malleable softer structure in between as it adapts to the surface during each full weight-bearing stride.

Figure 28.13 (left)
Leg length. Simple
measurement from anterior
superior iliac spine to
medial malleolus at ankle,
subject lying flat

Figure 28.14 (right)
Summary of foot
movements during running.
At heel-strike (a) in the gait
cycle, the rigid foot lands,
outer border first, in
supination. The inner side
of the foot rotates
(pronation) (b) as the
weight-bearing phase
develops. In the stance
phase (c) of full
weight-bearing, the foot is
fully pronated. As the body
passes over the grounded
foot, supination (d) follows
to prepare the more rigid
foot (e) for take-off in the
propulsive phase

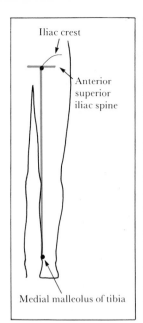

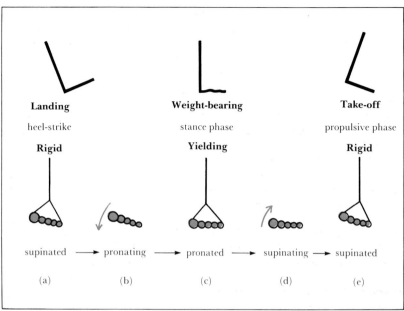

The normal foot is more rigid as it lands, outer side first, at heel-strike. As the rest of the foot is grounded, it rotates towards its inner side and relaxes so that it partially moulds itself to the surface. Meanwhile the rest of the body passes over the grounded foot in the stance phase of the gait cycle.

The rigid foot at landing is held in supination, the hallux (big toe) being highest in the line of the metatarsals at the ball of the foot. After heel-strike, the mid- and front-foot land in turn, accompanied by the downward rotation of the hallux relative to the outside of the foot. This rotation is called pronation and is a normal event.

The body passes over the grounded foot and the weight-bearing stance phase is followed by take-off. The heel rises first and the foot 'unwinds' the landing pronation with supination. This brings the foot back from the relatively lax state of pronation into the greater rigidity of full supination, thus ensuring the maximum efficiency of a rigid lever thrust-off into the next part of the gait cycle.

Pronation (*Figure 28.15*) is a normal and essential event in walking and running, but excessive pronation may be due to certain anatomical variations and leads to symptoms. Practice will acquaint the observer with the normal range of mid-foot pronation during exercise and this can be assessed clinically in consulting rooms, or a short corridor. The patient must, of course be bare-footed and bare-legged. It is useful to make him walk or run on the spot. A small treadmill may be used in limited space.

Certain anatomical conditions predispose to excessive mid-foot pronation. Leg-length difference has been mentioned above. Bowed tibia (tibial varus) changes the normal foot alignment towards pronation (*Figure 28.16*) so that further pronation may become excessive during the stance phase.

Heel stability Heel instability or deviation also leads to excessive pronation. *Figure 28.17* shows the different heel alignments.

If the calcaneum is inverted or everted the anatomical basis for mid-foot action is altered through the link at the subtalar joint with the bony chain of the foot skeleton. This may induce relative instability with consequent excessive pronation. An important function of the heel counter in shoes (*see* Chapter 29) is to hold the calcaneum stable in the landing phase of foot movement.

A further consequence of calcaneal deviation or instability is an enhanced risk of Achilles tendon pain. Instead of a relatively straight perpendicular movement of the tendon, up and down, the calcaneal movements from side-to-side induce bow-string-like movements in the Achilles tendon. In this case, correction of the foot alignment often relieves Achilles pain without further treatment.

The forefoot Similar instabilities of the forefoot may induce excessive pronation. *Figure 28.18* shows possible variations. The line of the metatarsal heads at the back of the foot is related to the perpendicular line of the heel. The normal right angle is compared with forefoot valgus (*Figure 28.18a*), hallux relatively down, and forefoot varus (*Figure 28.18c*), hallux relatively up.

Flat foot (pes planus) This common condition does not usually cause symptoms at any age. The mid-foot is placed lower than usual with consequent pronation (*Figure 28.19b*). Some athletes suffer foot pain after hard or prolonged exercise because of the excessive pronation induced.

Cavus foot A rigid high-arched foot may be due to neurological spasticity or innate skeletal structure. *Figure 28.19* compares the normal with the cavus foot with its characteristic high arch and often bulky mid-foot. There is often clawing of the toes and the sharply downward thrust of the metatarsal bones induces thick callus formation under the ball of the foot. This is a rigid supinated foot which cannot pronate adequately. Runners with cavus feet often show a short-striding, high-stepping gait, a natural

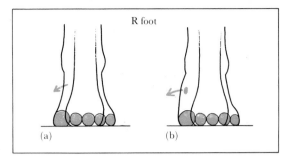

Figure 28.15
Pronation and overpronation.
(a) Normal, minimal pronation. (b) Excessive pronation with rotation inwards of mid-foot on full weight-bearing

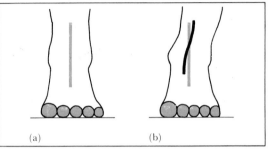

Figure 28.16
Tibial varus. (a) Normal alignment. (b) Tibial varus (curved tibia) with compensatory pronation, further increased during weight-bearing

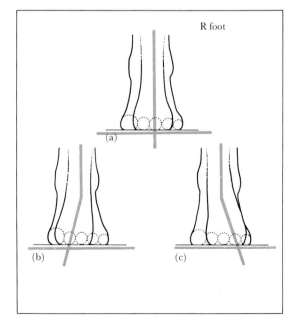

Figure 28.17
Heel alignments.
(a) Normal with midline of heel perpendicular to ground. (b) Calcaneal inversion (varus) with heel inverted relative to midline. (c) Calcaneal eversion (valgus) – heel turns out relative to midline

Figure 28.18
Forefoot alignments.
(a) Normal heel
perpendicular to ground
and line of metatarsal heads
(ball of foot). (b) Forefoot
valgus. (c) Forefoot varus

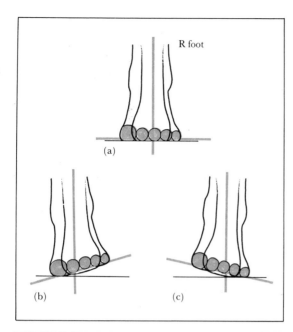

Figure 28.19
Arch form.
(a) Normal. (b) Flat foot
(pes planus). (c) High arch
(cavus type foot)

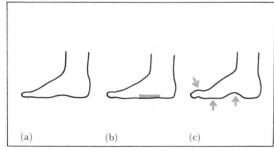

tissue is in the mid-foot, which is itself unusually raised. For some sportsmen with cavus foot, the only satisfactory solution may be to have custom-made shoes or boots incorporating extra shock absorption.

Cavus foot is often associated with Achilles pain due to tightness of the calf muscles. Stretching exercises are an essential remedial measure and should include hamstring stretching as these muscles tend also to be tight.

Orthoses

Excessive pronation and most of the above malalignments can be alleviated by suitable orthoses. While some simple orthoses are available over the counter it is strongly recommended that therapeutic orthoses are individually prescribed and professionally made.

There is a real danger that self-help with ready-made appliances may cause or aggravate injury by increasing, rather than correcting, malalignment if the wrong device is selected. Unfortunately, professional help is expensive.

Orthoses are made from a positive cast of the patient's foot from initial plaster impressions taken in the anatomically neutral position. Casting cannot be performed accurately unless this position is first correctly defined and set by the therapist.

Orthoses may be rigidly made in some form of plastic, or may consist of flexible materials. The simple cast of the patient's foot is 'countered' by stabilizing or tilting corrections in the form of wedges applied to the front or the back of the appliance. Orthoses usually run from the back of the heel to the mid-foot or the metatarsal heads.

It is essential that orthoses should be considered together with footwear. A common problem is that of accommodating both foot and orthotic appliance in a small shoe. For this reason, any necessary height adjustments, to compensate for leg shortening, are best added to the outer sole of the shoe. Unilateral addition of thick insoles may cause further difficulties in shoe fit.

adjustment to the need to land full-footedly because the foot is not flexible enough to follow the normal supination–pronation sequence.

Footwear presents problems because sports shoes almost invariably suit the 'normal' distribution of tissue in feet. As shoe size and fit (Chapter 29) are determined only by the overall length of the foot and its metatarsal head circumference, there is no clear way of denoting a shoe for the cavus foot. The size and fit give no indication that the main bulk of foot

The athlete should, after provision with orthoses, buy new shoes only if he can secure a good fit with all his adaptations. Until the recent introduction of wider fittings in certain makes of running shoes, some broad-footed athletes were unable to use their orthoses for sport.

It is not always possible to predict the athlete's tolerance of his orthoses. Some take immediately to their appliances with complete relief of pain, others need to wear them in slowly. Some can tolerate rigid orthoses in day shoes only, but not for running; others find relief with corrected day shoes, but not sports shoes. Many have soft orthoses for running. The relative need for orthoses may be modified by the construction of the sports shoe. A well-designed and fitted shoe with a good heel counter and sufficient midsole stability may diminish the need for appliances, as may an appropriate varus or valgus wedge built into the shoe sole itself (*warning – inappropriate selection of wedged shoes may double the trouble!*). Running surfaces vary; hard roads call for maximum support, while bare feet on sand need no help as the yielding ground effectively moulds the perfect orthosis for each stride.

Gradual wearing-in of new orthotic appliances or height adjustments should always be recommended. Overenthusiastic training with new appliances can cause all the symptoms which orthoses usually cure – the athlete used to his own alignment is in effect giving himself an acute mechanical derangement!

29 Footwear

Until very recently, sportsmen were presented with cheap, badly designed and often dangerously constructed footwear for what is actually the most demanding time in the life of their feet! While footwear design has improved considerably in the last few years, there still remain design faults and technical difficulties.

The sports shoe or boot must be suitable for its purpose. Economies are often false when it comes to, say, training on the wrong surfaces in match boots and so on. The sportsman must define the purpose of his footwear and buy accordingly. The runner, for instance, may need two or three different types of training shoe for different surfaces. The footballer may choose at least two different boots or types of studs for different ground conditions.

Fit

The first essential is that footwear should fit well. Most manufacturers offer sports footwear which is too narrow for the sporting foot. Fit is assessed in two ways (*Figure 29.1*). The shoe size in full or half numbers represents the length from heel to toe. The fit is an expression of circumference gauged around the metatarsal heads at the ball of the foot. The usual fault is that shoes and boots are too long and narrow and sportsmen with broad feet are forced either to squeeze into small shoes or to buy unnecessarily large sizes to make up some of the deficient fit. On the other hand, sportsmen are often their own worst enemies because it has been shown in surveys that many sportsmen prefer to use a rather tight-fitting shoe, possibly in the mistaken belief that a snug fit is more efficient and less likely to slip off.

The choice between boots and shoes (discussed in relation to ankle injuries on page 213) will depend on personal preference and ground circumstances as well as custom and requirements in different games. In general, higher-sided boots offer more direct protection to the ankle.

Lacing

The differences in individual foot structures must be emphasized – there is no such thing as a perfect boot or shoe, merely the best fit for the individual. Particular attention should be paid to comfort about the tongue, collar and heel-back of any footwear. Cushioning may feel comfortable initially but become macerated and hardened with the sweat and stretching of wear to cause tenosynovitis or blistering around the ankles. Some high-style tongues and lacings are uncomfortable on many feet. In general, it is more satisfactory to have a well-fitting one-piece toebox to a shoe with short lacing (*Figure 29.2*), than to make up a wide range of fittings with a very long lacing system which then tends to crinkle and cause blistering to the skin and tenosynovitis to the toe extensor tendons underneath.,

Heel-backs and Achilles tabs

The heel-back should be very carefully assessed. In recent years several brands have offered a so-called Achilles heel-protecting tab, a well-padded upward extension of the back of the heel (*Figure 29.3*). This may originally have been intended as a simple pull-on tab but, in its harder forms, provides harmful pressure directly into the back of the Achilles tendon, causing much injury (*see* page 205). If a pair of shoes is satisfactory in every other respect, suitable surgery to the shoe may be the answer! Cut the outer surface of the shoe at the back of the offending heel-tab, removing the contained padding and outer layer of leather or plastic. Then carefully fold over the surviving inner lining, glue and trim accordingly (*Figure 29.3*). A crude but effective alternative is to make single or double slits straight down the back of the heel-tab.

Uppers

The shoe upper may consist of leather, suede, plastic or nylon. Comfort and individual preference will guide the purchaser in most cases. Suede or leather reinforcements should be added at key points, especially around the front of the toes, the arch and heel-counter.

At the back a firm heel-counter is desirable. This consits of a built-in cup-shaped reinforcement to hold the heel in a stable position on landing during the stride. Without this, the athlete's heel tends to wobble slightly more on landing and this may accelerate overuse injury. The heel-flare also helps to stabilize landings (*Figure 29.4*).

Soles and heels

An adequate sole and heel are the basis of any sports shoe. The first essential is that the overall design and resilience be suitable for the game and purpose in

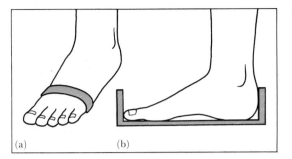

Figure 29.1
Foot fit (a) and size (b)

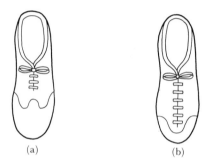

Figure 29.2
Lacing. Short lacing and one-piece shoe front (a) gives better fit than small front and long lacing (b) which adapts to different fittings but causes blisters from fabric folds

question. With the advent of highly resilient polyurethanes and foams, it is possible to produce durable and protective sports shoes for most purposes at relatively light weights, although expense remains a major problem.

For most purposes some degree of heel-raise is desirable, if for no other reason than that most people have been conditioned to use a heel-raise in all their footwear from early life and it would be unwise to remove this during the most strenuous action when stresses are multiplied. The degree of heel-raise preferred will vary from person to person, and should be tried out. Some shoes tend to slope in a continuous straight line from heel to toe and these should be tried most carefully before being purchased as this is not a normal configuration in footwear and may not be entirely satisfactory, particularly if there is any degree of hallux rigidus (page 220).

The heels should be rounded for most running shoes. This is because the heel itself is round and the rounding-off of the shoe eliminates the slight jarring

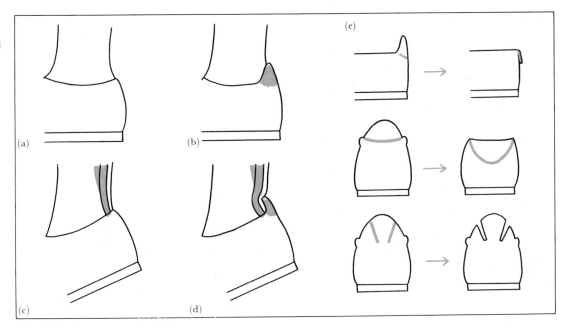

Figure 29.3
The notorious 'Achilles protector' tab. Conventional heel (a) and Achilles tab (b) standing and in thrusting position (c) and (d), where the 'tab' presses into the Achilles, but the simple heel does not. The remedy: (e) cut outer layers and bind over the lining or, more drastically, simply slit the shoe heel-tab open with two cuts

Figure 29.4
The heel-counter (a) and stabilizing flares (b). Flares are not suitable for court games (*see text*)

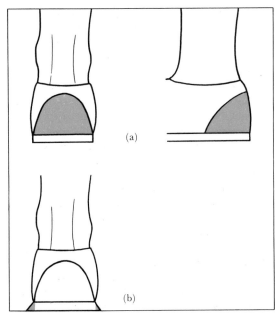

instability often present when sharply squared-off heels are used. Suitable flaring-out of a heel (*Figure 29.4*) enhances the stability so that the ideal running shoe (*Figure 29.5*) would have a slightly flared padded heel under a rounded edge and a firm heel-counter. At the front of the shoe, wear is often more satisfactory with similar rounding-off at the toe.

Training and road-running shoes have foam cushioning in single or multiple layers throughout the sole and heel. A hardwearing composition or rubber outer traction sole provides surface grip and should be chosen for the particular surface and sporting purpose required.

Warning – the right shoe for the right game!

A word of warning about using the wrong shoes. If a highly padded and flared running shoe is worn, for instance, on a squash court, injury risk is increased

243

because that shoe may be so stable that it is, in effect, too stable for the highly dynamic purposes required by the squash player. His need to roll his foot and turn rapidly may be frustrated by the very safety factors designed for running. The result may be that his simpler movements are frustrated while he is suddenly flipped over from one extreme of stability into a sudden severe inversion or eversion stress, thus risking injury. He needs a flatter, more flexible type of shoe for the purposes of his court game and this shoe will, in turn, be less than satisfactory for his stamina training in road runs.

It is unfortunate that shoe manufacturers have not paid sufficient attention to the broad foot, which is probably more common than average in serious sports players because of greater muscular development. There is a tendency for manufacturers to select the minimum required number of sole sizes for their sports wear and then to accommodate the different number of sizes by stitching on a range of different-sized uppers. Thus, two or three sizes of shoe may share a common-sized sole. The inevitable result of this is that the broad-footed player finds himself overhanging the sole-plate and risking impact injuries along the outer border of the foot on hard surfaces (*Figure 28.11*). A few minutes spent examining the sports shoes in any changing room will bring this fact home to the observer.

It is up to the sportsman to be utterly critical with his shoe suppliers and to refuse to purchase any sports shoe or boot which does not fit satisfactorily and which is not suitable for the exact sporting purpose for which it is being bought.

If it is worth buying good shoes for safety and good performance in sport, then it is equally important to take good care of them. Worn shoes become ineffective and lose their protective capacity. Worn spikes or studs create pressures on the undersurface of the foot and are dangerous in contact sports.

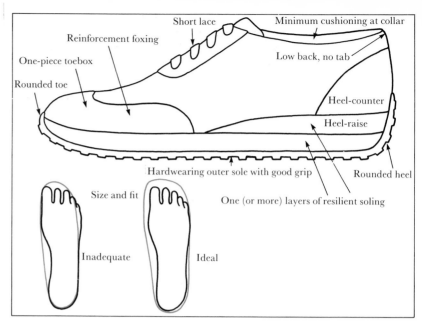

Figure 29.5
Running shoe – ideal features

Stud care

Contact game studs can be dangerous if neglected. While the laws of the game may require pre-game inspections, human nature often fails to conform. Certain nylon compounds sharpen up to a razor-like edge with wear and can cut other players dangerously. There is a particular danger in running across roads or similar surfaces to get to the pitch because this may sharpen up otherwise safe studs. Aluminium studs are safer than most nylon compounds because while they are hard their wear patterns do not create the sharp cutting edges of some nylons.

There are considerable technical difficulties in the manufacture of safe, effective, durable studs and in fixing them securely to sole-plates. Much technical development still has to be undertaken by manufacturers. An elementary safety measure is to remember that the checking of studs in contact sports must be made at the moment of entering the field of play, after all other surfaces have been crossed. Most manufacturers provide a template which indicates the correct and permissible stud dimensions and worn studs should be replaced before play is allowed.

Appendix 1:
Doping Control Regulations of the International Amateur Athletic Federation (as at 31st March 1982)

Reproduced by kind permission of the International Amateur Athletic Federation. Full unedited version available from IAAF, 3 Hans Crescent, London SW1.

The IAAF strongly condemns the use of 'dope' by athletes on both fair-play and health grounds. Apart from the immediate health hazards, there is considerable risk that the use of dope may have serious side effects on the athlete's health which will become apparent in later years.

Doping is, therefore, expressly forbidden, and any athlete offending the IAAF Doping Rule renders himself ineligible to take part in competitions under IAAF Rules.

There is provision under IAAF rules for an appeal to the Council for reinstatement. It should be noted, in this respect, however, that the Council has ruled that any such reinstatement may not come into force within 18 months of the offence.

Part 1 – IAAF Rule 144 – 'Doping'

1. Doping is strictly forbidden.
2. Doping is the use by or distribution to an athlete of certain substances which could have the effect of improving artificially the athlete's physical and/or mental condition and so augmenting his athletic performance.
3. Doping substances, for the purpose of this rule, comprise the following groups:

(a) *Psychomotor stimulant drugs:*

amphetamine	methylamphetamine
benzphetamine	methylphenidate
caffeine (quantitative analysis)	norpseudo ephedrine
cocaine	pemoline
diethylpropion	phendimetrazine
dimethylamphetamine	phenmetrazine
ethylamphetamine	phentermine
fencamfamin	pipradol
fenproporex	prolintane

and chemically or pharmacologically related compounds

(b) *Sympathomimetic amines:*
ephedrine methoxyphenamine methylephedrine and chemically or pharmacologically related compounds

(c) *Miscellaneous central nervous system stimulants:* e.g.

amiphenasole	micoren
bemigride	nikethamide
leptazol	strychnine

and chemically or pharmacologically related compounds

(d) *Narcotic analgesics:* e.g.

morphine	pethidine
heroin	dextromoramide
methadone	dipipanone

and chemically or pharmacologically related compounds

Note: Codeine is permitted for therapeutic uses

(e) *Anabolic steroids:* e.g.

clostebol	methandriol	stanolone
ethyloestrenol	methyltestosterone	stanozolol
fluoxymesterone	nandrolone	testosterone
methandienone	oxandrolone	and its esters
methenolone	oxymetholone	(quantitative analysis)

and chemically or pharmacologically related compounds

This list is not necessarily comprehensive. Cases of doubt as to other substances which may be regarded as doping substances shall be referred to the Medical Committee for decision.

BEFORE ANY PENALTIES ARE IMPOSED UNDER THIS RULE, THE ACTUAL DOPING SUBSTANCE MUST BE IDENTIFIED.

4. Doping controls conducted under IAAF Doping Control Regulations shall take place at specified meetings. In addition, doping controls shall be held if ordered by the IAAF, or by the area or national governing body responsible for organizing or sanctioning a meeting.

Doping controls shall be carried out under the supervision of a Doping Committee for the meeting which shall include:

(1) The Medical Delegate (Chairman)

(2) A member or representative of the IAAF Medical Committee

(3) A qualified medical officer of the organizing country.

Before the event, the criteria for selecting the athletes to be controlled shall be determined by the Doping Committee. This should be either on a final position basis and/or a random basis, but not by selection of named individuals. The total number of athletes tested may depend on the capacity of the Laboratory.

Additional controls may be ordered after the event at the discretion of the Doping Committee.

5. An athlete who takes part in a competition must, if so requested in writing by the responsible official, submit to a doping control. Refusal to do so will result in disqualification from the competition and the athlete will be deemed to have rendered himself ineligible for competition as if a positive result had been obtained. He shall be reported to the IAAF and his/her national governing body by the Doping Committee Chairman.

6. To facilitate the analysis, any form of medication administered by any route within two days of the start of the competition or event, must be declared to the Doping Committee on the Doping Control form.

7. A competitor found to have a doping substance or/and a metabolite of a doping substance present in his urine at an athletics meeting shall be disqualified from the competition and the case reported to the IAAF and his national governing body.

Likewise, any person assisting or inciting others to use doping substances shall be considered as having committed an offence against IAAF Rules, and thus exposes himself/herself to disciplinary action.

Any offences under this rule arising from competition at a national level shall be reported by the national governing body to the IAAF.

8. The detailed procedure for the conduct of tests, including the collection of urine samples, the method of analysis and the use of accredited laboratories, shall be determined by the Medical Committee of the IAAF. Copies of the current approved procedure shall be supplied on request by the IAAF to responsible organizing bodies for the information and guidance of the Doping Committees, athletes and officials.

Part II – Procedure for doping controls

1. General
(a) The Medical Delegate appointed for the meeting shall enter into contact with the Organizing Committee at least three months in advance.
(b) Meeting Organizers must ensure that adequate control-centre facilities are provided, e.g. waiting rooms, WCs, private rooms (secure from intruders) for registration etc. The Control Centre must be clearly marked and signposted from the Stadium for the benefit of athletes selected.
(c) No later than three days before a meeting, the members of the Doping Committee will ensure that all the necessary equipment is available in the doping control room. This will include control of IAAF standard bottles provided, their numbering and sealing methods.
(d) All officials concerned should inform themselves regarding the procedure, and team officials should ensure that athletes in their delegation are warned in advance that they may be required to undergo a doping control.
(e) Athletes selected for doping control must be handed a Notice as soon as possible after their event and, in any case, not later than 30 minutes after the event. The handing over of this Notice shall be carried out as discreetly as possible, and the athlete shall acknowledge receipt on the relevant section of the Notice.
2. Collection and registration of urine samples
(a) The athlete has to report to the Control Centre within one hour after the completion of his event and he may be accompanied by a team doctor or team official. There, the urine shall be collected for testing in the laboratory. The competitor shall have fulfilled his duty to submit to the doping control only after having delivered the necessary amount of urine, irrespective of the time required for this.

(b) In addition to the competitor and any accompanying person, only the following persons may be present in the Doping Control Centre:
– Members of the Doping Committee
– the officials in charge of the Centre
– the official in charge of taking samples
– an interpreter.
(c) At no time should there be more than one competitor in the room when urine is collected in the collecting vessel.
A minimum of 100 ml of urine must be collected from a competitor to be tested.
(d) The competitor shall be allowed the choice of two or three glass bottles from a number of clean unused bottles.
Note: Three bottles are necessary only if the control test for anabolic steroids is conducted in a laboratory different from that used for testing the other doping substances given above.
(e) The urine sample collected shall then be divided by an official in the presence of the competitor into the two or three chosen glass bottles, all of which must bear the same code, e.g.:
No:1 A (testing for doping substances except for anabolic steroids)   50 ml
No:1 B (anabolic steroid testing)   25 ml
No:1 R (reserve sample)   25 ml
or when only one laboratory is being used:
No:1 A (testing for doping substances including anabolic steroids)   75 ml
No:1 R (reserve sample)   25 ml
(f) The pH of the sample shall be measured using indicator paper and using the rest of the urine sample in the vessel in which it was collected. The result obtained is to be entered on the competitor's Doping Control Form.
(g) The two or three glass bottles shall be sealed in the presence of the competitor, who should check that the code on the bottle is the same as the official's entry against the competitor's name on the Doping Control Form. This code shall be etched or scratched on the bottles; any other method must receive prior approval from the

Chairman of the Medical Committee.

The sealing shall be carried out by the official in charge of the station using a special sealing apparatus and a seal which is provided either by the IAAF or by the Regional Association.

(h) The signatures of the competitor and an official of the Doping Control Centre must appear on the Doping Control Form showing that the above procedure has been carried out.

The Control Form should be so devised that two duplicate forms are produced at the same time.

(i) All Control Forms shall be given to the IAAF Medical Delegate. The top copy and first duplicate copy shall be placed in envelopes and immediately sealed at the end of the competition. The Medical Delegate shall retain the top copy, and transmit the first duplicate copy to the relevant authority (e.g. IAAF or Regional Association). The second duplicate Control Form shall be given to the controlled athlete.

(j) A separate record should be extracted from the Control Forms, listing against each bottle code number the quantity of urine, the pH and any drugs declared, but no other information. This record shall be passed to the laboratory when the samples are sent for testing.

3. Storage and disposal of samples

(a) Before the bottles containing the urine samples are packed, check that all samples taken are present and that the numbering is in accordance with the list of code numbers.

(b) The bottles shall be placed into a suitable container for submission to the analytical laboratory (laboratories). The reserve samples shall be placed in a separate container for storage in case of repeat analysis.

(c) After the completion of the Doping Controls, the container(s) containing the bottles for the laboratory (laboratories) and the container of reserve samples shall be sealed. At least two of the members of the Doping Committee shall be present when the samples are sealed in the containers.

The sealed container(s) shall not be opened during transit to the laboratory (laboratories).

(d) The samples for analysis shall be despatched as soon as possible after the end of the competition and by the quickest method, to the analytical laboratory (laboratories) designated by the IAAF.

(e) The Medical Delegate shall be responsible for the Reserve samples. He must store them in a refrigerator in case they are required for repeat analysis.

(f) The reserve samples may only be destroyed after the final results of the first analysis have been declared and it is confirmed that they are not required for repeat analysis.

(g) It is important that all samples of urine should be securely stored in a refrigerator before testing.

4. Analysis of samples

(a) Only laboratories accredited or approved by the IAAF on the advice of the Medical Committee may be used to carry out the analysis in connection with Doping Control.

Access to the laboratory during the analysis is restricted to members of the Doping Committee for the meeting and to members of the IAAF Medical Committee, and to the authorised observers (*see* 5(g)).

(b) The method of analysis is detailed in 'Requirements for accreditation of a doping control laboratory' obtainable from the IAAF Bureau.

5. Communication of results and protests

(a) The results of the control are strictly confidential and must be communicated to the Medical Delegate of the Doping Committee or his nominee in a sealed envelope.

(b) The evidence which has led to a definitive identification of a doping substance must be made available to the Medical Delegate or his nominee.

(c) If the Doping Committee decides that after the first analysis there is evidence of doping, the Federation concerned shall be informed; if possible, this shall be, in the first instance, via the team manager of the athlete. In any case, written notification to the Federation must follow by registered letter. The athlete concerned shall be informed as soon as possible.

(d) The competitor, or an official acting on his behalf, may, within 24 hours of being notified, challenge a positive result.

(e) If no challenge is received within 24 hours, the analysis of the corresponding reserve sample shall immediately be carried out in the same laboratory, but by different persons.

(f) If a challenge is received within the given time limit, the analysis of the corresponding reserve sample shall, as soon as possible, be carried out in the same laboratory, but by different persons. The National Federation concerned must be informed immediately, either directly by registered post, or through the Team Manager or other official representative, that the analysis is to take place and invited to attend.

(g) One or two of its representatives may be present during the retesting procedure and the analysis shall be carried out also in the presence of an international expert designated by the IAAF.

(h) Until the results of the analysis become known, all details connected with the investigation are to be treated as confidential by all persons connected with the Control.

(i) If the analysis of the reserve sample shows a positive result, this fact shall immediately be reported to the IAAF by the Chairman of the Doping Committee, who must also inform the Organizing Committee of the meeting that the athlete must be disqualified from the competition.

(j) The IAAF shall then inform the athlete's National Federation that the athlete is ineligible for competition under IAAF rules.

6. Subsequent action

(a) The athlete remains ineligible unless the IAAF Council reinstates him or her upon application by the Member responsible for the athlete. Such reinstatement may not come into force within 18 months of the offence.

(b) It is desirable that the athlete's National Federation should carry out an investigation to ascertain:
   (i) the source of the illegal substances
   (ii) any earlier use of illegal substances
   (iii) the identity of any person inciting him/her to take drugs.

A report of such findings should be made to the IAAF.

Appendix 2: Contents of medical bags

The contents will depend on the nature of the risks anticipated and the experience and skill of the owner. There are several attractively packaged bags on the market but they may stock inappropriate items for particular purposes unless the contents are individually selected. It is not necessary to own an expensive or elaborate bag – the most efficient ones are simple and cleanly stocked by the coach, therapist or doctor according to need. The following guidelines are suggested.

COACH'S BAG

Cleansing agents:	disinfectant (e.g. Savlon, Eusol, etc.); surgical spirit; cotton wool; tincture of iodine or merthiolate
Dressings:	lint; sterile dressings; triangular bandage (for arm sling); bandages – cotton, crepe; Elastoplast
Dressing strips:	Band aids; rolls of Elastoplast/zinc oxide plaster (N.B. allergy may occur, in which case either strap only over an intermediate layer of foam or tubigrip, or buy non-allergic tape)
Cold application:	ice; Thermos jug; cooling sachets; cold spray
Instruments:	eyebath, patch and cleansing solution; forceps (tweezers); scissors
Skin applications:	plain talc; antifungal talc; Vaseline
Skin protection:	padding, e.g. Sorbo, Plastazote, orthopaedic felt or foam
Pain-relieving tablets:	soluble aspirin; aspirin and codeine; paracetamol
Sport-specific items:	e.g. spare studs, spikes, resin for grip, laces
Bucket:	sponge; towel; smelling salts

CLUB BAG

In addition to the above, and according to sport-specific needs, the following may be added:
splinting materials, including inflatable limb
splints
stretcher
airway (*and* instructions beforehand in its use)

PHYSIOTHERAPIST'S BAG

In addition to the 'coach's bag', an airway and inflatable splint where appropriate, plus preferred treatment modalities, e.g.

cold: ice, Thermos (wide neck jugs); cooling packs
heat-retaining packs; hot water bottle
strapping, according to individual circumstances
electrical treatment equipment (check foreign
voltages and plugs, multi-adaptor plug and
extension lead)

Medication: **warning:** physiotherapists are not expected to prescribe 'POM' – 'prescription only medications' – nor to inject patients under any normal circumstances, either with systemic substances or with locally acting drugs. Doing so may lead to legal action for negligence.

DOCTOR'S BAG

Depends on particular sport and personal experience. If looking after a team with a physiotherapist, it is reasonable to share responsibilities so that the latter will take a full 'coach's' + 'physiotherapist's' bag while the medical practitioner takes care of medical and surgical supplies. Additional suggestions include the following.

Surgical: instruments for debridement and simple stitching
ophthalmoscope/otoscope
airway

Drugs: (*but see* Chapters 12 and 13)
pain relief: dysmenorrhoea, hangovers
anti-inflammatories
diarrhoea, e.g. codeine phosphate, Lomotil, loperamide
vomiting and travel sickness
sedative/tranquillizer
antibiotics, e.g. pencillin V, erythromycin
(for the penicillin-allergic),
a tetracycline, a
sulphonamide (mixture),
remembering urinary
infections in young women
and elderly male officials
the contraceptive pill (and tampons, both frequently 'forgotten' by anxious sportswomen)
ear wax solvents, e.g. cerumol, waxsol; to save weight a 5 or 10 ml syringe is adequate for ear syringing
injectables: according to circumstances
– general medication
– local steroid, anaesthetic

Index